Musculoskeletal Anatomy Coloring Book

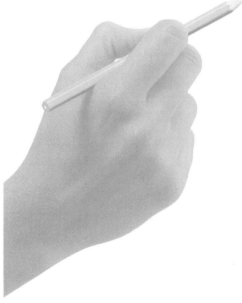

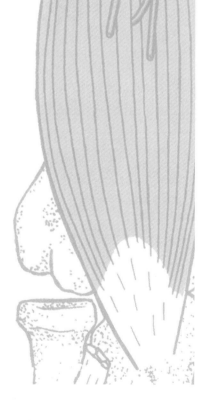

Musculoskeletal Anatomy Coloring Book

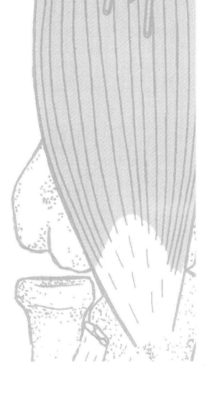

Joseph E. Muscolino, DC

Instructor, Connecticut Center
for Massage Therapy
Newington, Connecticut

Owner, www.LearnMuscles.com
Redding, Connecticut

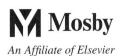

Mosby

An Affiliate of Elsevier

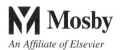

An Affiliate of Elsevier

11830 Westline Industrial Drive
St. Louis, Missouri 63146

MUSCULOSKELETAL ANATOMY COLORING BOOK

ISBN-13: 978-0-323-02522-5
ISBN-10:   0-323-02522-6

Publishing Director: Linda Duncan
Acquisitions Editor: Kellie White
Developmental Editor: Jennifer Watrous
Publishing Services Manager: Linda McKinley
Designer: Teresa McBryan
Editorial Assistant: Kendra Bailey

Printed in the United States of America

Last digit is the print number: 9 8 7 6 5

Preface

AND HOW TO USE THIS BOOK

Sciences have long been taught in a classroom format in which an instructor lectures to students and the students have textbooks to read at home. Unfortunately, lecture format and textbook reading do not cater to the kinesthetic element of learning that is present in all of us. Toward that end, coloring books of anatomy and physiology are useful tools for approaching and learning class material in a manner that is not possible via lecture and textbook format alone. However, I do not believe that coloring books should replace quality classroom instruction and quality textbooks; rather I believe that coloring books of anatomy and physiology are valuable adjunctive learning tools that should be used in conjunction with classroom learning and textbook reading.

For this reason, I recommend the *Musculoskeletal Anatomy Coloring Book* to aid you as you endeavor to learn the structure and function of the musculoskeletal system, as well as the other major systems of the human body. With regard to an adjunct textbook for learning muscles, I recommend *The Muscular System Manual: The Skeletal Muscles of the Human Body* (Mosby, 2003).

Beyond being simply a coloring book, this book is also designed to help the reader learn the information in a number of ways. First, regarding muscles, the two hurdles for the new student are learning the attachments (origins and insertions) and actions of the muscles. In the chapter on muscles (Chapter 2), the text information of the attachments is written next to the locations on the illustration where the actual muscle attachments are located. As you color the muscles from attachment to attachment, I recommend that you integrate this written information by saying the attachments out loud. To help learn the actions of the muscles, arrows that visually demonstrate the line(s) of pull of the muscle have been placed within the muscle. As you color in these arrows, note the actions that are caused by the

line of pull demonstrated by the arrows. Putting the attachment and action information together with the illustration, and kinesthetically coloring at the same time, allow for a fuller integration of the information that you need to learn!

This book is also designed to allow the student to quiz himself/herself. Throughout the book, wherever you find blank lead lines pointing to a structure, use that opportunity to quiz yourself on being able to identify the structure. The answer key is located on p. 423. On each right-hand page of a 2-page muscle spread in Chapter 2, there are illustrations showing the individual muscle being studied within its larger group of muscles. For another opportunity to quiz yourself, write in the directional terms around these illustrations (e.g., anterior, posterior, lateral, etc.). Check your answers by turning to the illustrations at the beginning or end of each section in Chapter 2.

While this book covers every major system of the human body, its emphasis is the musculoskeletal system. More specifically, the major emphasis of this book is the muscular system.

This book is organized into an introduction, six chapters, and an appendix. The introduction contains valuable text information toward understanding the systems that are covered in the six chapters. I strongly recommend reading the introductory text before you begin coloring. Chapters 1 through 3 cover the musculoskeletal system. Of these chapters, Chapter 2, which covers the major skeletal muscles of the body, is divided into 10 sections. For those of you who are also studying from *The Muscular System Manual,* you will find that the muscles are covered in the same order in both books. Chapters 4 and 5 cover the nervous system and arterial system, the understanding of which is important toward learning innervation and arterial supply to the skeletal muscles. Chapter 6 covers tissue structure and the other major systems of the human body.

The appendix includes the answer key to the self-testing pages that are included throughout the book.

Regarding the use of colors, of course you may use any that you like to color the various structures. However, there are certain colors standardly used for the anatomical structures of the human body, and I recommend the following to you as guidelines:

- Red is classically used for blood vessels that carry 'oxygenated' blood (arteries of the systemic circulation and veins of the pulmonic circulation) and blue is used for all blood vessels that carry 'deoxygenated' blood (veins of the systemic circulation and arteries of the pulmonic circulation).

- Red is also used for coloring the muscles of the body. Therefore, to make muscles distinct from blood vessels that have been colored red, perhaps a different shade (I recommend a lighter shade) of red can be used for the muscles.

- The attachments of muscles (tendons and aponeuroses) and other fibrous fascia are usually colored white; given that the page is already white, you may simply leave them uncolored. However, since this is a coloring book and the purpose of this book is to learn kinesthetically by coloring, I recommend that you do color them. A light shade of color would be best.

- Yellow is classically used for nerves.

- As for coloring bones, I recommend the following:

  1) When coloring the bones in Chapter 1, color the entire bone lightly with a light shade of color, different from those used above; a light yellow to beige color is most often used. Then use a darker color to color over the landmarks on the bone that you feel are important to you and you want to learn. This will help these landmarks to visually stand out as well as help root them kinesthetically.

  2) When coloring the bones in Chapter 2, I recommend that you use a different color for each of the muscle's two bony attachments (if there are more than two different bony attachments for a particular muscle, you may use more colors). Further, I recommend that you color the attachment of the muscle that is usually fixed (i.e., the origin) with a darker

color to convey upon it a feeling of being heavier and more stable. Conversely, I recommend that you use a lighter color for the attachment that usually moves (i.e., the insertion) to convey a feeling of being lighter and therefore more mobile.

- Cartilage is always lightly shaded; pale blue is usually used.

- When coloring the many systems of Chapter 6, beyond the conventionally used colors that are mentioned above, please note the following: the liver is usually a fairly dark brown, the gall bladder is usually green, fat is usually yellow, lymph is usually green, and the brain and spinal cord are usually a light brown.

- The purpose of this book is for you to learn by coloring, and hopefully enjoy yourself along the way. If you prefer to use colors different from those recommended above, and it will add to your enjoyment and learning, please do so. They are only guidelines. Most important is that you enjoy and learn!

Because this is a coloring book and not a textbook, the text in this book has been kept to a minimum. This has been done for two reasons: 1) excessive text tends to clutter the page and obscure visualization of the structures being colored and learned; and 2) the inclusion of text forces the illustrations to be smaller, which also makes visualization and coloring more difficult. Further, I feel that coloring books are best used as adjuncts to textbooks, not as a replacement. Although this coloring book can certainly stand on its own, in many ways it is a companion to *The Muscular System Manual: The Skeletal Muscles of the Human Body* (Mosby, 2003), which is strongly recommended for students wishing to learn more about the musculoskeletal system.

However, since an understanding of what is being colored is crucial, and the handiness of having some of that information accessible in the same book is helpful, this two-part introductory text section has been included. Part 1 is a brief overview of each of the major systems of the body. Part 2 is a very practical approach that gives you a method to understand how muscles work; the more you understand, the less you have to memorize! I strongly recommend reading this introductory text before diving into the coloring.

Introduction

PART 1: BRIEF OVERVIEW OF THE SYSTEMS OF THE BODY

The Cell

The cell is the basic structural and functional building block of the human body. While cells are diverse in structure (and function), there are certain essential elements of most cells. Cells essentially have two parts, an inner nucleus and the surrounding cytoplasmic fluid; both of these two structures have a semipermeable membrane around them. The nucleus contains DNA (the genetic blueprint) and the nucleolus (which makes ribosomes). In the cytoplasm, there are many organelles (small organs), each with a particular function. These organelles are held in place by fine filaments that are found in the cytoplasm; these filaments create a skeletal structure for the cell called the *cytoskeleton.*

The major cytoplasmic organelles are: ribosomes (they function to synthesize proteins), mitochondria (they turn glucose and oxygen into ATP molecules for energy), endoplasmic reticulum (there are two types, 'rough' and 'smooth'; they function as a transport system within the cell), golgi apparatus (which functions to refine and transport proteins), and lysosomes (which digest and break down intracellular substances).

There are also organelles that can be located on the outside membrane of the cell. These structures are called *cilia* and *flagella,* both of which function to create movement, either of the cell itself, or of substances along the surface of the cell. Usually, a cell has either one long flagellum or numerous shorter cilia.

Integumentary System

An integument is a covering; hence the integumentary system covers the body. The integumentary system is comprised of the cutaneous membrane, (i.e., the skin, and the accessory organs of the skin). The skin has two layers to it: the outer epidermis, which is stratified squamous epithelium, and the deeper dermis, which is fibrous connective tissue. The accessory organs are the hair follicles, arrector pili muscles, sebaceous glands, and eccrine and apocrine sweat glands. The main function of the skin is to provide a barrier between the inside of our body and the outside world. This barrier prevents pathogens (disease-causing microorganisms) from entering the body and keeps moisture and body contents from escaping. The skin also functions to help regulate internal body temperature by two processes: 1) sweating, and 2) dermal blood vessel dilation, which regulates the amount of blood that flows to the skin for exchange of heat with the outside world. Deep to the skin is subcutaneous fascia.

Cardiovascular System

The cardiovascular system is made up of the cardiac system and the vascular system. The cardiac system is comprised of the heart; the vascular system is comprised of blood vessels (i.e., the arteries, capillaries, and the veins).

The heart is essentially a double pump, having a left side and a right side (each side having two chambers: an atrium and a ventricle). The heart's left side pumps oxygen-rich/carbon dioxide–poor blood into vessels that bring the blood out to the cells and tissues of the body; this is called the *systemic circulation.* At the cellular/tissue level, these vessels give their oxygen (and other nutrients) to the cells so that the vital processes of metabolism can occur. These vessels also pick up carbon dioxide (and other waste products) from the cells and transport these substances back to the right side of the heart. The heart's right side then pumps this oxygen-poor/carbon dioxide–rich blood to the lungs, where it is oxygenated and loses much of its carbon dioxide; this is called the *pulmonic circulation.* This oxygen-rich/carbon dioxide–poor blood then returns back to the left side of the heart where it can be pumped out to the cells and tissues of the body once again.

It is the vessels of the cardiovascular system that carry the blood that is pumped by the heart. There are three types of blood vessels: arteries, capillaries, and veins. Arteries carry blood away from the heart. As they do so, arteries branch and diminish in size, eventually becoming capillaries. Capillaries are thin-walled vessels that do the essential job of exchange of oxygen and carbon dioxide (and other nutrients and waste products) with the cells. Capillaries then converge with each other to form veins, which carry the blood back to the heart. NOTE: Arteries in the systemic circulation carry 'oxygenated' blood; arteries in the pulmonic circulation carry 'deoxygenated' blood; veins in the systemic circulation carry 'de-oxygenated' blood; veins in the pulmonic circulation carry 'oxygenated' blood.

Hence, the cardiovascular system is a double circulation. The systemic circulation is created by the left side of the heart pumping to the cells/tissues of the body and the return of this blood to the right side of the heart; the pulmonic circulation is created by the right side of the heart pumping to the lungs and the return of this blood to the left side of the heart.

Lymphatic System

Not all the systemic blood that is pumped out to the tissues of the body by the arteries is returned back to the heart by the veins. A small amount of the fluid that leaves the capillaries at the tissue level is left behind in the tissues. If this extra intercellular tissue fluid is not removed, a build-up of fluid (swelling) will occur in the tissues of the body. It is the job of the lymphatic system to return this fluid back to the heart. The lymphatic system does this by carrying this fluid in lymphatic vessels (where it is termed 'lymph') back toward the heart. It actually deposits the lymph into a large vein; from there the venous system returns this fluid back to the right side of the heart. Along the way, the lymph in lymphatic vessels travels through lymph nodes that are high in white blood cells that filter the blood, attacking any foreign disease-causing pathogens. Hence, the lymphatic system has two purposes: to return extra tissue fluid back to the heart and to filter possible pathogens from the blood.

Respiratory System

Oxygen is one of the most important nutrients that the cardiovascular system circulates to the tissues of the body. It is the job of the respiratory system to bring oxygen into the body and place this oxygen into the cardiovascular system. The respiratory system may be divided into the passageways that carry oxygen to the lungs when we breathe in (inspiration), and the lungs themselves. The passageways include: the nose, nasal cavity, mouth, pharynx, larynx, and the trachea. The lungs contain the bronchial tree and the alveolar sacs. It is in the lungs that the blood that comes from the right side of the heart (pulmonic circulation) picks up oxygen to return to the left side of the heart where it can be pumped to the cells and tissues of the body (systemic circulation). The lungs also pick up the waste product carbon dioxide from the blood; this carbon dioxide is then transported out of the lungs to the outside world through the aforementioned passageways when we breathe out (expiration). Hence, the respiratory system has two purposes: to carry oxygen into the body and place it into the blood, and to eliminate carbon dioxide from the blood and carry it out of the body.

Urinary System

As the cardiovascular system circulates blood throughout the body, waste products from cellular metabolism accumulate within the blood. It is the job of the two kidneys of the urinary system to filter these waste products from the blood. The waste products that the kidneys filter from the blood form urine, which leaves each kidney through a long muscular tube called a *ureter;* the two ureters carry the urine to the urinary bladder. The urine is stored in the urinary bladder until a sufficient amount is present. The urine is then expelled from the urinary bladder through the urethra to the outside world. This process of expelling urine is called *urination* or *micturition.*

Gastrointestinal System

As we have said, the cells of the body must be constantly supplied with nutrients by the bloodstream. Other than oxygen that comes from the lungs, these nutrients come from the gastrointestinal system. The gastrointestinal system is comprised of two parts: a long passageway called the *alimentary canal* that begins at the mouth and ends at the anus, and the accessory organs that secrete substances (primarily enzymes) into the alimentary canal. The alimentary canal consists of the mouth, pharynx, esophagus, stomach, small intestine, and large intestine. The accessory organs are the salivary glands, pancreas, liver, and gall bladder. The gastrointestinal system essentially functions as follows: food enters at the mouth; as the food travels through the alimentary canal, whatever is digested and absorbed is taken into the bloodstream for use in the body (i.e., nutrients that the bloodstream carries to the cells); whatever substances are not digested and absorbed continue through the alimentary canal and exit through the anus as feces. The liver also functions to filter unwanted chemicals of the body (both created by metabolism and ingested from external sources) from the blood.

Immune System

"Immunity" means freedom. It is the function of your immune system to keep you free from disease. The immune system does this by fighting foreign microorganisms such as bacteria and viruses (pathogens) that might cause infection and disease. The most important cells of your body that do this are macrophages and a type of white blood cell called *lymphocytes.* There are two main types of lymphocytes, T-lymphocytes and B-lymphocytes (also known as *T cells* and *B cells*); each one of them attacks pathogens in a different manner. T-lymphocytes directly attack the pathogens, engaging in cell to cell contact, secreting substances that are toxic to the pathogen; further, T-lymphocytes help to activate B-lymphocytes. B-lymphocytes secrete antibodies (immunoglobulins) that attack the pathogens. Macrophages destroy pathogens by the process of phagocytosis, in which the pathogens are ingested into the macrophage and broken down by the lysosomes of the macrophage.

Endocrine System

The endocrine system is composed of structures that secrete hormones into the bloodstream. The major endocrine glands are the hypothalamus, pituitary, thyroid, parathyroid, adrenal, pancreas, testes, and ovaries. Other endocrine glands are the pineal and thymus. Generally, the hormones of the hypothalamus control the hormone production of the pituitary and the hormones of the pituitary then control the hormone secretions of other glands such as the thyroid, adrenal, testes, and ovaries. The function of hormones is to act as chemical messengers that regulate the metabolic processes of the body. The endocrine system is also intimately linked to the nervous system of the body; indeed the hypothalamus and pituitary (as well as the pineal gland) are structures of the brain.

Sensory System

The sensory system is the system of receptors in the body that allows us to sense the external world around us as well as sense the internal environment of our body. The senses are usually divided into the somatic senses and special senses. Somatic senses are touch, pressure, temperature, pain, and stretch receptors. Somatic sensory receptors are primarily located in the skin and around the joints. Special senses are smell, taste, vision, hearing, and equilibrium. Special sensory receptors are located in the nasal cavity, mouth, eyes, and ears. All sensory stimuli travel to the central nervous system where they are processed and interpreted. Given these sensory stimuli, the central nervous system determines the appropriate response(s) for our health, enjoyment, and safety.

Nervous System

The nervous system is the master controller of the body. The cells of the nervous system are called *nerve cells* or *neurons.* These neurons carry their messages by the transmission of electrical impulses. There are five types of neuroglial cells that support the neurons in various ways. Structurally, the nervous system can be divided into the central nervous system (CNS) and the peripheral nervous system (PNS). The central nervous system is in the center of your body; it is comprised of the brain and spinal cord. The brain can be further subdivided into the cerebral hemispheres, cerebellar hemispheres, diencephalon, midbrain, pons, and medulla oblongata. The peripheral nervous system is comprised of all nerves that are located peripheral to the central nervous system; these are the 12 pairs of cranial nerves and the 31 pairs of spinal nerves. Functionally, the neurons of the nervous system can carry three types of electrical messages: sensory, integrative, and motor. Sensory signals travel through peripheral sensory nerves to the central nervous system. The central nervous system then integrates these sensory stimuli and a response is determined. The order to execute this response then travels through peripheral motor nerves to whatever muscle or gland is being ordered to take action. The nervous system is a tremendously complex system that controls and coordinates virtually everything in the human body. Further, it is responsible for conscious thought, emotional feeling, memory, and movement, as well as unconscious control of our body.

Reproductive System

The reproductive system has the job of carrying on our species into the future by creating offspring. There are two reproductive systems: the male and female.

The male reproductive system functions to create sperm, maintain them, and then deliver them to the site of fertilization (the reproductive system of the female). The primary structures of the male reproductive system are the testes, which produce the sperm. The accessory organs of the male reproductive system function to maintain and deliver the sperm to the site of fertilization. The accessory reproductive organs can be divided into internal and external structures. The internal accessory reproductive organs are the epididymis, vas deference, seminal vesicle, prostate gland, and the bulbourethral glands. The external accessory reproductive organs are the scrotum and the penis.

The female reproductive system functions to create eggs, maintain and deliver them to the site of fertilization, and if fertilization occurs, provide a favorable environment for the developing offspring to grow and then deliver the offspring to the outside world. The primary structures of the female reproductive system are the ovaries, which produce the eggs. The accessory organs of the female reproductive system function to carry on the other activities as listed above. The internal accessory reproductive organs are the fallopian tubes, uterus, and the vagina. The external accessory reproductive organs are the labia majora, labia minora, clitoris, vestibular glands, and the vestibular bulb.

Overview of the Interrelationships of the Organ Systems of the Body - The Big Picture

The preceding was a brief overview of the major visceral organ systems of the body, each one described somewhat independently. However, understanding how each system of the body works without understanding the bigger picture of how these systems interrelate to create the smooth operation of the human body as a whole is like understanding what each piece of a jigsaw puzzle looks like without having any sense of what the bigger picture is that the puzzle creates. Toward that end, the following is a glimpse of the bigger picture of how the organ systems of the human interrelate to operate our body. Admittedly, it is a gross simplification, but is still useful for our purposes.

Our body is composed of trillions of cells, each one a living entity that requires two things: 1) nutri-ents to carry on its functions, and 2) its waste products to be carried away.

These two crucial jobs fall to the cardiovascular system, along with the aid of the lymphatic system (together, these two systems comprise the circulatory system). These two systems circulate fluid (blood and lymph) that carries the nutrients and wastes of the cells of the body. As the circulation of blood occurs, needed nutrients are used up. It is the job of the respiratory system to bring in needed oxygen to the blood and it is the job of the gastrointestinal system to bring in most every other needed nutrient. As the blood circulates, it also builds up waste products of metabolism and other undesired elements, and needs to be filtered. The blood is filtered by the lungs, lymph nodes, kidney, and liver.

The integumentary system provides a covering or barrier between the internal contents and the outside world. This barrier is especially important in preventing foreign microorganisms from entering our body and causing infection and disease. When pathogens do find entry into the body, the immune system functions to attack these foreign invaders. The endocrine system secretes hormones into the bloodstream that function to control the metabolism of the body. Sensory receptors gather sensory stimuli and carry these stimuli to the central nervous system of the body. The brain and spinal cord of the central nervous system then integrate and interpret these sensory stimuli and determine what response(s) the body will have. It is the responsibility of the reproductive system to see that our species is continued into the future by the birth of offspring.

For all movement of the body, the musculoskeletal system is involved. The musculoskeletal system is comprised of the bones of the skeleton, the joints located between the bones, and the muscles that move the bones at the joints of the body.

The Musculoskeletal System

Skeletal System

The skeletal system is composed of bones that create a skeletal structure for support of the body. On a tissue level, bones are made up of spongy bone (that as its name implies, has spaces like a sponge) and compact bone (that as its name implies, is tightly compacted tissue). Of primary importance to the musculoskeletal system is: bones provide rigid levers to which muscles can attach and these bones are located within body parts. When a muscle contracts, the muscle pulls on a bone and the body part that the bone is located within may move. Bones also function to protect internal organs, provide a reservoir of calcium, and house bone marrow that makes blood cells. Bones are usually divided into four major categories based upon their shape. These categories are: long and short bones, flat bones, round bones, and irregular bones.

Joints

Structurally, a joint is where two or more bones are joined together by soft (connective) tissue; functionally, a joint allows movement. There are three types of joints in the body: fibrous, cartilaginous, and synovial. Fibrous joints are united by tough fibrous tissue and cartilaginous joints are united by cartilaginous tissue. However, the most movement is allowed by synovial joints, which is the only type of joint that has a joint cavity. A typical synovial joint is a joint in which the two bones are connected by a double-layered capsule of soft tissue. This joint capsule has an outer fibrous layer that is lined with an inner synovial membrane. The joint capsule encloses a joint cavity that has synovial fluid within it; the synovial fluid is created by the synovial membrane. The joint (articular) surfaces of the bones are covered with cartilage for cushioning. Synovial joints are often classified based on the number of axes about which they permit motion. There are uniaxial, biaxial, triaxial, and nonaxial synovial joints. Outside of the joint (defined as being outside of the joint capsule) are ligaments that connect the two bones to each other. These ligaments function to hold the bones in proper alignment by limiting movement and preventing dislocation. There are also muscles located outside of the joint. These muscles attach to the bones via their tendons, crossing the joint that is located between the bones. When a muscle contracts, it can create movement.

Muscle Cell Structure and Function

A muscle is an organ made up of many muscle cells that are longitudinal in shape (long and thin). For this reason, a muscle cell is also known as a *muscle fiber.* These muscle fibers are arranged into groups known as *fascicles.* Fibrous fascia connective tissue encases each individual muscle fiber (endomysium), each fascicle (perimysium), and the entire muscle (epimysium). It is the continuation of this fibrous fascia that creates the tendon (or aponeurosis) that attaches a muscle to a bone. Each muscle fiber is composed of myofibrils that run longitudinally within the fiber. These myofibrils are divided into sarcomeres that are arranged end to end. Each sarcomere is in turn composed of longitudinally oriented protein filaments known as *actin* and *myosin;* actin filaments are thin and myosin filaments are thick. The actin filaments are attached to the boundaries of the sarcomere, known as *Z lines;* the myosin filaments are located in the center of the sarcomere. When a stimulus comes from the nervous system, this stimulus travels into the interior of the muscle fiber via the transverse ("T") tubules. This message to contract causes stored calcium ions in the sarcoplasmic reticulum (endoplasmic reticulum) of the muscle fiber to be released into the sarcoplasm (cytoplasm). The calcium ions bond to the actin, exposing active sites on the actin to which the myosin heads attach, forming cross-bridges. These myosin cross-bridges then bend, thereby pulling the actin filaments in toward the center (NOTE: this sliding of the actin filament along the myosin filament gives the name to this process, the *sliding filament theory*); this causes the sarcomere to shorten. When the sarcomeres shorten, the myofibril shortens. When the myofibrils shorten, the muscle fiber shortens. When enough muscle fibers shorten, the muscle shortens, creating a pulling force on its attachments. If this pulling force is sufficient, motion of the body parts to which the muscle is attached will occur.

PART 2 - LEARNING HOW MUSCLES FUNCTION

A BRIEF SKETCH OF THE BIG PICTURE OF LEARNING HOW MUSCLES FUNCTION

The Basics of Muscle Structure and Function

A muscle attaches, via its tendons, from one bone to another bone. In so doing, a muscle crosses the joint that is located between the two bones (see Figure 1).

When a muscle contracts, it attempts to shorten toward its center. If the muscle is successful in shortening toward its center, then the two bones that it is attached to will have a force exerted on them that will pull them toward each other (see Figure 2).

Since the bony attachments of the muscle are within body parts, if the muscle moves a bone, then the body part that the bone is within is moved. In this way, muscles can cause movement of parts of the body. When a muscle contracts and shortens as described here, this type of contraction is called a *concentric contraction* and the muscle that is concentrically contracting is called a "mover."

It is worth noting that whether or not a muscle is successful in shortening toward its center is determined by the strength of the pulling force of the muscle compared with the force necessary to actually move one or both body parts that the muscle is attached to. The force necessary to move a body part is usually the force necessary to move the weight of the body part. However, other forces may be involved.

What Happens When a Muscle Concentrically Contracts?

Assuming that a muscle contracts with sufficient strength to shorten toward its center, let's look at the possible scenarios that can occur. If we call one of the attachments of the muscle "Bone A" and

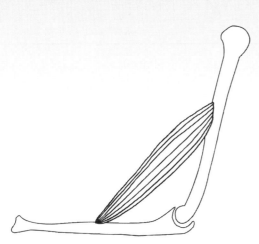

Figure 1. The location of a muscle is shown; it attaches from one bone to another bone and crosses the joint that is located between the two bones.

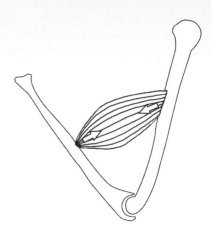

Figure 2. A muscle is shown contracting and shortening (a concentric contraction).

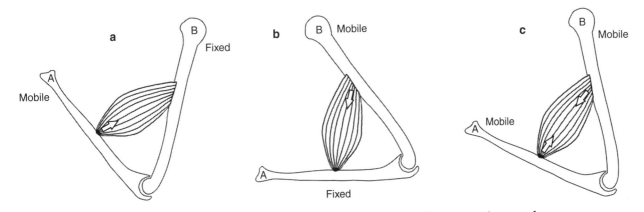

Figure 3. The three scenarios of a muscle concentrically contracting are shown.
In Figure 3a, Bone A moves toward Bone B.
In Figure 3b, Bone B moves toward Bone A.
In Figure 3c, Bone A and Bone B both move toward each other.

the other attachment of the muscle "Bone B," then we see that there are three possible scenarios (see Figure 3):

1. Bone A will be pulled toward Bone B.

2. Bone B will be pulled toward Bone A.

3. Both Bone A and Bone B will be pulled toward each other.

In this manner, a muscle creates a joint action. To fully describe this joint action, we must state which body part has moved and we also must state at which joint the movement has occurred.

As an example to illustrate these concepts, let's look at the brachialis muscle. One attachment of the brachialis is onto the humerus of the arm and the other attachment of the brachialis is onto the ulna of the forearm. In attaching to the arm and the forearm, the brachialis crosses the elbow joint that is located between these two body parts (see Figure 4).

When the brachialis contracts, it attempts to shorten toward its center and exerts a pulling force on the forearm and the arm.

Scenario 1: The usual result of the brachialis contracting is that the forearm will be pulled toward the arm. This is because the forearm is lighter than the arm and therefore would be likely to move before the arm would. (Additionally, if the arm were to move, the trunk would have to move as well, which makes it even less likely that the arm will be the attachment that will move.) To fully describe this action, we call it *flexion of the forearm at the elbow joint* (see Figure 5a). In this scenario, the arm is the attachment that is fixed and the forearm is the attachment that is mobile.

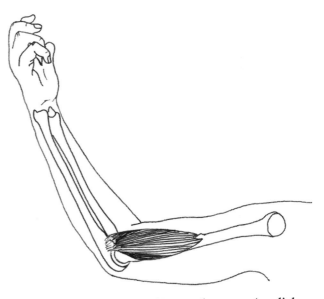

Figure 4. The right brachialis muscle at rest (medial view).

Scenario 2: However, it is possible for the arm to move toward the forearm. If the forearm were to be fixed in place, perhaps because the hand is holding on to an immovable object, then the arm would have to move instead. This action is called *flexion of the arm at the elbow joint* (see Figure 5b). In this scenario, the forearm is the attachment that is fixed and the arm is the attachment that is mobile. This scenario can be called a "reverse action" because the attachment that is usually fixed, the arm, is now mobile, and the attachment that is usually mobile, the forearm, is now fixed.

Figure 5a: Flexion of the forearm at the elbow joint. The arm is fixed and the forearm is mobile, moving toward the arm.

Figure 5b: Flexion of the arm at the elbow joint. The forearm is fixed (in our illustration, the hand is holding onto an immovable bar) and the arm is mobile, moving toward the forearm.

Figure 5c: Flexion of the forearm and the arm at the elbow joint. Neither attachment is fixed so both are mobile, moving toward each other.

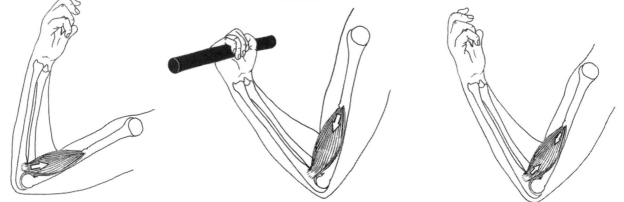

Figure 5. The three scenarios that can result from a concentric contraction of the brachialis muscle.

Scenario 3: Since the contraction of the brachialis exerts a pulling force on the forearm and the arm, it is possible for both of these bones to move. When this occurs, there are two actions: flexion of the forearm at the elbow joint and flexion of the arm at the elbow joint (see Figure 5c). In this case, both bones are mobile and neither one is fixed.

It is important to realize that the brachialis does not intend nor choose which attachment will move, or if both attachments will move. When a muscle contracts, it merely exerts a pulling force toward its center. Which attachment moves is determined by other factors. The relative weight of the body parts is the most common factor. However, another common determinant is when the central nervous system directs another muscle in the body to contract. The contraction of this second muscle "fixes" (stops from moving) one of the attachments of our mover muscle. (If this occurs, this second muscle that contracts to fix a body part would be called a "fixator" or "stabilizer" muscle.) It follows that if one attachment is fixed, then the other attachment would be mobile.

Beginning the Process of Learning Muscles

Essentially, when learning about muscles, there are two major aspects that must be learned: the attachments and actions of the muscle.

Generally speaking, attachments of a muscle must be memorized. However, there are times when clues are given about the attachments of a muscle by the muscle's name. For example, the name *coracobrachialis* tells us that the muscle has one attachment on the coracoid process of the scapula and that its other attachment is on the brachium (i.e., the humerus). Similarly, the name *zygomaticus major* tells us that this muscle attaches onto the zygomatic bone (and that there must be another muscle called the *zygomaticus minor*).

Unlike muscle attachments, muscle actions do not have to be memorized. Instead, by understanding the simple concept that a muscle pulls at its attachments to move a body part, the action or actions of a muscle can be reasoned out.

5-Step Approach to Learning Muscles

When first confronted with having to study and learn about a muscle, I recommend the following approach:

1. Look at the name of the muscle to see if it gives you any "free information" that saves you from having to memorize attachments or actions of the muscle.

2. Learn the general location of the muscle well enough to be able to visualize the muscle on your body. At this point, you need only know it well enough to know: 1) which joint it crosses, 2) where it crosses the joint, and 3) how it crosses the joint, i.e., what direction its fibers are running.

3. Use this general knowledge of the muscle's location to figure out the actions of the muscle.

4. Go back and learn (memorize, if necessary) the specific attachments of the muscle.

5. Now look at the relationship of this muscle to other muscles (and other soft tissue structures) of the body. Look at the following: Is this muscle superficial or deep? And, what other muscles (and other soft tissue structures) are located near this muscle?

Figuring Out a Muscle's Actions (Step 3)

Once you have a general familiarity with a muscle's location on your body, then it is time to begin the process of reasoning out the actions of the muscle. The most important thing that you must look at is:

the direction of the muscle fibers relative to the joint that it crosses.

By doing this, you can see:

the line of pull of the muscle relative to the joint.

This line of pull will determine the actions of the muscle, i.e., how the contraction of the muscle will cause the body parts to move at that joint.

The approach that I like to have my students follow is to ask the following three questions of themselves:

1. *What joint does the muscle cross?*

2. *Where does the muscle cross the joint?*

3. *How does the muscle cross the joint?*

Question 1 - What Joint Does the Muscle Cross?

I always recommend to my students that the first question to ask and answer in figuring out the actions of a muscle is to simply know what joint it crosses. The following rule applies: If a muscle crosses a joint, then it will have an action at that joint. For example, if we look at the coracobrachialis, knowing that it crosses the shoulder joint tells us that it must have an action at the shoulder joint. We may not know what the exact action of the coracobrachialis is yet, but at least we now know at what joint it has its actions. To figure out exactly what these actions are, we need to look at the next two questions. (It is worth pointing out that the converse of this rule is also true, that is: if a muscle does not cross a joint, then it will not have an action at that joint.)

Questions 2 and 3: - Where Does the Muscle Cross the Joint?   and   How Does the Muscle Cross the Joint?

These two questions must be looked at together. The "where" of a muscle crossing a joint is whether it crosses the joint anteriorly, posteriorly, medially, or laterally. It is helpful to place a muscle into one of these broad groups because the following general rules apply: muscles that cross a joint anteriorly will usually flex a body part at that joint, and muscles that cross a joint posteriorly will usually extend a body part at that joint*; muscles that cross a joint laterally will usually abduct or laterally flex a body part at that joint, and muscles that cross a joint medially will usually adduct a body part at that joint. The "how" of a muscle crossing a joint is whether it crosses the joint with its fibers running vertically or horizontally. This is also very important.

To illustrate this idea, lets look at the pectoralis major muscle. The pectoralis major has two parts, a clavicular head and a sternocostal head. The "where" of these two heads of the pectoralis major crossing the shoulder joint is the same, that is, they both cross the shoulder joint anteriorly. But the "how" of these two heads crossing the shoulder joint is very different. The clavicular head crosses the shoulder joint with its fibers running vertically, therefore it flexes the arm at the shoulder joint (because it pulls the arm upward in the sagittal plane, which is flexion). However, the sternocostal head crosses the shoulder joint with its fibers running horizontally, therefore it adducts the arm at the shoulder joint (because it pulls the arm from lateral to medial in the frontal plane, which is adduction).

With a muscle that has a horizontal direction to its fibers, there is another factor that must be considered when looking at "how" this muscle crosses the joint. That is whether the muscle attaches to the first place on the bone that it reaches, or whether the muscle wraps around the bone before attaching to it. Muscles that run horizontally (in the transverse plane) and wrap around the bone before attaching to it create a rotation action when they contract and pull on the attachment. For example, the sternocostal head of the pectoralis major does not attach to the first point on the humerus that it reaches. Instead, it continues to wrap around the shaft of the humerus to attach onto the lateral lip of the bicipital groove of

---

* Flexion is nearly always an anterior movement of a body part and extension is nearly always a posterior movement of a body part. However, from the knee joint and further distal, flexion is a posterior movement and extension is an anterior movement of the body part.

the humerus. When the sternocostal head pulls, it medially rotates the arm at the shoulder joint (in addition to adducting it).

In essence, by asking the three questions: What joint does a muscle cross?, Where does the muscle cross the joint?, and How does the muscle cross the joint?, we are trying to determine the direction of the muscle fibers relative to the joint. Determining this will give us the line of pull of the muscle relative to the joint and that will give us the actions of the muscle, saving us the trouble of having to memorize this information!

Functional Groups Approach

The best method for approaching and learning each and every action of a new muscle that you first encounter to learn is to use the reasoning of step 3 of the 5-step approach. You have learned that for each aspect of the direction of fibers for a muscle, you apply the questions of where and how the muscle crosses the joint. This reasoning is solid and will lead you to reason out all actions of the muscle that is being studied. However, it can be very repetitive and time consuming as you apply this method to muscle after muscle after muscle that all cross the same joint in the same manner.

Therefore, once you are very comfortable with applying the questions of step 3 for learning the actions of each muscle individually, I recommend that you begin to use your understanding of how muscles function and apply it on a larger scale. Instead of looking at each muscle individually and going through all of the questions of step 3 for that muscle, take a step back and look at the broad functional groups of muscles at each joint. For example, instead of individually using the questions of step 3 to learn that the brachialis flexes the forearm at the elbow joint, and then that the biceps brachii flexes the forearm at the elbow joint, and then that the pronator teres flexes the forearm at the elbow joint, and also the flexor carpi radialis, palmaris longus, etc., etc., it is a simpler and more elegant approach to look at the functional groups of muscles that cross this joint. In other words, the bigger picture is to see that ALL muscles that cross the elbow joint anteriorly flex the forearm at the elbow joint. Looking at the body this way, when you encounter yet another muscle that crosses the elbow joint anteriorly, you can automatically place it into the group of forearm flexors at the elbow joint.

For each joint of the human body, look for the functional groups. In the case of the elbow joint, since it is a pure hinge, uniaxial joint, it is very simple; there are only two functional groups, anterior muscles that flex and posterior muscles that extend. Triaxial joints such as the shoulder or hip joint will have more functional groups (flexors, extensors, abductors, adductors, medial rotators, and lateral rotators) but the concepts will always be the same. Once you clearly see this concept, the learning of the actions of muscles of the body can be greatly simplified and streamlined.

Reminder About Reverse Actions

Please remember that the reverse actions of a muscle are always possible, even if they have not been specifically listed in this book. For some examples of reverse actions, please see Appendix C in the *Muscular System Manual.*

A Visual and Kinesthetic Exercise for Learning a Muscle's Actions

The Rubber Band Exercise

An excellent method for learning the actions of a muscle is to place a large colorful rubber band (or large colorful shoelace or string) on your body, or the body of a partner, in the same location that the muscle you are studying is located. Hold one end of the rubber band at one of the attachment sites of the muscle and hold the other end of the rubber band at the other attachment site of the muscle. Make sure that you have the rubber band running/oriented in the same direction as the direction of the fibers of the muscle. If it is not uncomfortable, you may even loop or tie the rubber band (or shoelace) around the body parts that are the attachments of the muscle.

Once you have the rubber band in place, pull one of the ends of the rubber band toward the center of the rubber band to see the action that the rubber band/muscle has upon that body part's attachment; return the attachment of the rubber band to where it began and then pull the other end of the rubber band toward the center of the rubber band to see the action that the rubber band/muscle has upon the other body part's attachment.

By placing the rubber band on your body or your partner's body, you are simulating the direction of the muscle's fibers relative to the joint that it crosses. By pulling either end of the rubber band toward the center, you are simulating the line of pull of the muscle relative to the joint that it crosses. The resultant movements that occur are the actions that the muscle would have. This is an excellent exercise to both visually see the actions of a muscle and to kinesthetically experience the actions of a muscle. This exercise can be used to learn all muscle actions, and can be especially helpful for determining actions that may be a little more difficult to visualize, such as rotation actions.

NOTE: I recommend the use of a large colorful rubber band more than a shoelace or string because when you stretch out a rubber band and place it in the location that a muscle would be, the natural elasticity of a rubber band creates a pull on the attachment sites that nicely simulates the pull of a muscle on its attachments when it contracts. If you can, I recommend that you work with a partner to do this exercise. Have your partner hold one of the "attachments" of the rubber band while you hold the other "attachment." This leaves one of your hands free to pull the rubber band attachment sites toward the center.

A FURTHER NOTE OF CAUTION: If you are using a rubber band, be careful that you do not accidently let go and have the rubber band hit you or your partner. For this reason, it would be preferable to use a shoelace instead of a rubber band when working near the face.

Acknowledgments

I would like to begin by thanking Barry Antoniow of Kiné-Concept Schools in Canada for first giving me the idea to develop a musculoskeletal anatomy coloring book. It has been long needed and I appreciate Barry's insight.

Since so much of the artwork for this coloring book has come from the *Muscular System Manual,* I would like to acknowledge the beautiful, crisp, and clear illustrations drawn by the artists of that book: the principal artist, Jean Luciano; and the additional artists, Rosa Cervoni, Barbara Haeger, and J.C. Muscolino. The quality of these illustrations greatly aids the reader in learning musculoskeletal anatomy.

I also must thank the entire crew over at Mosby, Elsevier Science: Kellie White, who made this project become a possibility; Jennifer Watrous, who worked with me each step of the way in developing it; and Linda McKinley and her team, who spent a tremendous amount of time in actually assembling and creating this book.

I must thank my entire family for their unending support as I spent hour after hour at the computer working on this book. Without their unconditional support, none of this would have been possible.

Lastly, I would like to say that studying by using coloring books has to be one of the more creative and fun ways to learn anatomy. For this reason, I would like to dedicate this book to my children, Randi and J.C., who have consistently taught me to try to keep creativity and fun in my approach to life.

Contents

PREFACE AND HOW TO USE THIS BOOK, v

INTRODUCTION, vii

CHAPTER 1—THE SKELETAL SYSTEM, 1

Bones of the Head
Anterior View of the Bones and Bony Landmarks of the Head, 3
Lateral View of the Bones and Bony Landmarks of the Head, 4
Inferior View of the Bones and Bony Landmarks of the Head, 5

Bones of the Neck
Anterior View of the Bones and Bony Landmarks of the Neck, 6
Posterior View of the Bones and Bony Landmarks of the Neck, 7

Bones of the Trunk
Anterior View of the Bones and Bony Landmarks of the Trunk, 8
Posterior View of the Bones and Bony Landmarks of the Trunk, 9

Bones of the Pelvis and Thigh
Anterior View of the Bones and Bony Landmarks of the Right Pelvis, 10
Anterior View of the Bones and Bony Landmarks of the Right Thigh, 11
Posterior View of the Bones and Bony Landmarks of the Right Pelvis, 12
Posterior View of the Bones and Bony Landmarks of the Right Thigh, 13

Bones of the Leg
Anterior View of the Bones and Bony Landmarks of the Right Leg, 14
Posterior View of the Bones and Bony Landmarks of the Right Leg, 15

Bones of the Foot
Dorsal View of the Bones and Bony Landmarks of the Right Foot, 16
Plantar View of the Bones and Bony Landmarks of the Right Foot, 17

Bones of the Scapula/Arm
Anterior View of the Bones and Bony Landmarks of the Right Scapula/Arm, 18
Posterior View of the Bones and Bony Landmarks of the Right Scapula/Arm, 19

Bones of the Forearm
Anterior View of the Bones and Bony Landmarks of the Right Forearm, 20
Posterior View of the Bones and Bony Landmarks of the Right Forearm, 21

Bones of the Hand
Palmar View of the Bones and Bony Landmarks of the Right Hand, 22
Dorsal View of the Bones and Bony Landmarks of the Right Hand, 23

CHAPTER 2—THE MUSCULAR SYSTEM, 25

Muscles of the Head
Occipitofrontalis, 28
Temporoparietalis, 30
Auricularis Anterior, Superior, and Posterior, 30
Orbicularis Oculi, 32

Levator Palpebrae Superioris, 32
Corrugator Supercilii, 34
Procerus, 34
Nasalis, 36
Depressor Septi Nasi, 36
Levator Labii Superioris Alaeque Nasi, 38
Levator Labii Superioris, 38
Zygomaticus Minor, 40
Zygomaticus Major, 40
Levator Anguli Oris, 42
Risorius, 42
Depressor Anguli Oris, 44
Depressor Labii Inferioris, 44
Mentalis, 46
Buccinator, 46
Orbicularis Oris, 48
Temporalis, 50
Masseter, 50
Lateral Pterygoid, 52
Medial Pterygoid, 52

Muscles of the Neck
Trapezius ("The Traps"), 62
Splenius Capitis, 64
Splenius Cervicis, 64
Levator Scapulae, 66
Rectus Capitis Posterior Major, 68
Rectus Capitis Posterior Minor, 68
Obliquus Capitis Inferior, 70
Obliquus Capitis Superior, 70
Platysma, 72
Sternocleidomastoid ("SCM"), 74
Sternohyoid, 76
Sternothyroid, 76
Thyrohyoid, 78
Omohyoid, 78
Digastric, 80
Stylohyoid, 80
Mylohyoid, 82
Geniohyoid, 82
Anterior Scalene, 84
Middle Scalene, 84
Posterior Scalene, 86
Longus Colli, 88
Longus Capitis, 88
Rectus Capitis Anterior, 90
Rectus Capitis Lateralis, 90

Muscles of the Trunk
Latissimus Dorsi ("The Lats"), 104
Rhomboids Major and Minor, 106
Serratus Anterior, 108
Serratus Posterior Superior, 110
Serratus Posterior Inferior, 110

The Erector Spinae Group, 112
Iliocostalis, 114
Longissimus, 114
Spinalis, 116
The Transversospinalis Group, 118
Semispinalis, 120
Multifidus, 120
Rotatores, 122
Quadratus Lumborum, 124
Interspinales, 126
Intertransversarii, 126
Levatores Costarum, 128
Subcostales, 128
Pectoralis Major, 130
Pectoralis Minor, 132
Subclavius, 132
External Intercostals, 134
Internal Intercostals, 136
Rectus Abdominis, 138
External Abdominal Oblique, 140
Internal Abdominal Oblique, 140
Transversus Abdominis, 142
Transversus Thoracis, 142
Diaphragm, 144

Muscles of the Pelvis
Psoas Major, 156
Iliacus, 158
Psoas Minor, 160
Gluteus Maximus, 162
Gluteus Medius, 164
Gluteus Minimus, 166
Piriformis, 168
Superior Gemellus, 170
Obturator Internus, 170
Inferior Gemellus, 172
Obturator Externus, 174
Quadratus Femoris, 176

Muscles of the Thigh
Tensor Fasciae Latae ("TFL"), 188
Sartorius, 190
Rectus Femoris, 192
Vastus Lateralis, 194
Vastus Medialis, 194
Vastus Intermedius, 196
Articularis Genus, 196
Pectineus, 198
Gracilis, 198
Adductor Longus, 200
Adductor Brevis, 202
Adductor Magnus, 204
Biceps Femoris, 206
Semitendinosus, 208
Semimembranosus, 208

Muscles of the Leg
Tibialis Anterior, 222
Extensor Hallucis Longus, 224
Extensor Digitorum Longus, 226
Fibularis Tertius, 226
Fibularis Longus, 228
Fibularis Brevis, 228
Gastrocnemius ("Gastrocs"), 230
Soleus, 230
Plantaris, 232
Popliteus, 232
Tibialis Posterior, 234
Flexor Digitorum Longus, 236
Flexor Hallucis Longus, 238

Intrinsic Muscles of the Foot
Extensor Digitorum Brevis, 250
Extensor Hallucis Brevis, 250
Abductor Hallucis, 252
Abductor Digiti Minimi Pedis, 252
Flexor Digitorum Brevis, 254
Quadratus Plantae, 256
Lumbricals Pedis, 256
Flexor Hallucis Brevis, 258
Flexor Digiti Minimi Pedis, 258
Adductor Hallucis, 260
Plantar Interossei, 262
Dorsal Interossei Pedis, 262

Muscles of the Scapula/Arm
Supraspinatus, 276
Infraspinatus, 276
Teres Minor, 278
Subscapularis, 278
Teres Major, 280
Deltoid, 282
Coracobrachialis, 284
Biceps Brachii, 286
Brachialis, 286
Triceps Brachii, 288

Muscles of the Forearm
Pronator Teres, 306
Pronator Quadratus, 306
Flexor Carpi Radialis, 308
Palmaris Longus, 308
Flexor Carpi Ulnaris, 310
Brachioradialis, 312
Flexor Digitorum Superficialis, 314
Flexor Digitorum Profundus, 314
Flexor Pollicis Longus, 316
Anconeus, 318
Extensor Carpi Radialis Longus, 320
Extensor Carpi Radialis Brevis, 320

Extensor Carpi Ulnaris, 322
Extensor Digitorum, 324
Extensor Digiti Minimi, 324
Supinator, 326
Abductor Pollicis Longus, 328
Extensor Pollicis Brevis, 328
Extensor Pollicis Longus, 330
Extensor Indicis, 330

Muscles of the Hand
Abductor Pollicis Brevis, 344
Flexor Pollicis Brevis, 344
Opponens Pollicis, 346
Opponens Digiti Minimi, 346
Abductor Digiti Minimi Manus, 348
Flexor Digiti Minimi Manus, 348
Palmaris Brevis, 350
Adductor Pollicis, 352
Lumbricals Manus, 352
Palmar Interossei, 354
Dorsal Interossei Manus, 354

CHAPTER 3—OTHER SKELETAL MUSCLES, 361

Anterior Views of the Other Muscles of the Abdomen, 363
Views of the Muscles of the Perineum, 364
Views of the Muscles of the Tongue, 365
View of the Muscles of the Palate, 366
View of the Muscles of the Pharynx, 367
Views of the Muscles of the Larynx, 368
Views of the Muscles of the Larynx, 369
Views of the Extrinsic Muscles of the Right Eye, 370
View of the Muscles of the Tympanic Cavity, 371

CHAPTER 4—THE NERVOUS SYSTEM, 373

Cranial Nerves, 374
View of Spinal Nerve Organization, 375
View of the Cervical Plexus, 376
View of the Brachial Plexus, 377
View of the Lumbar Plexus, 378
Views of the Sacral and Coccygeal Plexuses, 379
Views of Innervation to the Right Lower Extremity, 380
Anterior View of Innervation to the Right Upper Extremity, 381

CHAPTER 5—THE ARTERIAL SYSTEM, 383

Lateral View of Arterial Supply to the Head and Neck, 384
Anterior View of Arterial Supply to the Trunk and Pelvis, 385

Anterior View of Arterial Supply to the Right Lower
  Extremity, 386
Anterior View of Arterial Supply to the Right Upper
  Extremity, 387

CHAPTER 6—OTHER STRUCTURES AND
SYSTEMS OF THE BODY, 388

The Cell, 390
Bone Tissue, 392
Muscle Tissue, 394
Nerve Tissue, 396
Joints, 398
Integumentary System, 400
Cardiac System, 402

Venous System, 404
Lymphatic System, 406
Respiratory System, 408
Urinary System, 410
Gastrointestinal System, 412
Immune System, 414
Endocrine System, 416
Sensory System, 418
Reproductive System, 420

ANSWER KEY, 422

CREDITS, 454

Musculoskeletal
Anatomy
Coloring Book

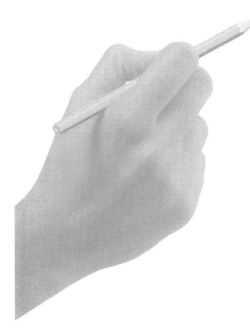

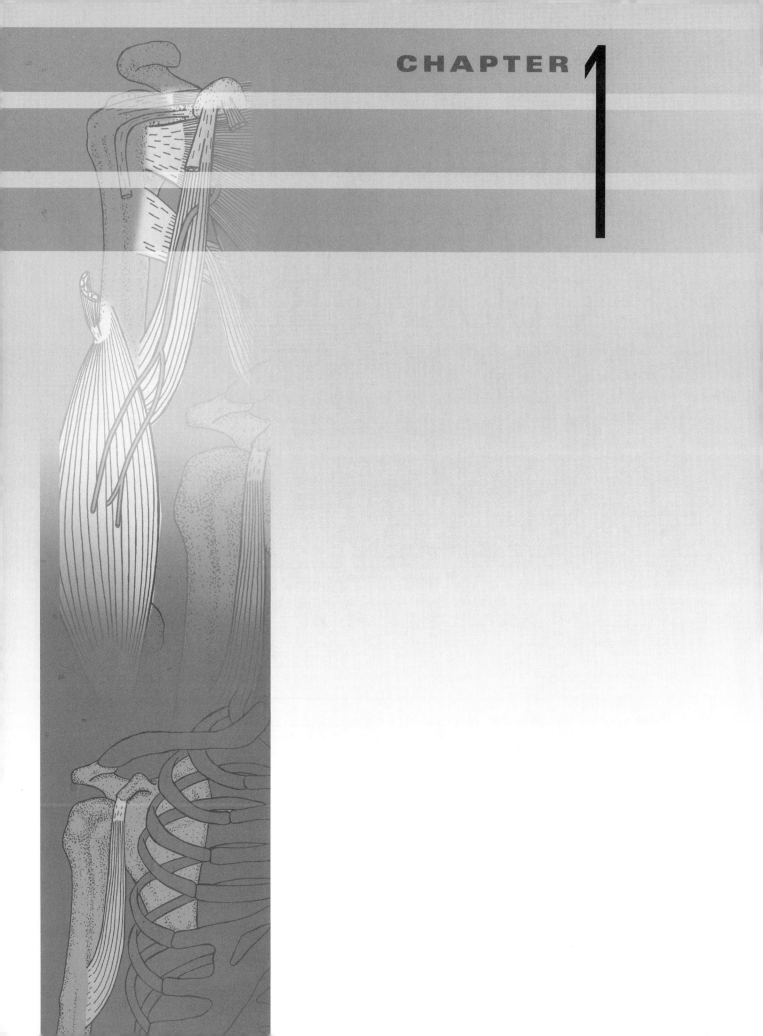

CHAPTER 1

The Skeletal System

GET READY TO EXPLORE:

Bones of the Head
Anterior View of the Bones and Bony Landmarks of the Head, 3
Lateral View of the Bones and Bony Landmarks of the Head, 4
Inferior View of the Bones and Bony Landmarks of the Head, 5

Bones of the Neck
Anterior View of the Bones and Bony Landmarks of the Neck, 6
Posterior View of the Bones and Bony Landmarks of the Neck, 7

Bones of the Trunk
Antrerior View of the Bones and Bony Landmarks of the Trunk, 8
Posterior View of the Bones and Bony Landmarks of the Trunk, 9

Bones of the Pelvis and Thigh
Anterior View of the Bones and Bony Landmarks of the Right Pelvis, 10
Anterior View of the Bones and Bony Landmarks of the Right Thigh, 11
Posterior View of the Bones and Bony Landmarks of the Right Pelvis, 12
Posterior View of the Bones and Bony Landmarks of the Right Thigh, 13

Bones of the Leg
Anterior View of the Bones and Bony Landmarks of the Right Leg, 14
Posterior View of the Bones and Bony Landmarks of the Right Leg, 15

Bones of the Foot
Dorsal View of the Bones and Bony Landmarks of the Right Foot, 16
Plantar View of the Bones and Bony Landmarks of the Right Foot, 17

Bones of the Scapula/Arm
Anterior View of the Bones and Bony Landmarks of the Right Scapula/Arm, 18
Posterior View of the Bones and Bony Landmarks of the Right Scapula/Arm, 19

Bones of the Forearm
Anterior View of the Bones and Bony Landmarks of the Right Forearm, 20
Posterior View of the Bones and Bony Landmarks of the Right Forearm, 21

Bones of the Hand
Palmar View of the Bones and Bony Landmarks of the Right Hand, 22
Dorsal View of the Bones and Bony Landmarks of the Right Hand, 23

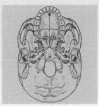

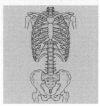

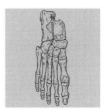

An asterisk (*) following a number indicates that the structure is a bony landmark rather than a bone.

ANTERIOR VIEW OF THE BONES AND BONY LANDMARKS OF THE HEAD

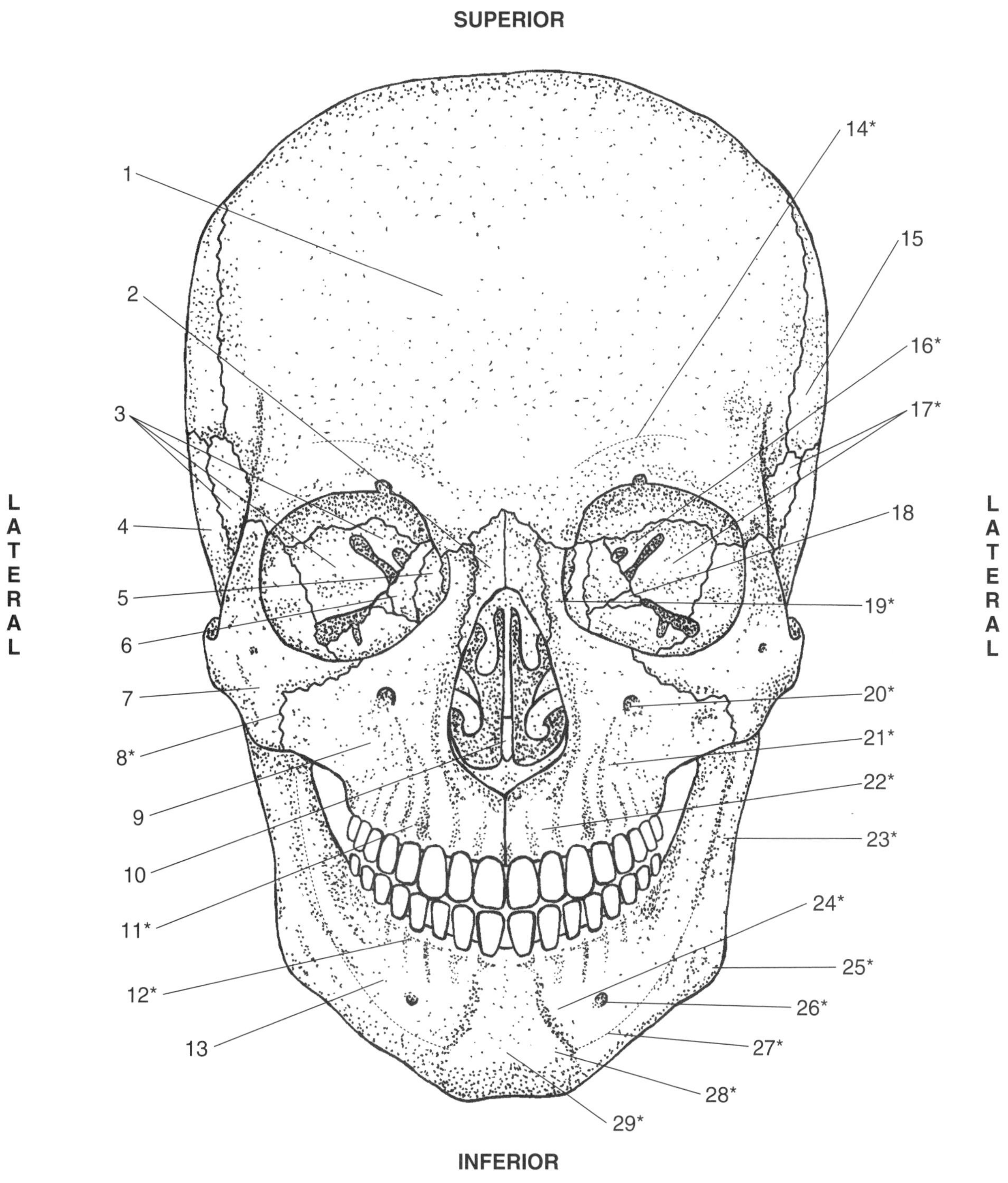

SUPERIOR

1

2

3

4

5

6

7

8*

9

10

11*

12*

13

14*

15

16*

17*

18

19*

20*

21*

22*

23*

24*

25*

26*

27*

28*

29*

LATERAL

LATERAL

INFERIOR

LATERAL VIEW OF THE BONES AND BONY LANDMARKS
OF THE HEAD

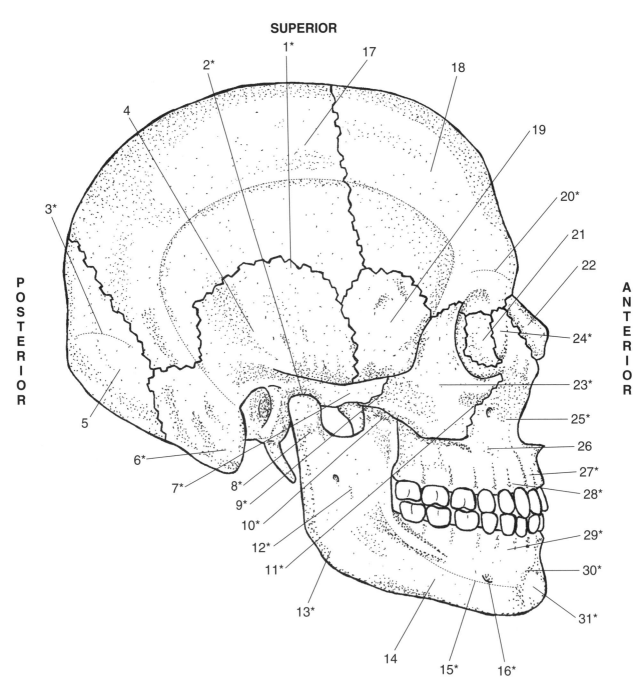

SUPERIOR

POSTERIOR

ANTERIOR

INFERIOR

INFERIOR VIEW OF THE BONES AND BONY LANDMARKS OF THE HEAD

ANTERIOR

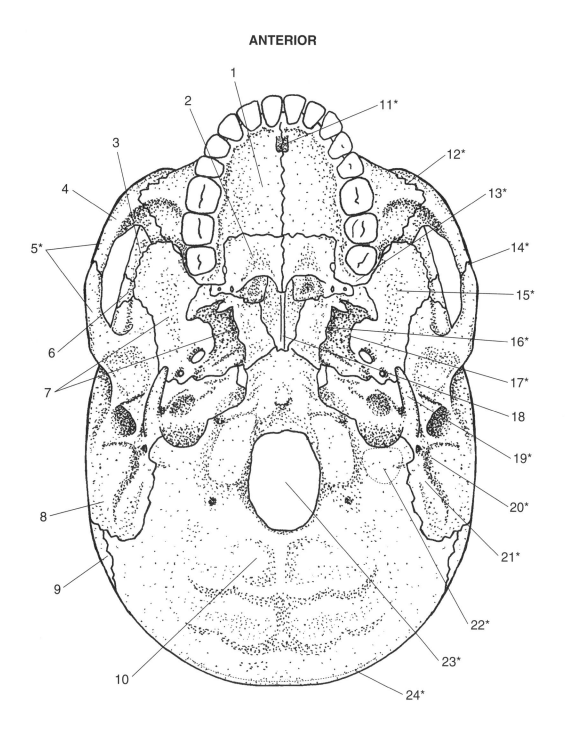

LATERAL

LATERAL

POSTERIOR

ANTERIOR VIEW OF THE BONES AND BONY LANDMARKS OF THE NECK

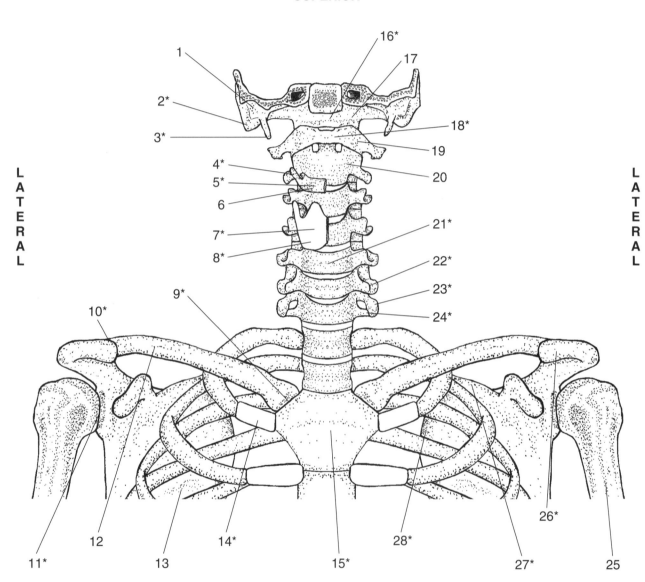

SUPERIOR

LATERAL

LATERAL

INFERIOR

POSTERIOR VIEW OF THE BONES AND BONY LANDMARKS OF THE NECK

SUPERIOR

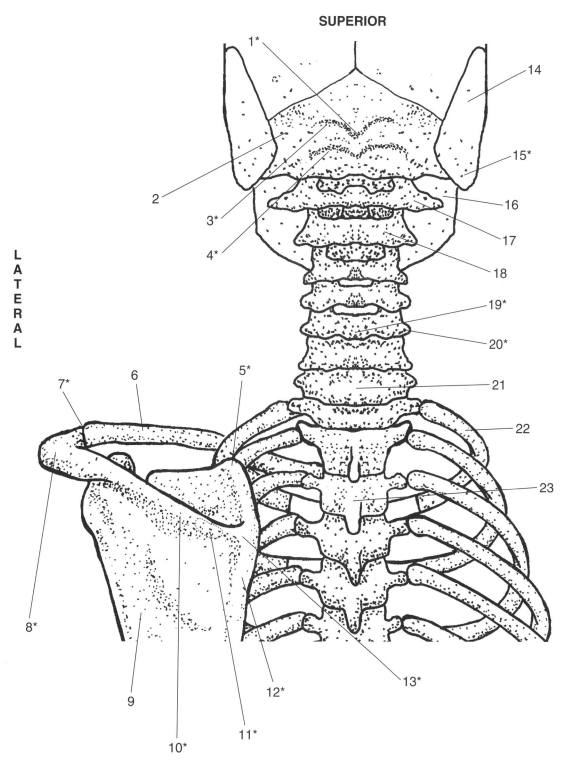

LATERAL

LATERAL

INFERIOR

ANTERIOR VIEW OF THE BONES AND BONY LANDMARKS
OF THE TRUNK

SUPERIOR

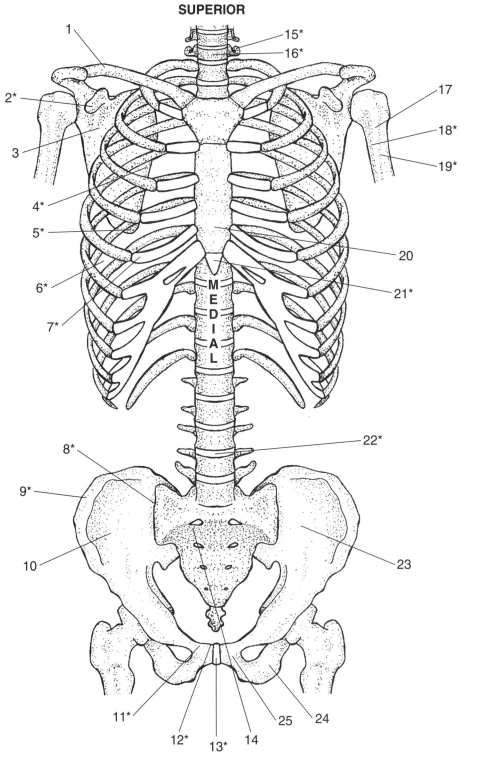

LATERAL

MEDIAL

LATERAL

1

15*
16*

2*

3

17

18*

19*

4*

5*

20

6*

21*

7*

8*

9*

22*

10

23

11*

12* 13* 14

25 24

INFERIOR

POSTERIOR VIEW OF THE BONES AND BONY LANDMARKS OF THE TRUNK

SUPERIOR

LATERAL

MEDIAL

LATERAL

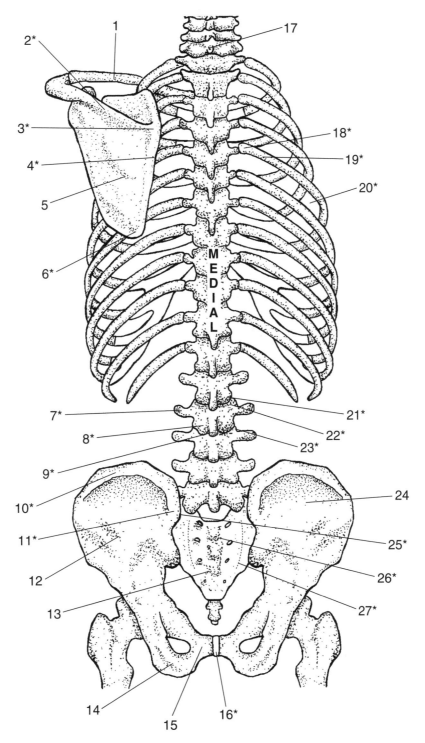

INFERIOR

ANTERIOR VIEW OF THE BONES AND BONY LANDMARKS OF THE RIGHT PELVIS

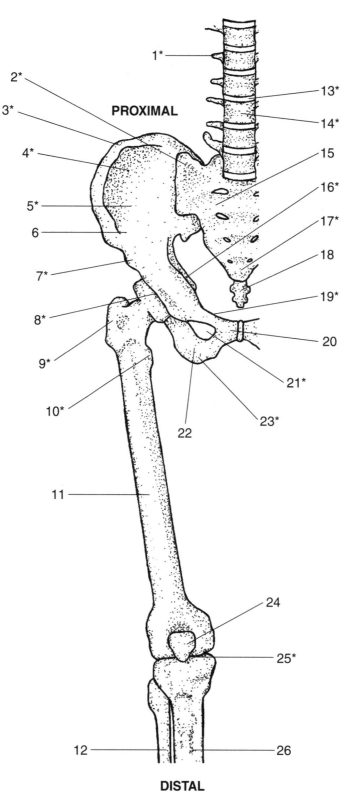

PROXIMAL

LATERAL

MEDIAL

DISTAL

ANTERIOR VIEW OF THE BONES AND BONY LANDMARKS OF THE RIGHT THIGH

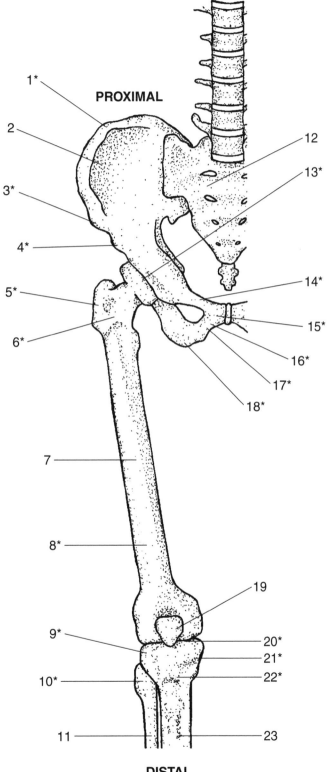
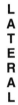

PROXIMAL

1*

2

3*

4*

5*

6*

7

8*

9*

10*

11

12

13*

14*

15*

16*

17*

18*

19

20*

21*

22*

23

LATERAL

MEDIAL

DISTAL

POSTERIOR VIEW OF THE BONES AND BONY LANDMARKS OF THE RIGHT PELVIS

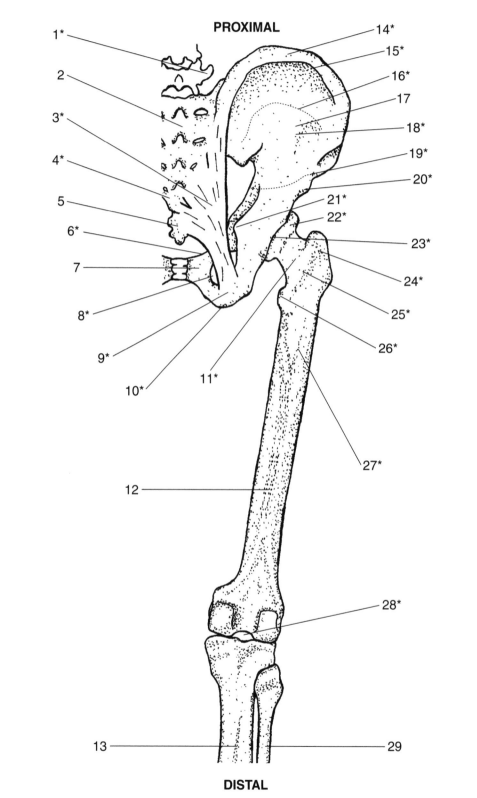

PROXIMAL

1*

2

3*

4*

5

6*

7

8*

9*

10*

11*

14*

15*

16*

17

18*

19*

20*

21*

22*

23*

24*

25*

26*

27*

MEDIAL

LATERAL

12

13

28*

29

DISTAL

POSTERIOR VIEW OF THE BONES AND BONY LANDMARKS OF THE RIGHT THIGH

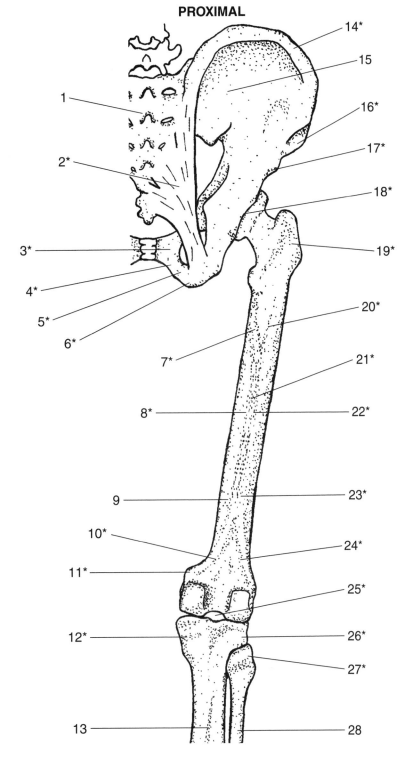

PROXIMAL

MEDIAL

LATERAL

DISTAL

ANTERIOR VIEW OF THE BONES AND BONY LANDMARKS OF THE RIGHT LEG

PROXIMAL

1*

2*

3*

4*

5*

6

7*

8

9

10*

11

12

13

14

15*

16

17*

18*

19*

20

21

22

23

24

25

26

27

LATERAL

MEDIAL

DISTAL

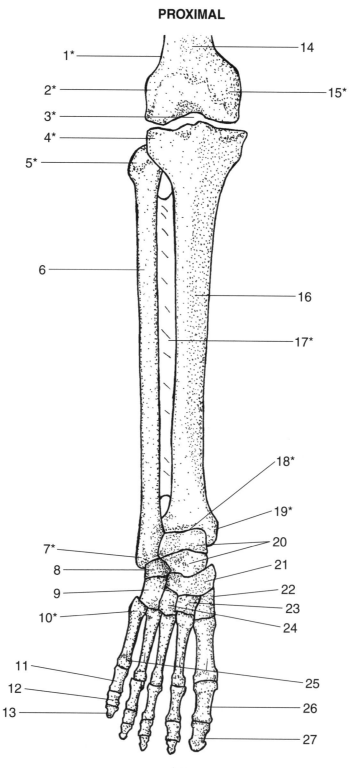

POSTERIOR VIEW OF THE BONES AND BONY LANDMARKS
OF THE RIGHT LEG

PROXIMAL

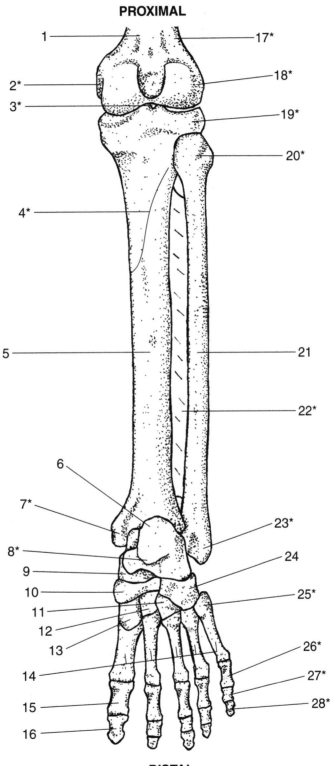

1

17*

2*

18*

3*

19*

20*

4*

MEDIAL

LATERAL

5

21

22*

6

7*

23*

8*

24

9

10

25*

11

12

13

26*

14

27*

15

28*

16

DISTAL

DORSAL VIEW OF THE BONES AND BONY LANDMARKS
OF THE RIGHT FOOT

PROXIMAL

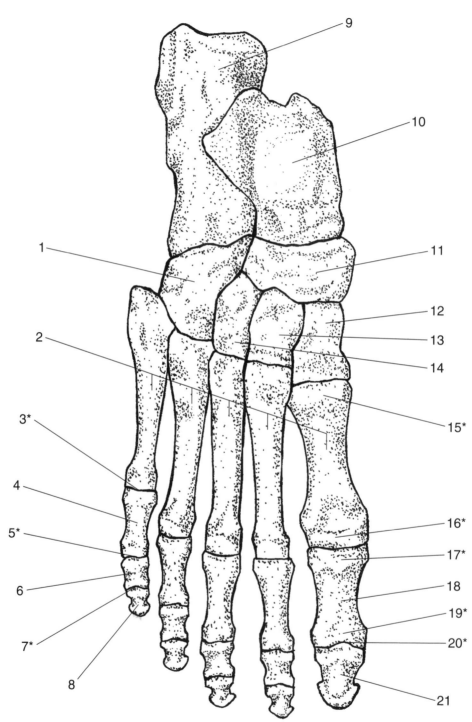

L
A
T
E
R
A
L

M
E
D
I
A
L

DISTAL

PLANTAR VIEW OF THE BONES AND BONY LANDMARKS OF THE RIGHT FOOT

PROXIMAL

MEDIAL

LATERAL

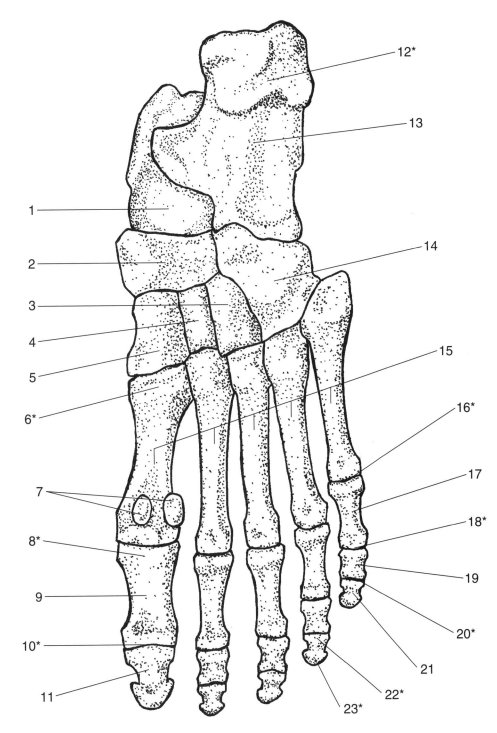

DISTAL

ANTERIOR VIEW OF THE BONES AND BONY LANDMARKS OF THE RIGHT SCAPULA/ARM

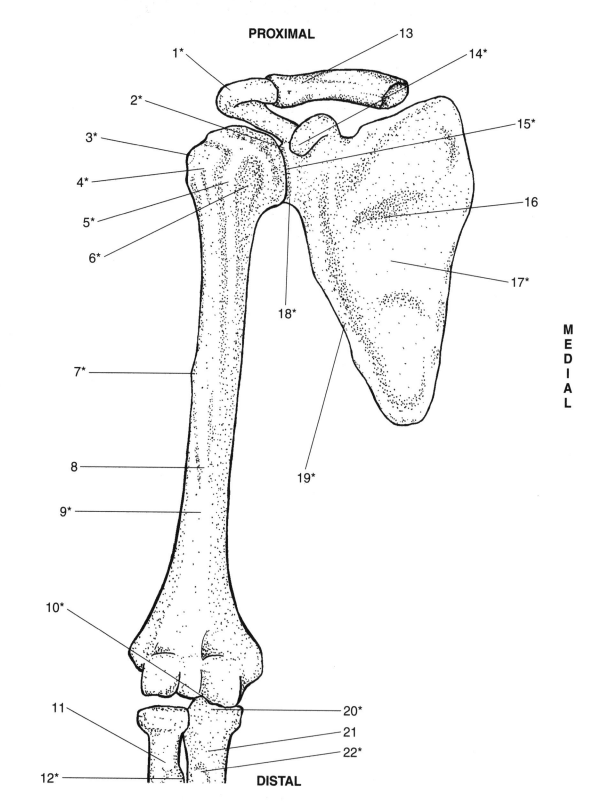

POSTERIOR VIEW OF THE BONES AND BONY LANDMARKS OF THE RIGHT SCAPULA/ARM

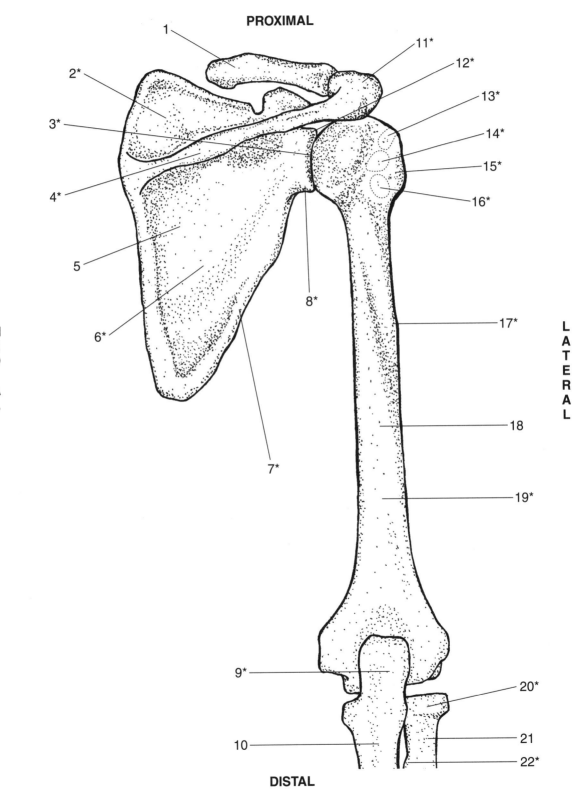

PROXIMAL

1

2*

3*

4*

5

6*

7*

8*

11*

12*

13*

14*

15*

16*

17*

18

19*

9*

10

20*

21

22*

MEDIAL

LATERAL

DISTAL

ANTERIOR VIEW OF THE BONES AND BONY LANDMARKS OF THE RIGHT FOREARM

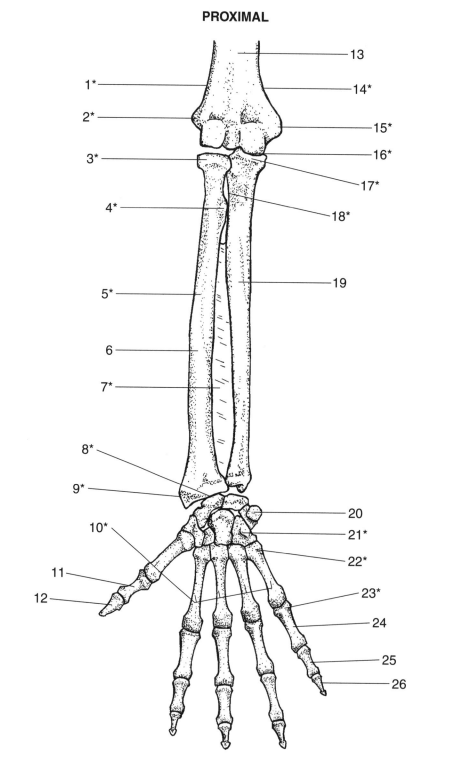

PROXIMAL

13

1*

14*

2*

15*

3*

16*

17*

4*

18*

19

5*

6

7*

8*

9*

20

10*

21*

22*

11

12

23*

24

25

26

LATERAL   RADIAL

ULNAR   MEDIAL

DISTAL

POSTERIOR VIEW OF THE BONES AND BONY LANDMARKS OF THE RIGHT FOREARM

PROXIMAL

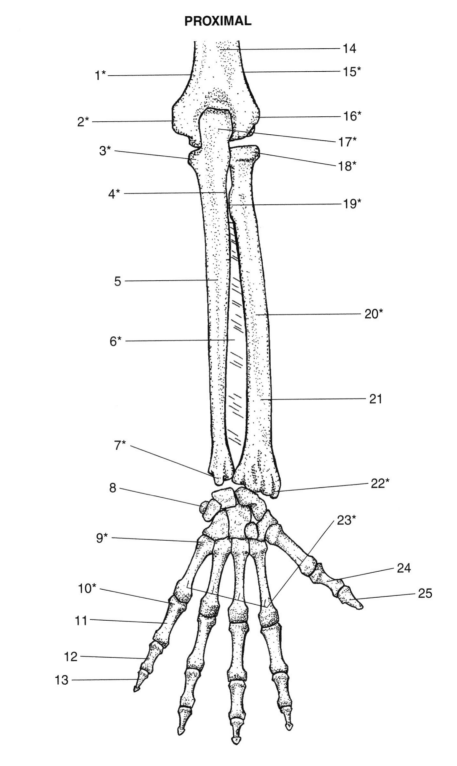

MEDIAL ULNAR

RADIAL LATERAL

DISTAL

PALMAR VIEW OF THE BONES AND BONY LANDMARKS
OF THE RIGHT HAND

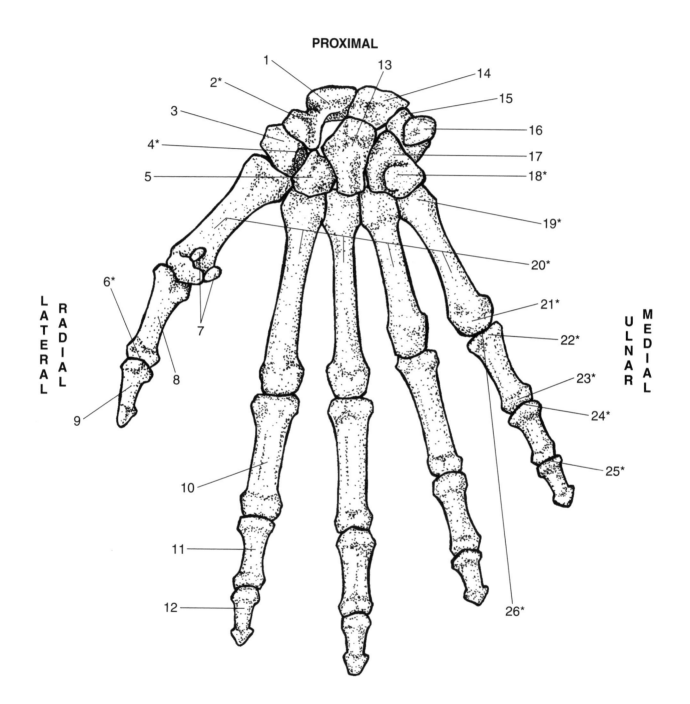

PROXIMAL

1
2*
3
4*
5
6*
7
8
9
10
11
12
13
14
15
16
17
18*
19*
20*
21*
22*
23*
24*
25*
26*

LATERAL RADIAL

ULNAR MEDIAL

DISTAL

DORSAL VIEW OF THE BONES AND BONY LANDMARKS
OF THE RIGHT HAND

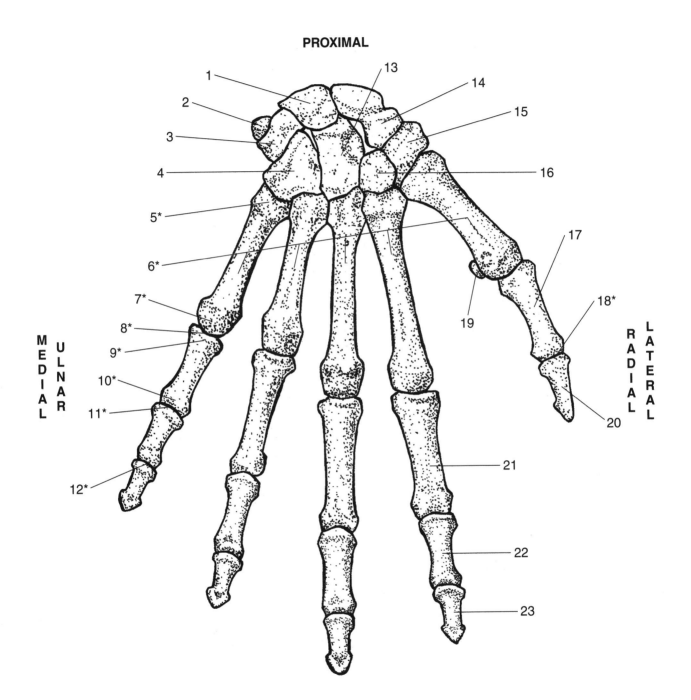

PROXIMAL

MEDIAL

ULNAR

RADIAL

LATERAL

DISTAL

CHAPTER 2

GET READY TO EXPLORE:

Muscles of the Head
Occipitofrontalis, 28
Temporoparietalis, 30
Auricularis Anterior, Superior, and Posterior, 30
Orbicularis Oculi, 32
Levator Palpebrae Superioris, 32
Corrugator Supercilii, 34
Procerus, 34
Nasalis, 36
Depressor Septi Nasi, 36
Levator Labii Superioris Alaeque Nasi, 38
Levator Labii Superioris, 38
Zygomaticus Minor, 40
Zygomaticus Major, 40
Levator Anguli Oris, 42
Risorius, 42
Depressor Anguli Oris, 44
Depressor Labii Inferioris, 44
Mentalis, 46
Buccinator, 46
Orbicularis Oris, 48
Temporalis, 50
Masseter, 50
Lateral Pterygoid, 52
Medial Pterygoid, 52

Muscles of the Neck
Trapezius ("The Traps"), 62
Splenius Capitis, 64
Splenius Cervicis, 64
Levator Scapulae, 66
Rectus Capitis Posterior Major, 68
Rectus Capitis Posterior Minor, 68
Obliquus Capitis Inferior, 70
Obliquus Capitis Superior, 70
Platysma, 72
Sternocleidomastoid ("SCM"), 74
Sternohyoid, 76
Sternothyroid, 76
Thyrohyoid, 78
Omohyoid, 78
Digastric, 80
Stylohyoid, 80
Mylohyoid, 82
Geniohyoid, 82

Anterior Scalene, 84
Middle Scalene, 84
Posterior Scalene, 86
Longus Colli, 88
Longus Capitis, 88
Rectus Capitis Anterior, 90
Rectus Capitis Lateralis, 90

Muscles of the Trunk
Latissimus Dorsi ("The Lats"), 104
Rhomboids Major and Minor, 106
Serratus Anterior, 108
Serratus Posterior Superior, 110
Serratus Posterior Inferior, 110
The Erector Spinae Group, 112
Iliocostalis, 114
Longissimus, 114
Spinalis, 116
The Transversospinalis Group, 118
Semispinalis, 120
Multifidus, 120
Rotatores, 122
Quadratus Lumborum, 124
Interspinales, 126
Intertransversarii, 126
Levatores Costarum, 128
Subcostales, 128
Pectoralis Major, 130
Pectoralis Minor, 132
Subclavius, 132
External Intercostals, 134
Internal Intercostals, 136
Rectus Abdominis, 138
External Abdominal Oblique, 140
Internal Abdominal Oblique, 140
Transversus Abdominis, 142
Transversus Thoracis, 142
Diaphragm, 144

Muscles of the Pelvis
Psoas Major, 156
Iliacus, 158
Psoas Minor, 160
Gluteus Maximus, 162
Gluteus Medius, 164

The Muscular System

Gluteus Minimus, 166
Piriformis, 168
Superior Gemellus, 170
Obturator Internus, 170
Inferior Gemellus, 172
Obturator Externus, 174
Quadratus Femoris, 176

Muscles of the Thigh
Tensor Fasciae Latae ("TFL"), 188
Sartorius, 190
Rectus Femoris, 192
Vastus Lateralis, 194
Vastus Medialis, 194
Vastus Intermedius, 196
Articularis Genus, 196
Pectineus, 198
Gracilis, 198
Adductor Longus, 200
Adductor Brevis, 202
Adductor Magnus, 204
Biceps Femoris, 206
Semitendinosus, 208
Semimembranosus, 208

Muscles of the Leg
Tibialis Anterior, 222
Extensor Hallucis Longus, 224
Extensor Digitorum Longus, 226
Fibularis Tertius, 226
Fibularis Longus, 228
Fibularis Brevis, 228
Gastrocnemius ("Gastrocs"), 230
Soleus, 230
Plantaris, 232
Popliteus, 232
Tibialis Posterior, 234
Flexor Digitorum Longus, 236
Flexor Hallucis Longus, 238

Intrinsic Muscles of the Foot
Extensor Digitorum Brevis, 250
Extensor Hallucis Brevis, 250
Abductor Hallucis, 252

Abductor Digiti Minimi Pedis, 252
Flexor Digitorum Brevis, 254
Quadratus Plantae, 256
Lumbricals Pedis, 256
Flexor Hallucis Brevis, 258
Flexor Digiti Minimi Pedis, 258
Adductor Hallucis, 260
Plantar Interossei, 262
Dorsal Interossei Pedis, 262

Muscles of the Scapula/Arm
Supraspinatus, 276
Infraspinatus, 276
Teres Minor, 278
Subscapularis, 278
Teres Major, 280
Deltoid, 282
Coracobrachialis, 284
Biceps Brachii, 286
Brachialis, 286
Triceps Brachii, 288

Muscles of the Forearm
Pronator Teres, 306
Pronator Quadratus, 306
Flexor Carpi Radialis, 308
Palmaris Longus, 308
Flexor Carpi Ulnaris, 310
Brachioradialis, 312
Flexor Digitorum Superficialis, 314
Flexor Digitorum Profundus, 314
Flexor Pollicis Longus, 316
Anconeus, 318
Extensor Carpi Radialis Longus, 320
Extensor Carpi Radialis Brevis, 320
Extensor Carpi Ulnaris, 322
Extensor Digitorum, 324
Extensor Digiti Minimi, 324
Supinator, 326
Abductor Pollicis Longus, 328
Extensor Pollicis Brevis, 328
Extensor Pollicis Longus, 330
Extensor Indicis, 330

Muscles of the Hand
Abductor Pollicis Brevis, 344
Flexor Pollicis Brevis, 344
Opponens Pollicis, 346
Opponens Digiti Minimi, 346
Abductor Digiti Minimi Manus, 348
Flexor Digiti Minimi Manus, 348
Palmaris Brevis, 350
Adductor Pollicis, 352
Lumbricals Manus, 352
Palmar Interossei, 354
Dorsal Interossei Manus, 354

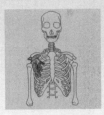

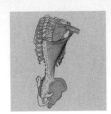

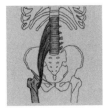

Muscle attachments are indicated by italics.

Muscles of the Head

ANTERIOR VIEW OF THE HEAD

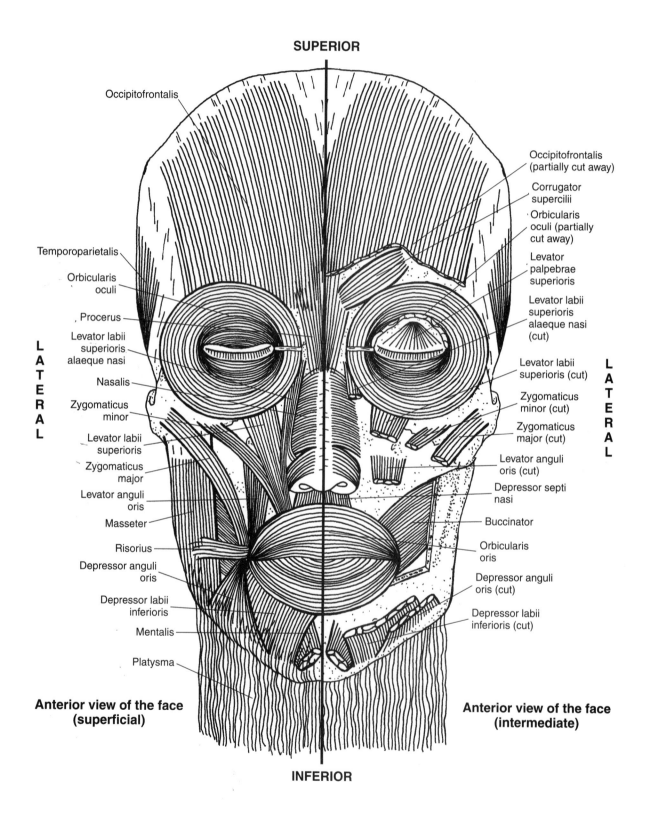

SUPERIOR

Occipitofrontalis

Occipitofrontalis
(partially cut away)

Corrugator
supercilii

Orbicularis
oculi (partially
cut away)

Levator
palpebrae
superioris

Levator labii
superioris
alaeque nasi
(cut)

Temporoparietalis

Orbicularis
oculi

Procerus

Levator labii
superioris
alaeque nasi

Levator labii
superioris (cut)

Nasalis

Zygomaticus
minor (cut)

Zygomaticus
minor

Zygomaticus
major (cut)

Levator labii
superioris

Levator anguli
oris (cut)

Zygomaticus
major

Depressor septi
nasi

Levator anguli
oris

Buccinator

Masseter

Orbicularis
oris

Risorius

Depressor anguli
oris

Depressor anguli
oris (cut)

Depressor labii
inferioris

Depressor labii
inferioris (cut)

Mentalis

Platysma

LATERAL

LATERAL

**Anterior view of the face
(superficial)**

**Anterior view of the face
(intermediate)**

INFERIOR

Muscles of the Head

LATERAL VIEW OF THE HEAD

SUPERIOR

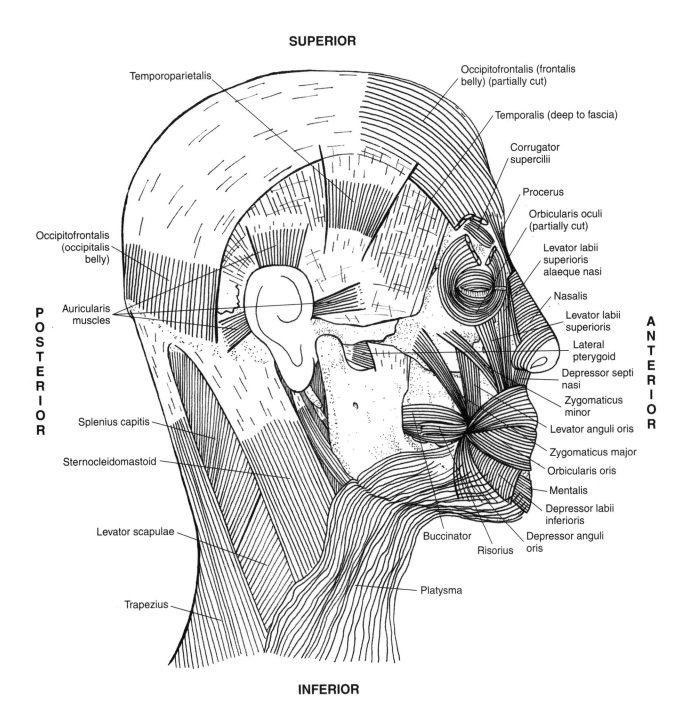

Temporoparietalis

Occipitofrontalis (frontalis belly) (partially cut)

Temporalis (deep to fascia)

Corrugator supercilii

Procerus

Orbicularis oculi (partially cut)

Occipitofrontalis (occipitalis belly)

Levator labii superioris alaeque nasi

Nasalis

Auricularis muscles

Levator labii superioris

Lateral pterygoid

Depressor septi nasi

Zygomaticus minor

Splenius capitis

Levator anguli oris

Sternocleidomastoid

Zygomaticus major

Orbicularis oris

Mentalis

Depressor labii inferioris

Levator scapulae

Depressor anguli oris

Buccinator

Risorius

Trapezius

Platysma

P O S T E R I O R

A N T E R I O R

INFERIOR

Muscles of the Head

OCCIPITOFRONTALIS

(PART OF THE EPICRANIUS)

ok-**sip**-i-to-fron-**ta**-lis

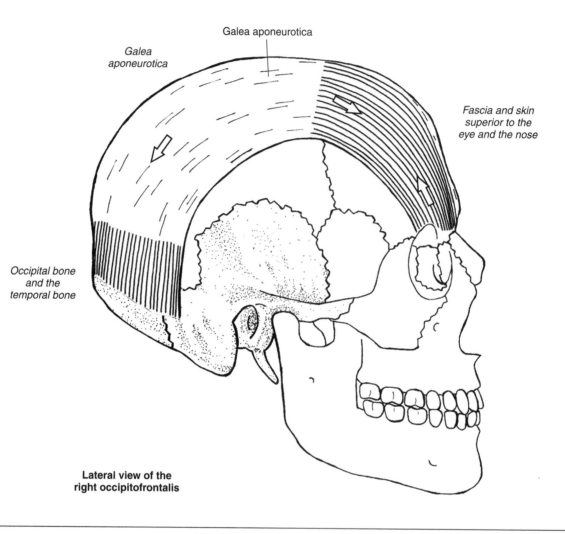

Galea aponeurotica

Galea aponeurotica

Fascia and skin superior to the eye and the nose

Occipital bone and the temporal bone

Lateral view of the right occipitofrontalis

Actions	**Innervation**	**Arterial Supply**
Draws the scalp posteriorly (occipitalis)	The facial nerve (CN VII)	Occipitalis: the occipital and posterior auricular arteries
Draws the scalp anteriorly (frontalis)		Frontalis: supraorbital and supratrochlear branches of the ophthalmic artery
Elevates the eyebrows (frontalis)		

Muscles of the Head

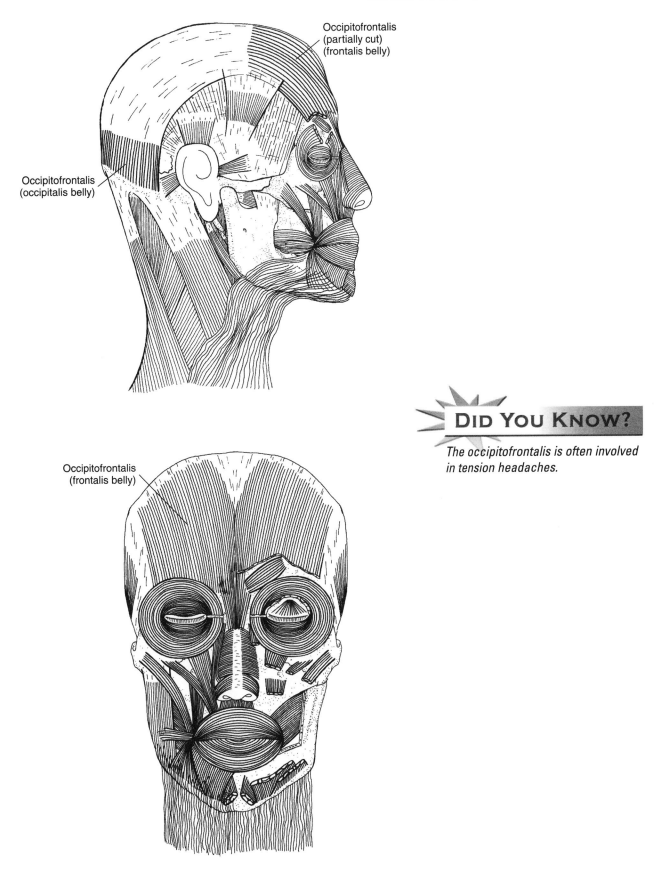

Occipitofrontalis
(partially cut)
(frontalis belly)

Occipitofrontalis
(occipitalis belly)

Occipitofrontalis
(frontalis belly)

DID YOU KNOW?

The occipitofrontalis is often involved in tension headaches.

Muscles of the Head

TEMPOROPARIETALIS
(PART OF THE EPICRANIUS)

tem-po-ro-pa-**ri**-i-**tal**-is

Actions
Elevates the ear
Tightens the scalp

Innervation
The facial nerve (CN VII)

Arterial Supply
The superficial temporal
and posterior auricular
arteries

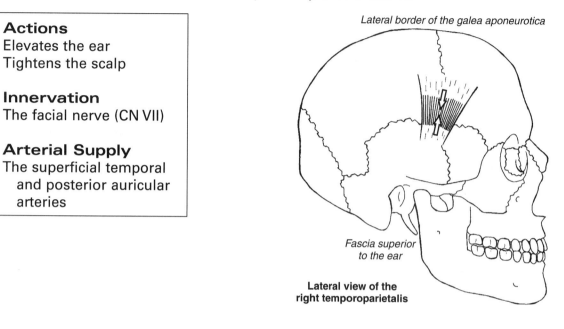

Lateral border of the galea aponeurotica

*Fascia superior
to the ear*

**Lateral view of the
right temporoparietalis**

AURICULARIS ANTERIOR, SUPERIOR, AND POSTERIOR

aw-**rik**-u-la-ris an-**tee**-ri-or, sue-**pee**-ri-or, pos-**tee**-ri-or

Actions
Draws the ear anteriorly
(auricularis anterior)
Elevates the ear (auricu-
laris superior)
Draws the ear posteriorly
(auricularis posterior)
Tightens and moves the
scalp (auricularis
anterior and superior)

Innervation
The facial nerve (CN VII)

Arterial Supply
The superficial temporal
and posterior auricular
arteries

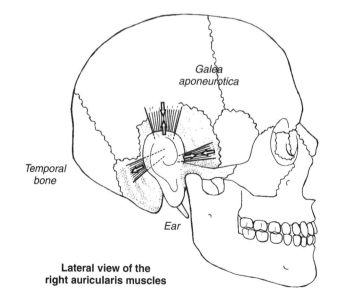

*Galea
aponeurotica*

*Temporal
bone*

Ear

**Lateral view of the
right auricularis muscles**

Muscles of the Head

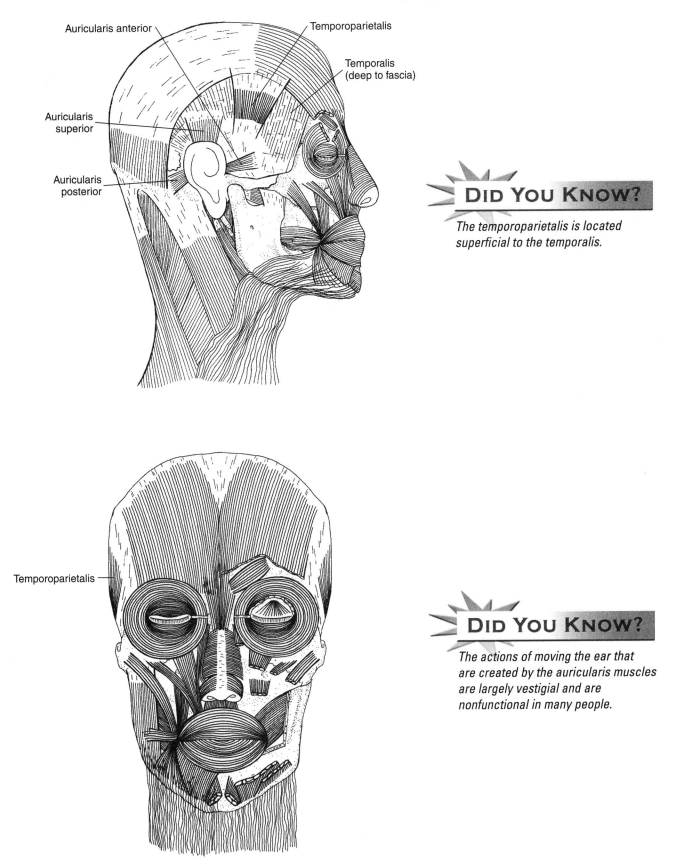

Auricularis anterior

Temporoparietalis

Temporalis
(deep to fascia)

Auricularis
superior

Auricularis
posterior

Temporoparietalis

DID YOU KNOW?

The temporoparietalis is located superficial to the temporalis.

DID YOU KNOW?

The actions of moving the ear that are created by the auricularis muscles are largely vestigial and are nonfunctional in many people.

Muscles of the Head

ORBICULARIS OCULI

or-**bik**-you-la-ris **ok**-you-lie

Actions
Closes and squints the
  eye (orbital part)
Depresses the upper
  eyelid (palpebral part)
Elevates the lower eyelid
  (palpebral part)
Assists tear transport
  and drainage (lacrimal
  part)

Innervation
The facial nerve (CN VII)

Arterial Supply
The branches of the
  facial artery and
  superficial temporal
  artery

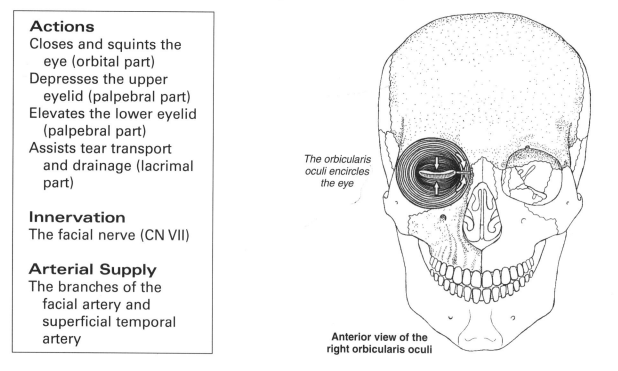

The orbicularis oculi encircles the eye

**Anterior view of the
right orbicularis oculi**

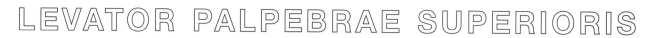

LEVATOR PALPEBRAE SUPERIORIS

le-vay-tor pal-**pee**-bree su-**pee**-ri-**or**-is

Action
Elevates the upper eyelid

Innervation
The oculomotor nerve
  (CN III)

Arterial Supply
The ophthalmic artery

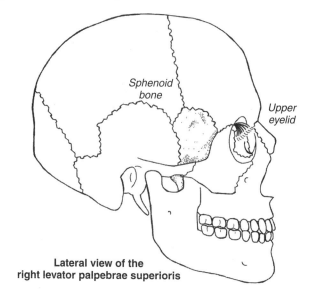

Sphenoid bone

Upper eyelid

**Lateral view of the
right levator palpebrae superioris**

Muscles of the Head

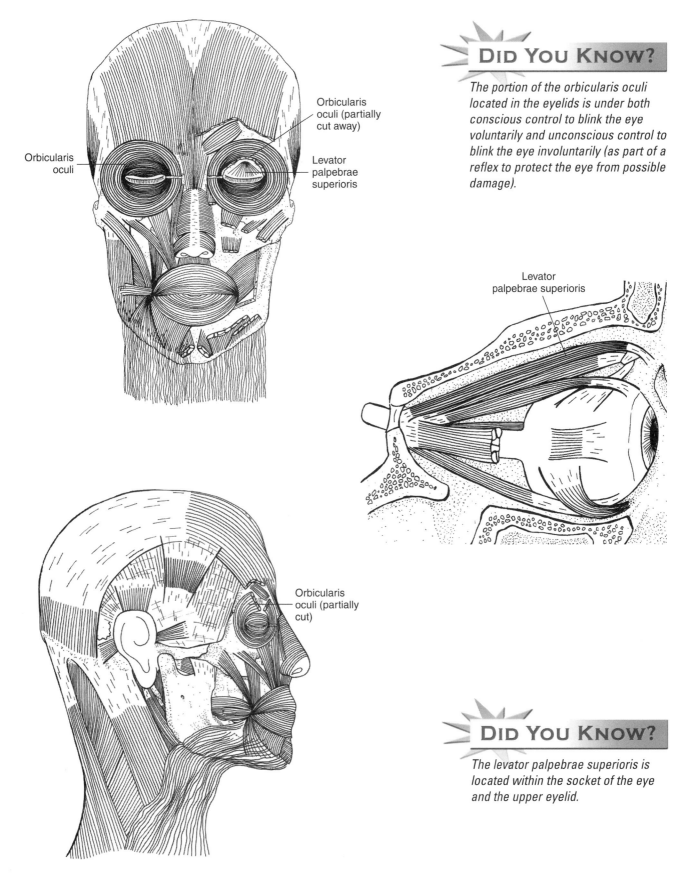

Orbicularis oculi (partially cut away)

Orbicularis oculi

Levator palpebrae superioris

DID YOU KNOW?

The portion of the orbicularis oculi located in the eyelids is under both conscious control to blink the eye voluntarily and unconscious control to blink the eye involuntarily (as part of a reflex to protect the eye from possible damage).

Levator palpebrae superioris

Orbicularis oculi (partially cut)

DID YOU KNOW?

The levator palpebrae superioris is located within the socket of the eye and the upper eyelid.

Muscles of the Head

CORRUGATOR SUPERCILII

kor-u-gay-tor su-per-**sil**-i-eye

Action
Draws eyebrow inferiorly and medially

Innervation
The facial nerve (CN VII)

Arterial Supply
The supratrochlear and supraorbital arteries

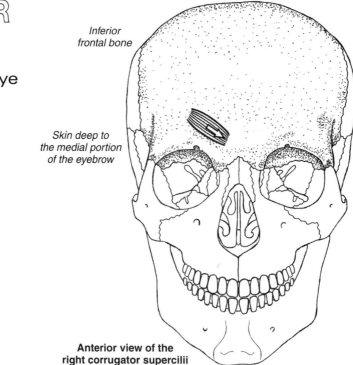

Inferior frontal bone

Skin deep to the medial portion of the eyebrow

Anterior view of the right corrugator supercilii

PROCERUS

pro-**se**-rus

Actions
Draws down the medial eyebrow
Wrinkles the skin of the nose

Innervation
The facial nerve (CN VII)

Arterial Supply
The facial artery

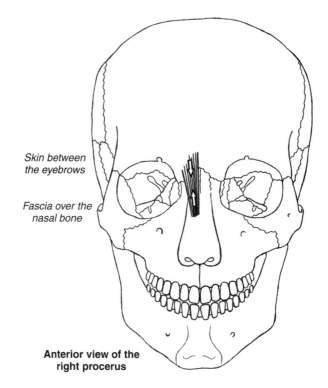

Skin between the eyebrows

Fascia over the nasal bone

Anterior view of the right procerus

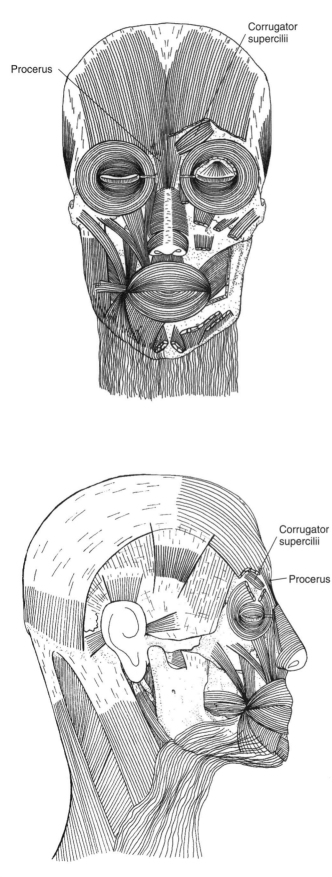

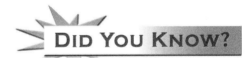

DID YOU KNOW?

Contraction of the corrugator supercilii contributes to frowning and also assists in shielding the eyes from bright sunlight.

DID YOU KNOW?

Procerus in Latin means 'chief noble' or 'prince'; hence the action of the procerus creates an expression that conveys a look of superiority.

Muscles of the Head

NASALIS

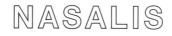

nay-**sa**-lis

Action
Flares the nostril
Innervation
The facial nerve (CN VII)
Arterial Supply
The facial artery

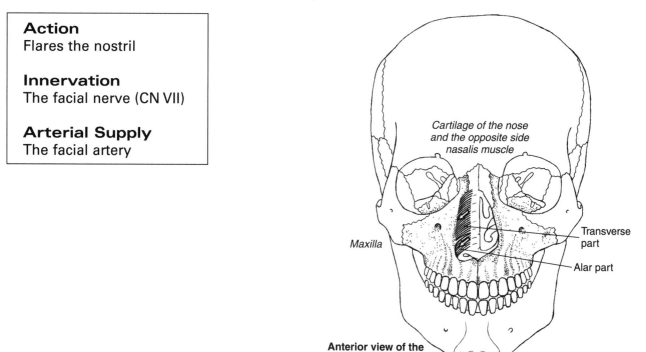

Cartilage of the nose
and the opposite side
nasalis muscle

Maxilla

Transverse
part

Alar part

**Anterior view of the
right nasalis**

DEPRESSOR SEPTI NASI

dee-**pres**-or **sep**-ti **nay**-zi

Action
Constricts the nostril
Innervation
The facial nerve (CN VII)
Arterial Supply
The facial artery

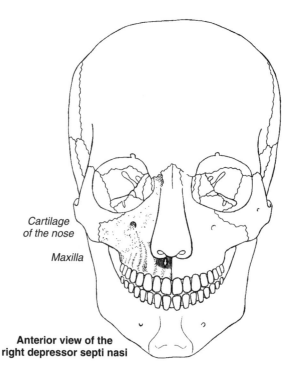

Cartilage
of the nose

Maxilla

**Anterior view of the
right depressor septi nasi**

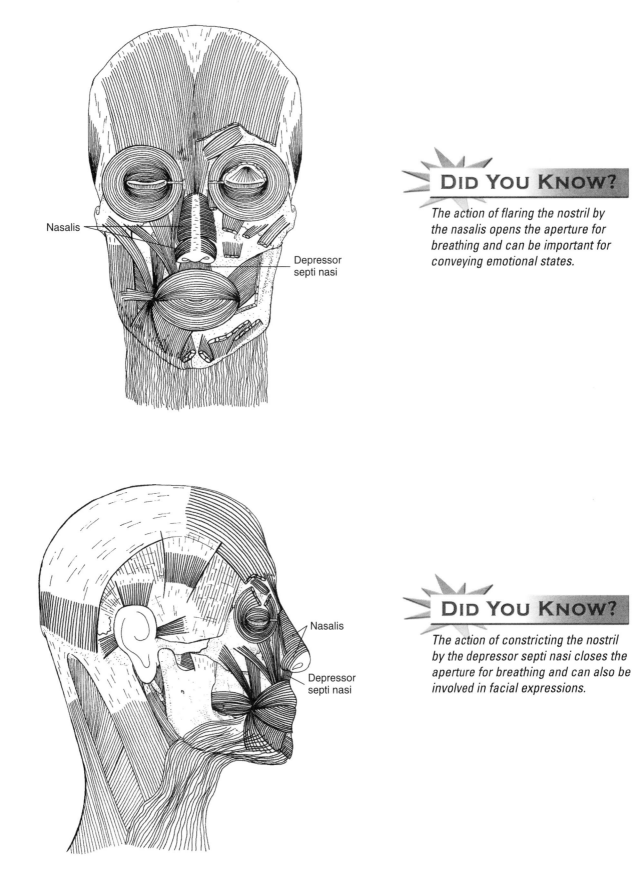

DID YOU KNOW?

The action of flaring the nostril by the nasalis opens the aperture for breathing and can be important for conveying emotional states.

DID YOU KNOW?

The action of constricting the nostril by the depressor septi nasi closes the aperture for breathing and can also be involved in facial expressions.

LEVATOR LABII SUPERIORIS ALAEQUE NASI

le-**vay**-tor **lay**-be-eye
soo-**pee**-ri-o-ris
a-**lee**-kwe **nay**-si

Actions
Elevates the upper lip
Flares the nostril
Everts the upper lip

Innervation
The facial nerve (CN VII)

Arterial Supply
The infraorbital artery

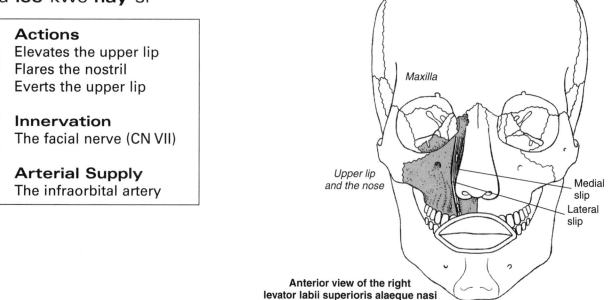

Maxilla

Upper lip and the nose

Medial slip

Lateral slip

**Anterior view of the right
levator labii superioris alaeque nasi**

LEVATOR LABII SUPERIORIS

le-**vay**-tor **lay**-be-eye
soo-**pee**-ri-**o**-ris

Actions
Elevates the upper lip
Everts the upper lip

Innervation
The facial nerve (CN VII)

Arterial Supply
The facial artery

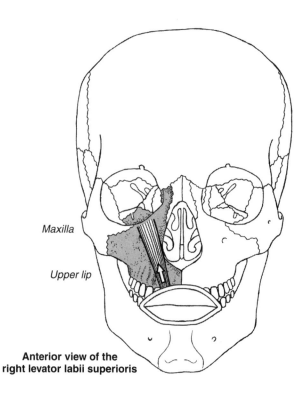

Maxilla

Upper lip

**Anterior view of the
right levator labii superioris**

Muscles of the Head

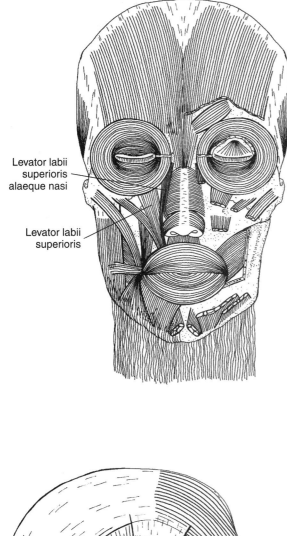

Levator labii superioris alaeque nasi

Levator labii superioris

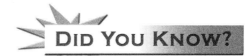

The levator labii superioris alaeque nasi is a muscle of facial expression that, as its name describes, can move both the mouth and the nose.

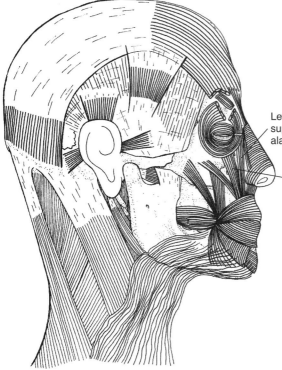

Levator labii superioris alaeque nasi

Levator labii superioris

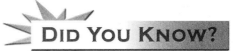

Contraction of the levator labii superioris muscles lifts the upper lip, which exposes the upper teeth. This action can contribute to a number of facial expressions.

Muscles of the Head

ZYGOMATICUS MINOR

zi-go-**mat**-ik-us **my**-nor

Actions
Elevates the upper lip
Everts the upper lip

Innervation
The facial nerve (CN VII)

Arterial Supply
The facial artery

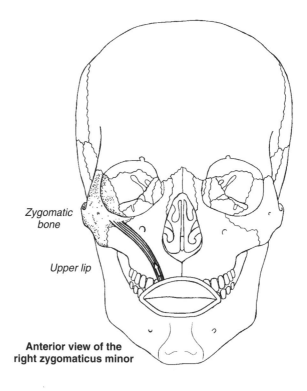

Zygomatic bone

Upper lip

Anterior view of the right zygomaticus minor

ZYGOMATICUS MAJOR

zi-go-**mat**-ik-us **may**-jor

Actions
Elevates the angle of the mouth
Draws laterally the angle of the mouth

Innervation
The facial nerve (CN VII)

Arterial Supply
The facial artery

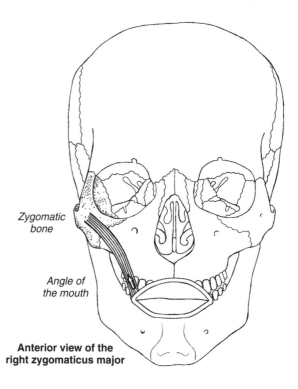

Zygomatic bone

Angle of the mouth

Anterior view of the right zygomaticus major

Muscles of the Head

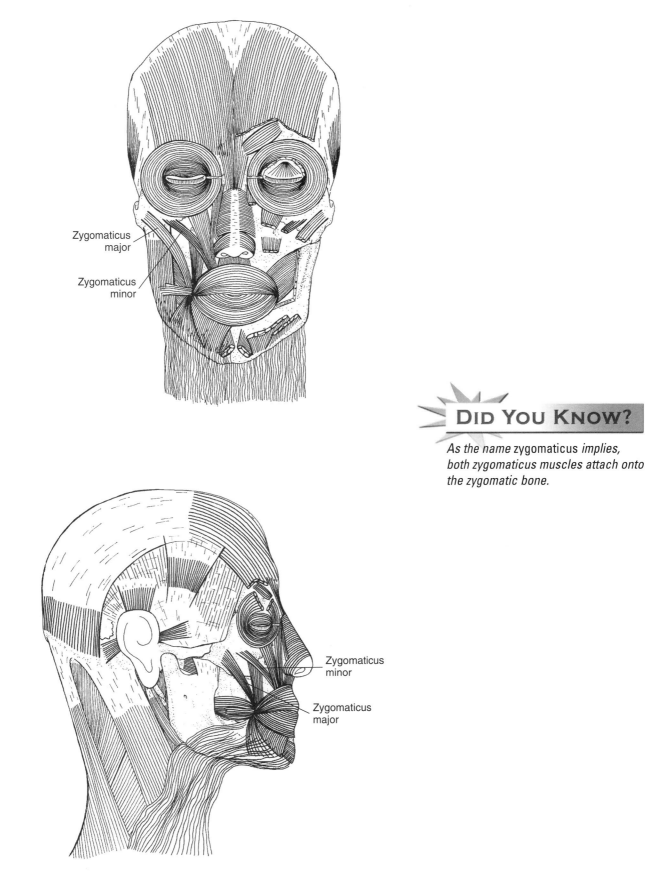

Zygomaticus major

Zygomaticus minor

DID YOU KNOW?

As the name zygomaticus *implies, both zygomaticus muscles attach onto the zygomatic bone.*

Zygomaticus minor

Zygomaticus major

Muscles of the Head

LEVATOR ANGULI ORIS

le-**vay**-tor **ang**-you-lie **o**-ris

Action Elevates the angle of the mouth **Innervation** The facial nerve (CN VII) **Arterial Supply** The facial artery

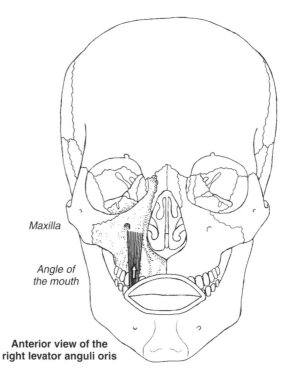

Maxilla

Angle of the mouth

Anterior view of the right levator anguli oris

RISORIUS

ri-**so**-ri-us

Action Draws laterally the angle of the mouth **Innervation** The facial nerve (CN VII) **Arterial Supply** The facial artery

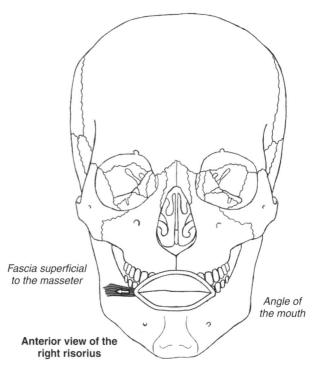

Fascia superficial to the masseter

Angle of the mouth

Anterior view of the right risorius

Muscles of the Head

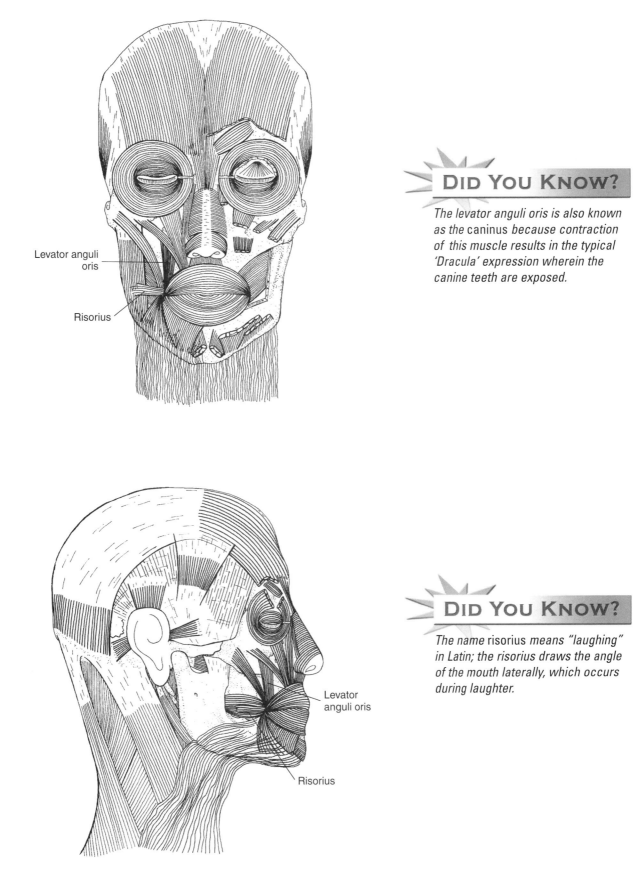

Levator anguli oris

Risorius

DID YOU KNOW?

The levator anguli oris is also known as the caninus *because contraction of this muscle results in the typical 'Dracula' expression wherein the canine teeth are exposed.*

Levator anguli oris

Risorius

DID YOU KNOW?

The name risorius *means "laughing" in Latin; the risorius draws the angle of the mouth laterally, which occurs during laughter.*

Muscles of the Head

DEPRESSOR ANGULI ORIS

dee-**pres**-or
ang-you-lie **o**-ris

Actions
Depresses the angle of
  the mouth
Draws laterally the angle
  of the mouth

Innervation
The facial nerve (CN VII)

Arterial Supply
The facial artery

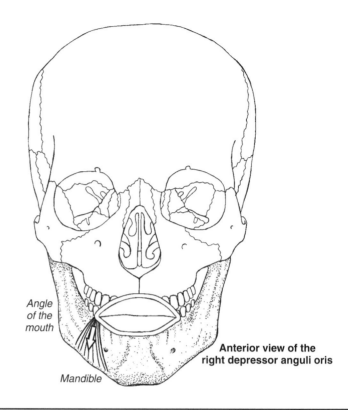

*Angle
of the
mouth*

**Anterior view of the
right depressor anguli oris**

Mandible

DEPRESSOR LABII INFERIORIS

dee-**pres**-or **lay**-be-eye
in-**fee**-ri-**o**-ris

Actions
Depresses the lower lip
Draws laterally the lower
  lip
Everts the lower lip

Innervation
The facial nerve (CN VII)

Arterial Supply
The facial artery

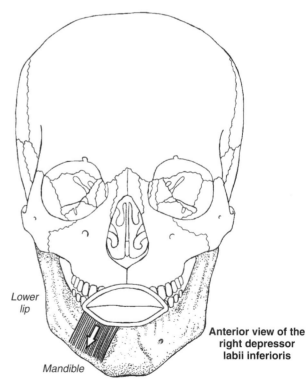

*Lower
lip*

**Anterior view of the
right depressor
labii inferioris**

Mandible

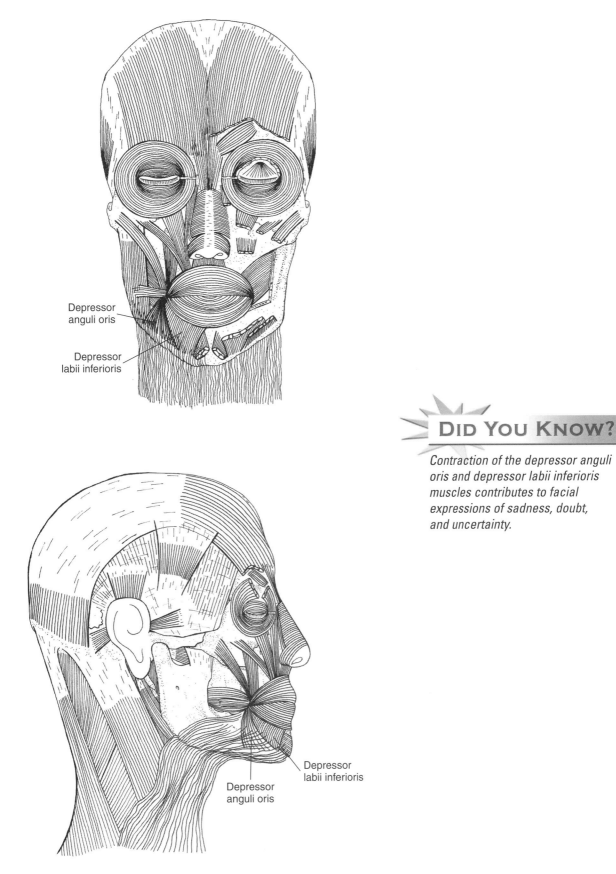

Depressor
anguli oris

Depressor
labii inferioris

Depressor
labii inferioris

Depressor
anguli oris

DID YOU KNOW?

Contraction of the depressor anguli oris and depressor labii inferioris muscles contributes to facial expressions of sadness, doubt, and uncertainty.

Muscles of the Head

MENTALIS

men-**ta**-lis

Actions
Elevates the lower lip
Everts and protracts the
    lower lip
Wrinkles the skin of the
    chin

Innervation
The facial nerve (CN VII)

Arterial Supply
The facial artery

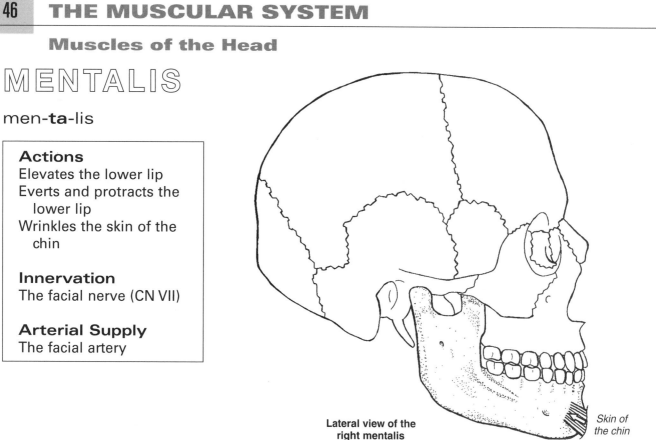

**Lateral view of the
right mentalis**

*Skin of
the chin*

Mandible

BUCCINATOR

buk-sin-**a**-tor

Action
Compresses the cheeks
    (against the teeth)

Innervation
The facial nerve (CN VII)

Arterial Supply
The maxillary and facial
    arteries

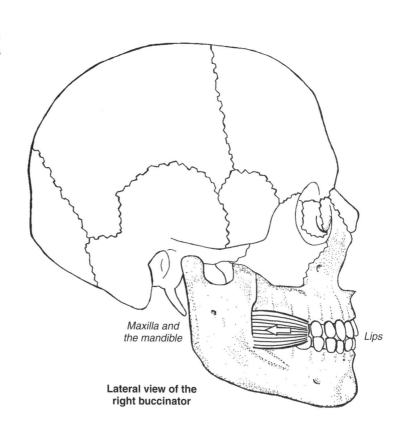

*Maxilla and
the mandible*

Lips

**Lateral view of the
right buccinator**

Muscles of the Head

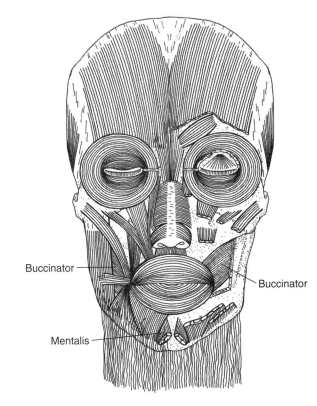

Buccinator

Buccinator

Mentalis

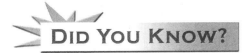

Strong contraction of the mentalis muscles can make the lower lip stick out, creating the facial expression of pouting.

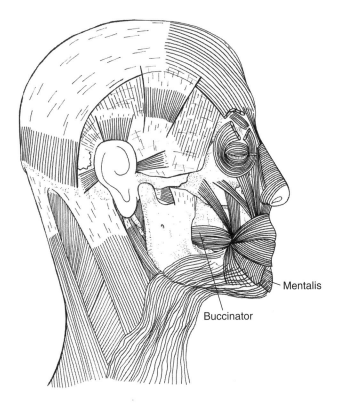

Mentalis

Buccinator

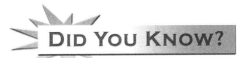

Contraction of the buccinator muscles is necessary for whistling, blowing up a balloon, and blowing into a brass or woodwind instrument.

Muscles of the Head

ORBICULARIS ORIS

or-**bik**-you-**la**-ris **o**-ris

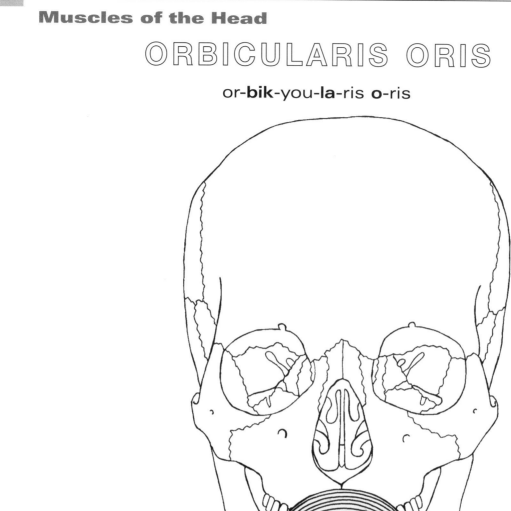

The orbicularis oris encircles the mouth

Anterior view of the orbicularis oris

Actions	Innervation	Arterial Supply
Closes the mouth	The facial nerve (CN VII)	The facial artery
Protracts the lips		

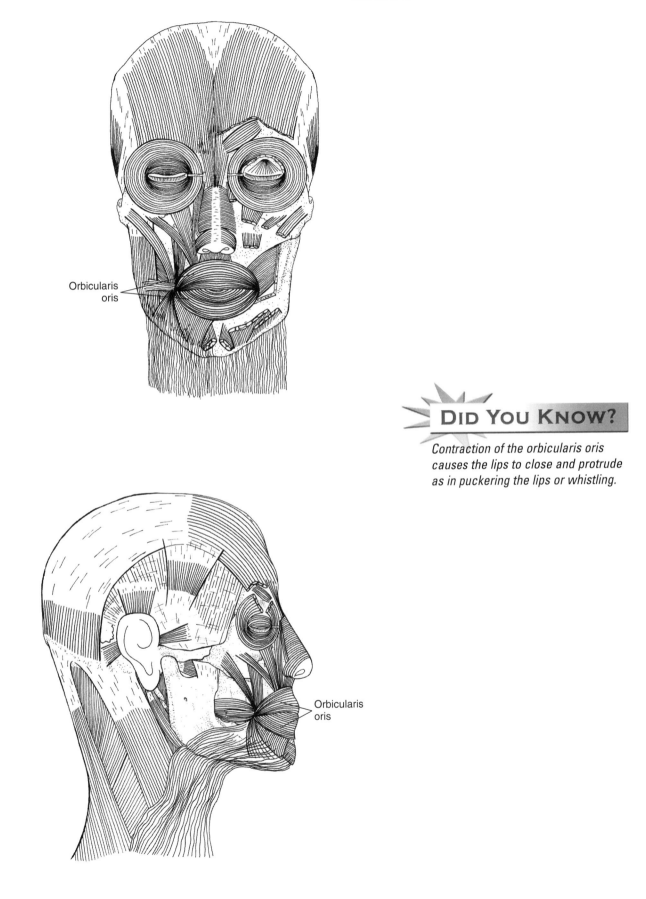

Orbicularis oris

Orbicularis oris

DID YOU KNOW?

Contraction of the orbicularis oris causes the lips to close and protrude as in puckering the lips or whistling.

Muscles of the Head

TEMPORALIS

tem-po-**ra**-lis

Actions
Elevates the mandible
at the temporoman-
dibular joint
Retracts the mandible at
the temporomandib-
ular joint

Innervation
The trigeminal nerve
(CN V)

Arterial Supply
The maxillary and
superficial temporal
arteries

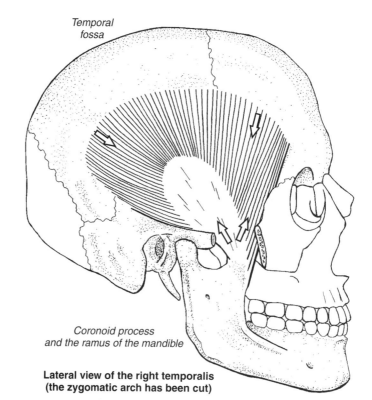

Temporal fossa

*Coronoid process
and the ramus of the mandible*

**Lateral view of the right temporalis
(the zygomatic arch has been cut)**

MASSETER

ma-sa-ter

Actions
Elevates the mandible
at the temporoman-
dibular joint
Protracts the mandible
at the temporoman-
dibular joint
Retracts the mandible at
the temporomandib-
ular joint

Innervation
The trigeminal nerve
(CN V)

Arterial Supply
The maxillary artery

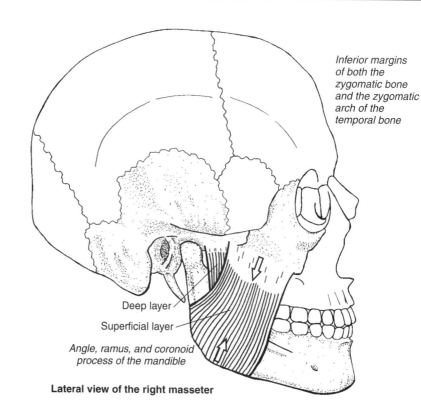

*Inferior margins
of both the
zygomatic bone
and the zygomatic
arch of the
temporal bone*

Deep layer
Superficial layer

*Angle, ramus, and coronoid
process of the mandible*

Lateral view of the right masseter

Muscles of the Head

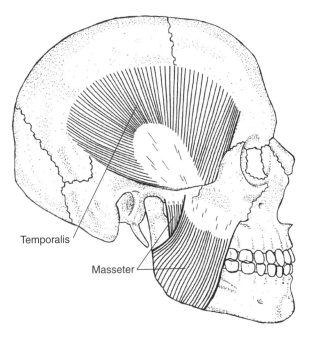

Temporalis

Masseter

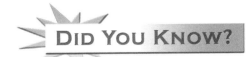
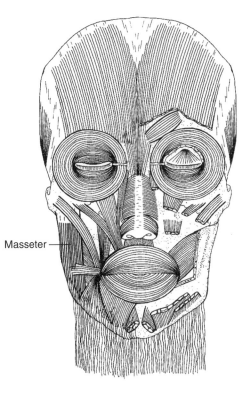

DID YOU KNOW?

The temporalis is often involved in tension headaches and temporomandibular joint (TMJ) dysfunction.

Masseter

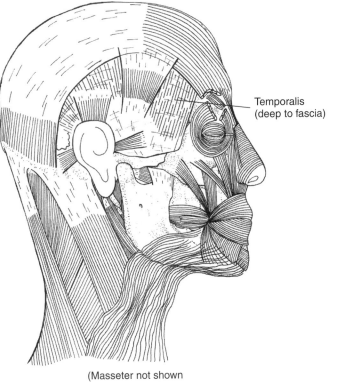

Temporalis (deep to fascia)

(Masseter not shown in this view)

DID YOU KNOW?

Proportional to its size, the masseter is considered to be the strongest muscle in the human body.

Muscles of the Head

LATERAL PTERYGOID

lat-er-al **ter**-i-goyd

Actions
Protracts the mandible at the temporomandibular joint
Contralaterally deviates the mandible at the temporomandibular joint

Innervation
The trigeminal nerve (CN V)

Arterial Supply
The maxillary artery

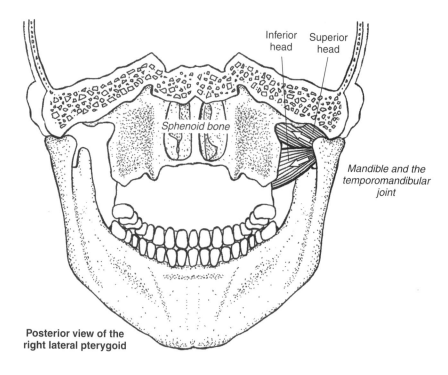

Inferior head   Superior head

Sphenoid bone

Mandible and the temporomandibular joint

Posterior view of the right lateral pterygoid

MEDIAL PTERYGOID

mee-dee-al **ter**-i-goyd

Actions
Elevates the mandible at the temporomandibular joint
Protracts the mandible at the temporomandibular joint
Contralaterally deviates the mandible at the temporomandibular joint

Innervation
The trigeminal nerve (CN V)

Arterial Supply
The maxillary artery

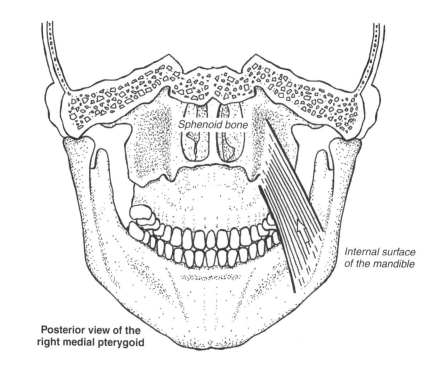

Sphenoid bone

Internal surface of the mandible

Posterior view of the right medial pterygoid

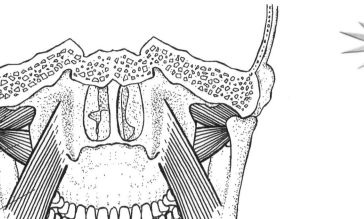

Lateral
pterygoid

Medial
pterygoid

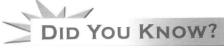

DID YOU KNOW?

The lateral pterygoid has an attachment directly into the capsule and articular disc of the TMJ, making this muscle likely to be involved in TMJ dysfunction.

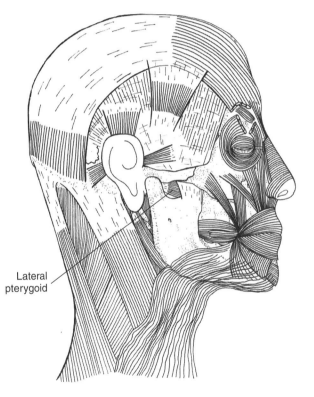

Lateral
pterygoid

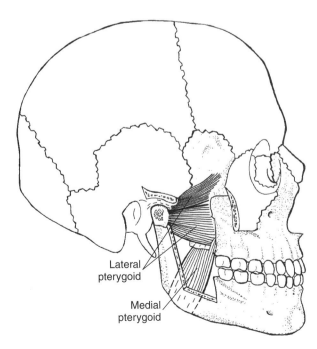

Lateral
pterygoid

Medial
pterygoid

DID YOU KNOW?

The direction of fibers of the medial pterygoid is essentially identical to the masseter, except that the medial pterygoid is deep to the mandible and the masseter is superficial to the mandible.

Muscles of the Head

ANTERIOR VIEW OF THE HEAD

SUPERIOR

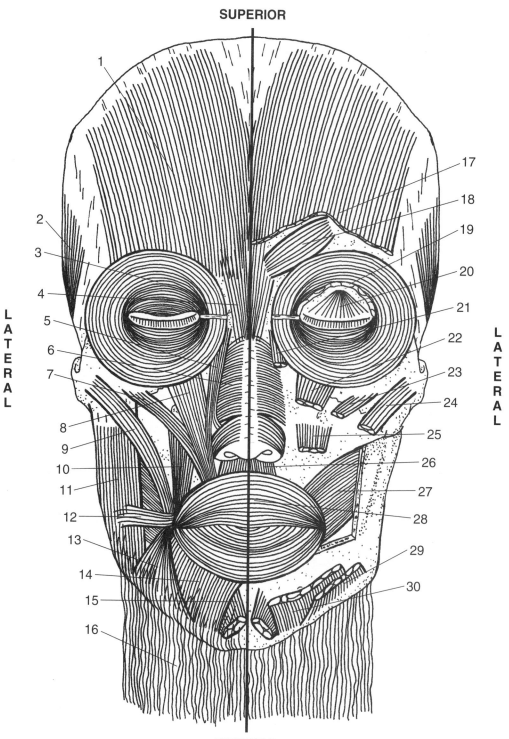

LATERAL

LATERAL

INFERIOR

LATERAL VIEW OF THE HEAD

SUPERIOR

POSTERIOR

ANTERIOR

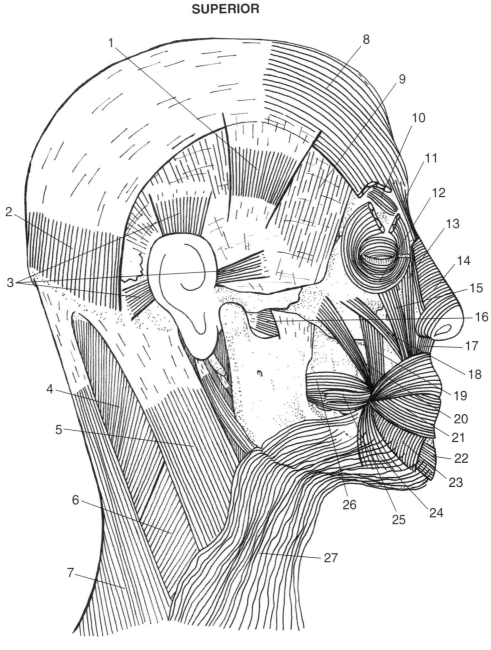

INFERIOR

Muscles of the Neck

ANTERIOR VIEW OF THE NECK (SUPERFICIAL)

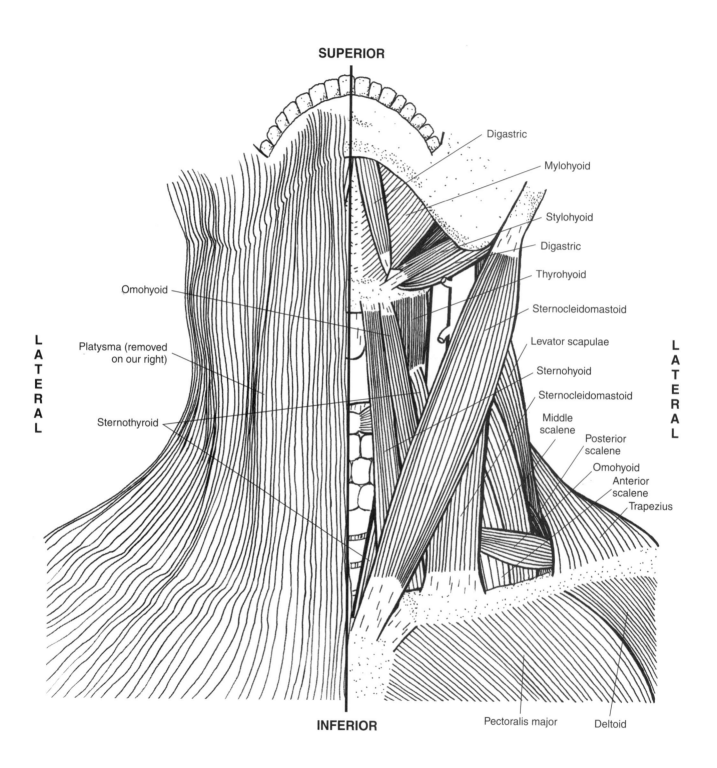

SUPERIOR

Digastric

Mylohyoid

Stylohyoid

Digastric

Thyrohyoid

Omohyoid

Sternocleidomastoid

Levator scapulae

Platysma (removed on our right)

Sternohyoid

Sternocleidomastoid

L A T E R A L

L A T E R A L

Middle scalene

Posterior scalene

Omohyoid

Sternothyroid

Anterior scalene

Trapezius

INFERIOR

Pectoralis major

Deltoid

ANTERIOR VIEW OF THE NECK (INTERMEDIATE)

SUPERIOR

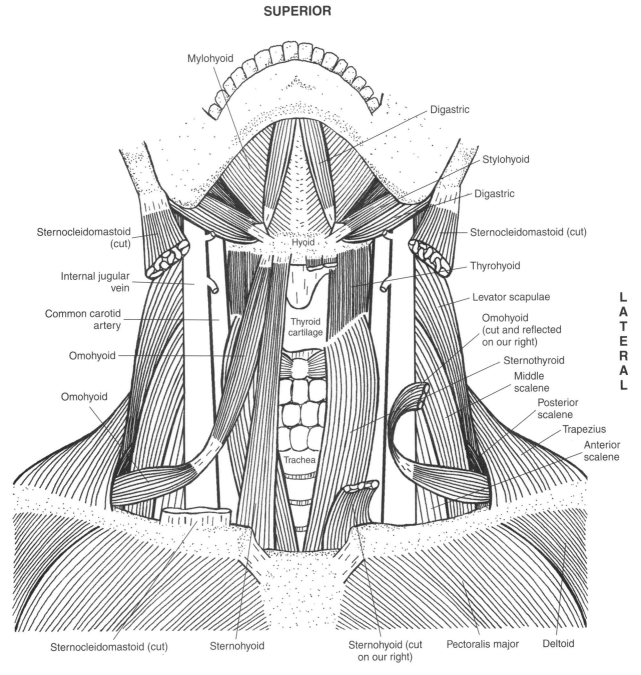

Mylohyoid

Digastric

Stylohyoid

Digastric

Sternocleidomastoid (cut)

Sternocleidomastoid (cut)

Hyoid

Thyrohyoid

Internal jugular vein

Levator scapulae

Common carotid artery

Thyroid cartilage

Omohyoid (cut and reflected on our right)

Sternothyroid

Omohyoid

Middle scalene

Posterior scalene

Omohyoid

Trapezius

Anterior scalene

Trachea

LATERAL

LATERAL

Sternocleidomastoid (cut)

Sternohyoid

Sternohyoid (cut on our right)

Pectoralis major

Deltoid

INFERIOR

ANTERIOR VIEW OF THE NECK (DEEP)

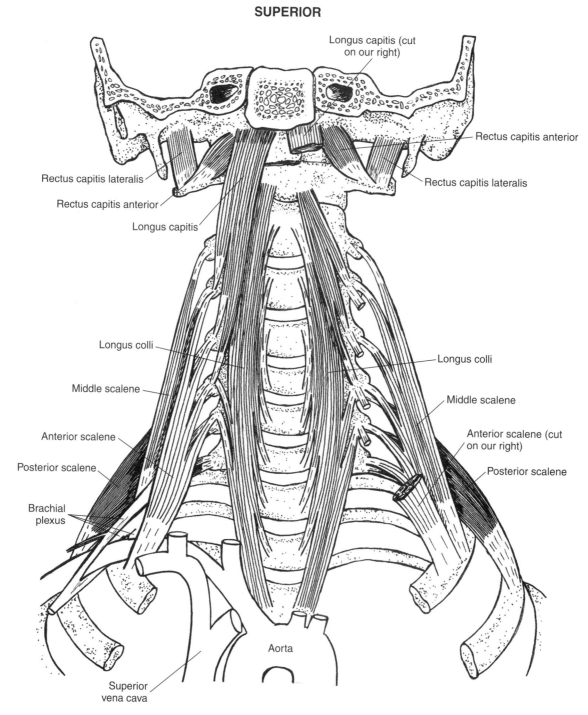

SUPERIOR

Longus capitis (cut on our right)

Rectus capitis anterior

Rectus capitis lateralis

Rectus capitis lateralis

Rectus capitis anterior

Rectus capitis lateralis

Longus capitis

LATERAL

LATERAL

Longus colli

Longus colli

Middle scalene

Middle scalene

Anterior scalene

Anterior scalene (cut on our right)

Posterior scalene

Posterior scalene

Brachial plexus

Aorta

Superior vena cava

INFERIOR

Muscles of the Neck

LATERAL VIEW OF THE NECK

SUPERIOR

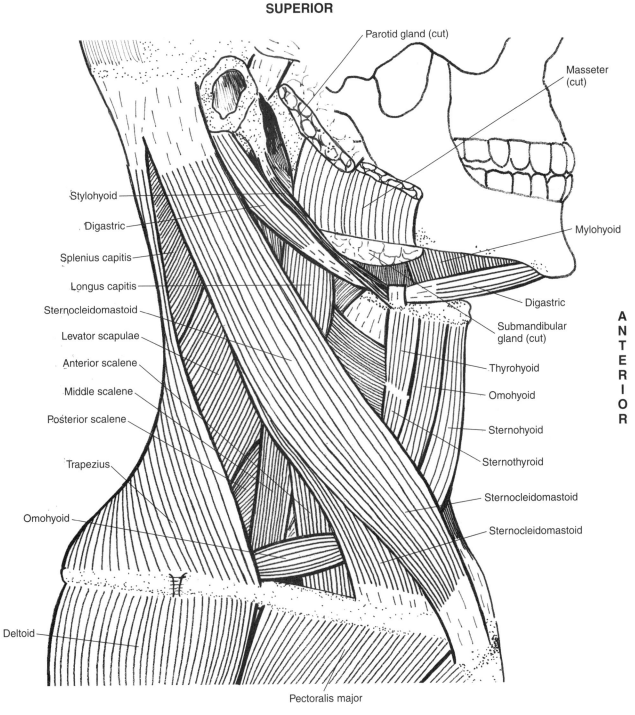

Parotid gland (cut)

Masseter (cut)

Stylohyoid

Digastric

Splenius capitis

Longus capitis

Sternocleidomastoid

Levator scapulae

Anterior scalene

Middle scalene

Posterior scalene

Trapezius

Omohyoid

Deltoid

Mylohyoid

Digastric

Submandibular gland (cut)

Thyrohyoid

Omohyoid

Sternohyoid

Sternothyroid

Sternocleidomastoid

Sternocleidomastoid

POSTERIOR

ANTERIOR

Pectoralis major

INFERIOR

POSTERIOR VIEW OF THE NECK
(SUPERFICIAL AND INTERMEDIATE)

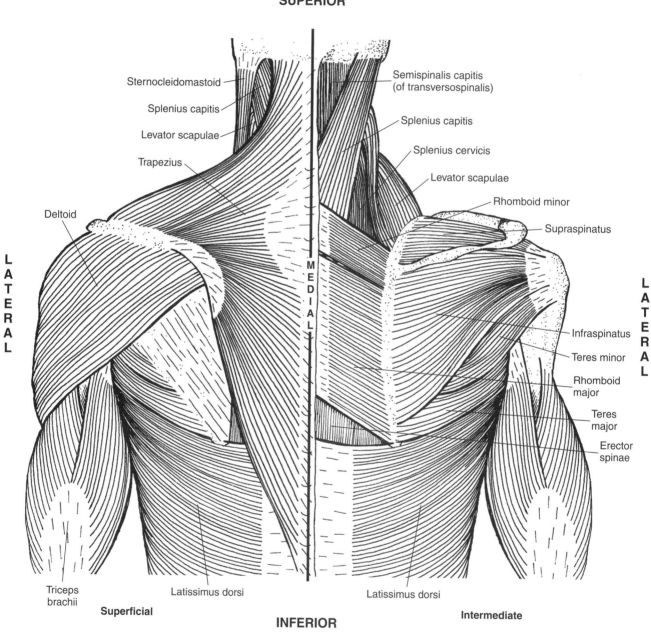

SUPERIOR

Sternocleidomastoid

Splenius capitis

Levator scapulae

Trapezius

Deltoid

LATERAL

Semispinalis capitis
(of transversospinalis)

Splenius capitis

Splenius cervicis

Levator scapulae

Rhomboid minor

Supraspinatus

Infraspinatus

Teres minor

Rhomboid major

Teres major

Erector spinae

LATERAL

MEDIAL

Triceps brachii

Latissimus dorsi

Superficial

Latissimus dorsi

Intermediate

INFERIOR

POSTERIOR VIEW OF THE NECK
(INTERMEDIATE AND DEEP)

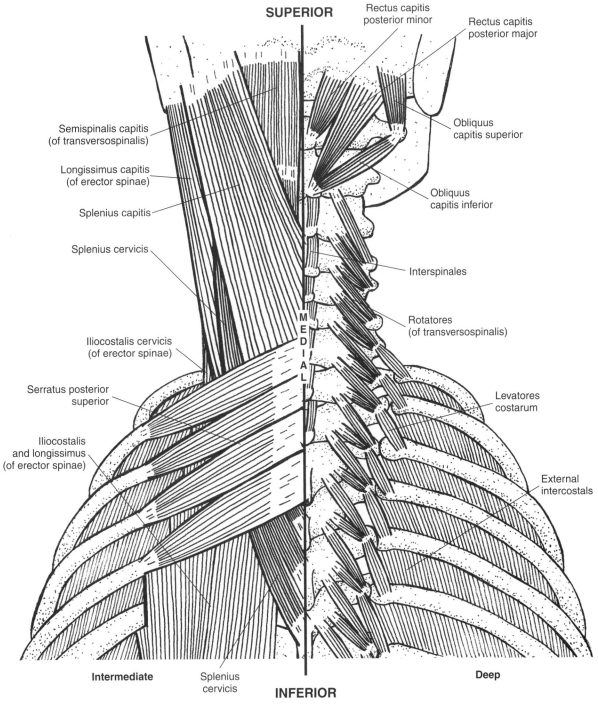

SUPERIOR

Rectus capitis
posterior minor

Rectus capitis
posterior major

Semispinalis capitis
(of transversospinalis)

Obliquus
capitis superior

Longissimus capitis
(of erector spinae)

Obliquus
capitis inferior

Splenius capitis

Splenius cervicis

Interspinales

LATERAL

MEDIAL

LATERAL

Iliocostalis cervicis
(of erector spinae)

Rotatores
(of transversospinalis)

Serratus posterior
superior

Levatores
costarum

Iliocostalis
and longissimus
(of erector spinae)

External
intercostals

Intermediate

Splenius
cervicis

Deep

INFERIOR

Muscles of the Neck

TRAPEZIUS (THE "TRAP")

tra-**pee**-zee-us

Actions
Lateral flexion of the neck and the head at the spinal joints (upper)

Extension of the neck and the head at the spinal joints (upper)

Contralateral rotation of the neck and the head at the spinal joints (upper)

Elevation of the scapula at the scapulocostal joint (upper)

Retraction (adduction) of the scapula at the scapulocostal joint (entire muscle)

Depression of the scapula at the scapulocostal joint (lower)

Upward rotation of the scapula at the scapulocostal joint (upper and lower)

Extension of the trunk at the spinal joints (middle and lower)

Innervation
Spinal accessory nerve (CN XI)

Arterial Supply
The transverse cervical artery and the dorsal scapular artery

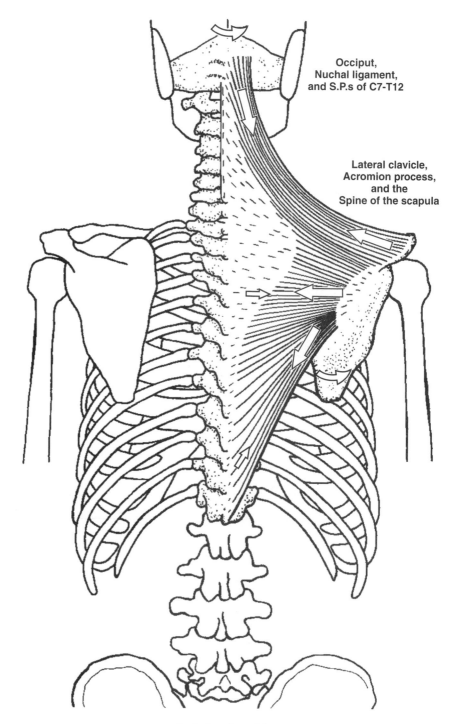

Occiput, Nuchal ligament, and S.P.s of C7-T12

Lateral clavicle, Acromion process, and the Spine of the scapula

Posterior view of the right trapezius

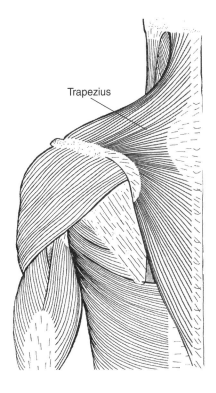

Trapezius

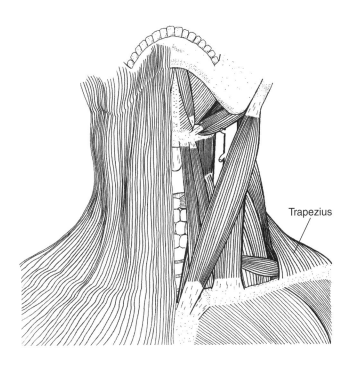

Trapezius

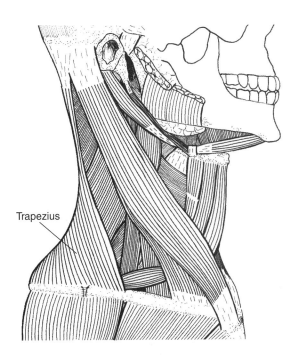

Trapezius

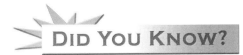

DID YOU KNOW?

The trapezius is considered to have three functional parts: upper, middle, and lower. This muscle is extremely important as it is involved in both postural stabilization and active movement of the head, neck, trunk, and shoulder girdle.

Muscles of the Neck

SPLENIUS CAPITIS

splee-nee-us **kap**-i-tis

Actions
Extension of the head and the neck at the spinal joints
Lateral flexion of the head and the neck at the spinal joints
Ipsilateral rotation of the head and the neck at the spinal joints

Innervation
Cervical spinal nerves

Arterial Supply
The occipital artery

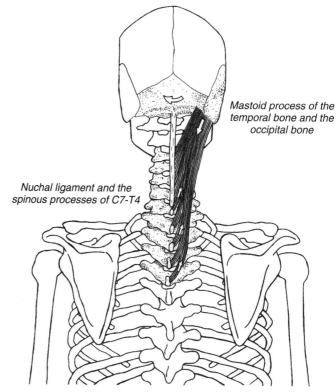

Mastoid process of the temporal bone and the occipital bone

Nuchal ligament and the spinous processes of C7-T4

Posterior view of the right splenius capitis

SPLENIUS CERVICIS

splee-nee-us **ser**-vi-sis

Actions
Extension of the neck at the spinal joints
Lateral flexion of the neck at the spinal joints
Ipsilateral rotation of the neck at the spinal joints

Innervation
Cervical spinal nerves

Arterial Supply
The occipital artery and the dorsal branches of the upper posterior intercostal arteries

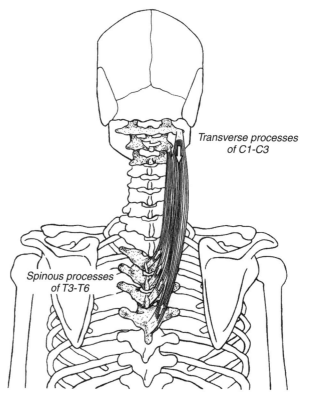

Transverse processes of C1-C3

Spinous processes of T3-T6

Posterior view of the right splenius cervicis

Muscles of the Neck

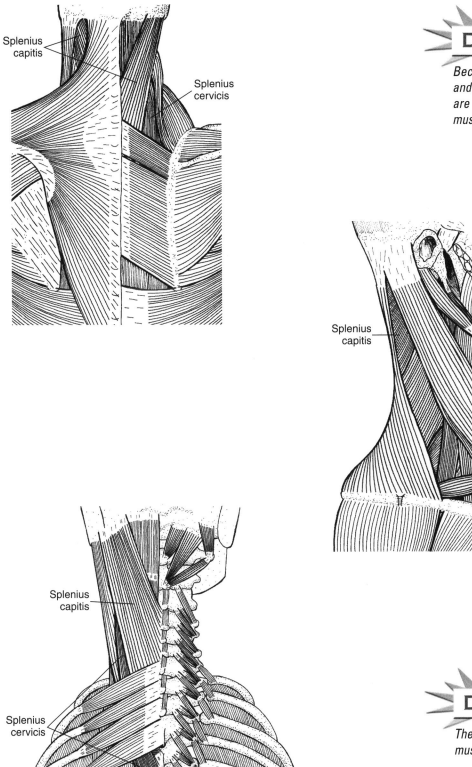

Splenius capitis

Splenius cervicis

Splenius capitis

Splenius cervicis

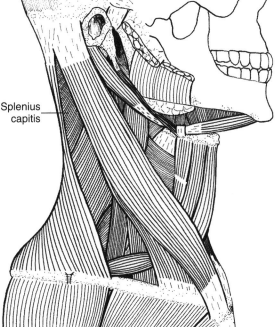

Splenius capitis

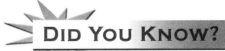

DID YOU KNOW?

Because of their 'V' shape, the left and right splenius capitis muscles are sometimes called the 'golf tee' muscles.

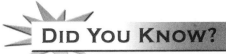

DID YOU KNOW?

The left and right splenius cervicis muscles also form a 'V' shape.

Muscles of the Neck

LEVATOR SCAPULAE

le-**vay**-tor **skap**-you-lee

Actions
Elevation of the scapula
  at the scapulocostal
  joint
Extension of the neck at
  the spinal joints
Lateral flexion of the
  neck at the spinal
  joints
Ipsilateral rotation of the
  neck at the spinal
  joints
Downward rotation of
  the scapula at the
  scapulocostal joint
Retraction (adduction) of
  the scapula at the
  scapulocostal joint

Innervation
Dorsal scapular nerve

Arterial Supply
The dorsal scapular
  artery

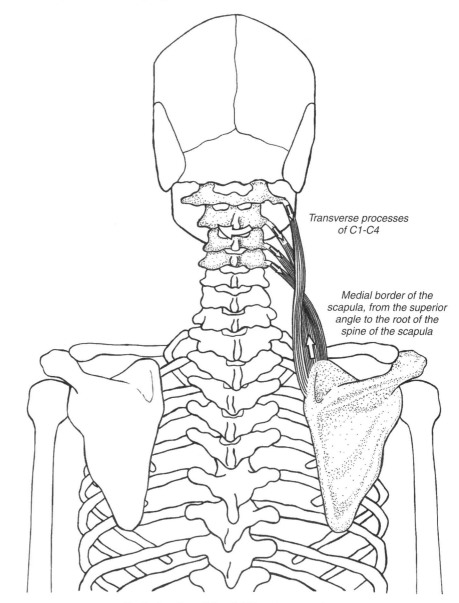

*Transverse processes
of C1-C4*

*Medial border of the
scapula, from the superior
angle to the root of the
spine of the scapula*

Posterior view of the right levator scapulae

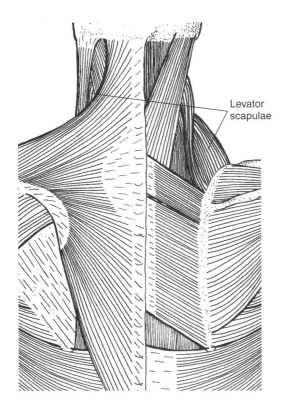

Levator
scapulae

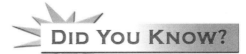

DID YOU KNOW?

The levator scapulae has a twist in its fibers so that the most superior fibers on the scapula attach the most inferiorly on the spine, and vice versa.

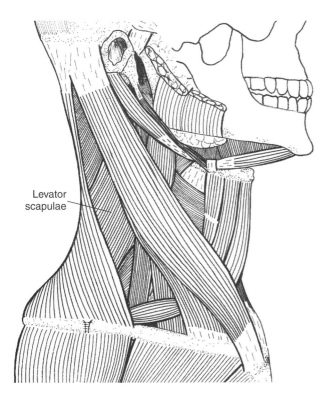

Levator
scapulae

Muscles of the Neck

RECTUS CAPITIS POSTERIOR MAJOR
(OF THE SUBOCCIPITAL GROUP)

rek-tus **kap**-i-tis
pos-**tee**-ri-or
may-jor

Actions
Extension of the head at
the atlanto-occipital
joint
Lateral flexion of the
head at the atlanto-
occipital joint
Ipsilateral rotation of the
head at the atlanto-
occipital joint
Extension and ipsilateral
rotation of the atlas at
the atlantoaxial joint

Innervation
The suboccipital nerve

Arterial Supply
The occipital artery and
the deep cervical
artery

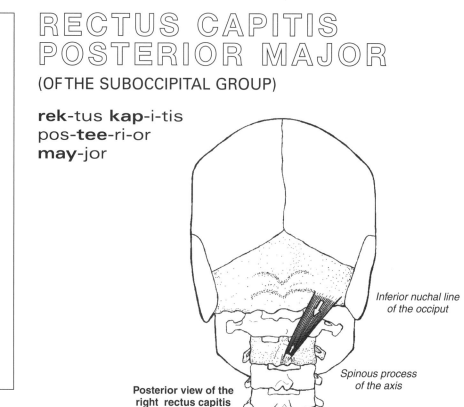

Inferior nuchal line of the occiput

Spinous process of the axis

Posterior view of the right rectus capitis posterior major

RECTUS CAPITIS POSTERIOR MINOR
(OF THE SUBOCCIPITAL GROUP)

rek-tus **kap**-i-tis pos-**tee**-ri-or **my**-nor

Action
Extension of the head at
the atlanto-occipital
joint

Innervation
The suboccipital nerve

Arterial Supply
The occipital artery and
muscular branches of
the vertebral artery

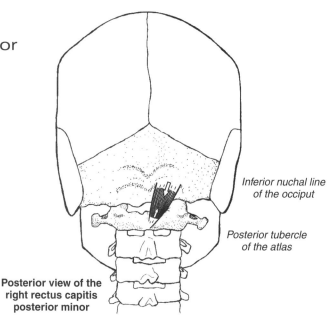

Inferior nuchal line of the occiput

Posterior tubercle of the atlas

Posterior view of the right rectus capitis posterior minor

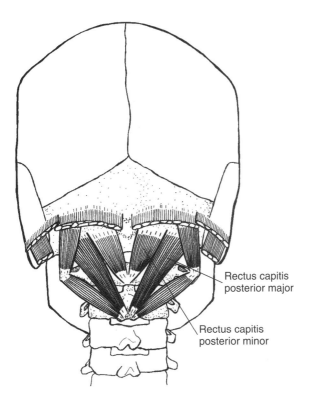

Rectus capitis
posterior major

Rectus capitis
posterior minor

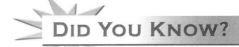

DID YOU KNOW?

The rectus capitis posterior major is the largest of the suboccipital group. The suboccipital group is primarily important as the postural stabilizer of the head.

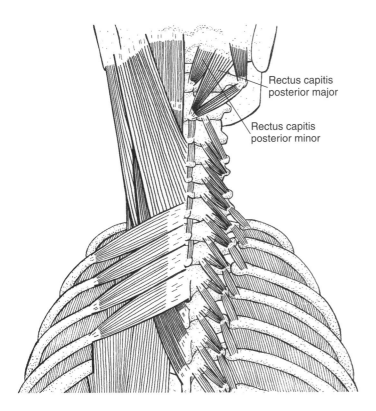

Rectus capitis
posterior major

Rectus capitis
posterior minor

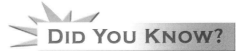

DID YOU KNOW?

The rectus capitis posterior minor has an additional attachment directly into the dura mater, making this muscle extremely likely to cause headaches when it is tight.

Muscles of the Neck

OBLIQUUS CAPITIS INFERIOR
(OF THE SUBOCCIPITAL GROUP)

ob-**lee**-kwus **kap**-i-tis in-**fee**-ri-or

Action
Ipsilateral rotation of
the atlas at the
atlantoaxial joint

Innervation
The suboccipital nerve

Arterial Supply
The deep cervical artery
and the descending
branch of the occipital
artery

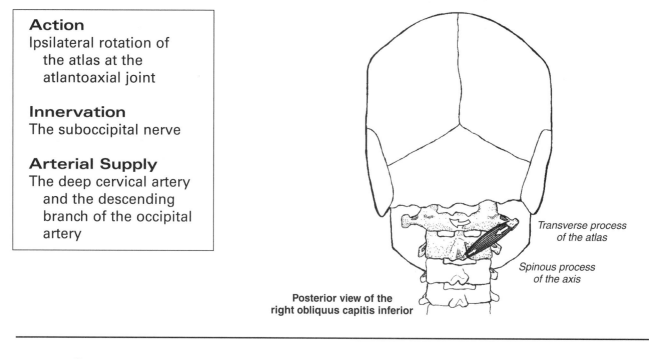

Transverse process
of the atlas

Spinous process
of the axis

**Posterior view of the
right obliquus capitis inferior**

OBLIQUUS CAPITIS SUPERIOR
(OF THE SUBOCCIPITAL GROUP)

ob-**lee**-kwus **kap**-i-tis sue-**pee**-ri-or

Actions
Extension of the head at
the atlanto-occipital
joint
Lateral flexion of the
head at the atlanto-
occipital joint

Innervation
The suboccipital nerve

Arterial Supply
The occipital artery and
the deep cervical
artery

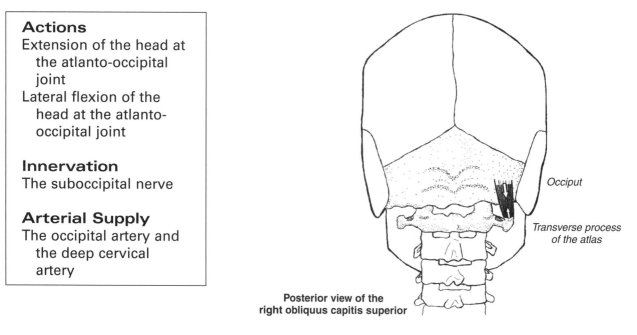

Occiput

Transverse process
of the atlas

**Posterior view of the
right obliquus capitis superior**

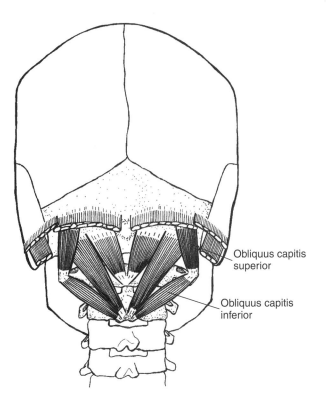

Obliquus capitis
superior

Obliquus capitis
inferior

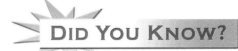

DID YOU KNOW?

*The obliquus capitis inferior is the
only one of the four suboccipital
muscles that does not cross the
atlanto-occipital joint to attach onto
the head.*

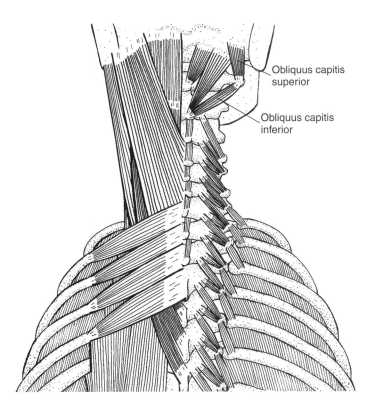

Obliquus capitis
superior

Obliquus capitis
inferior

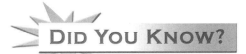

DID YOU KNOW?

*The obliquus capitis superior attaches
the most superiorly on the occiput.*

Muscles of the Neck

PLATYSMA

pla-**tiz**-ma

Actions
Draws up the skin of the
  superior chest and
  neck, creating ridges
  of skin in the neck
Depresses and draws
  the lower lip laterally
Depression of the
  mandible at the
  temporomandibular
  joint

Innervation
Facial nerve (CN VII)

Arterial Supply
The facial artery

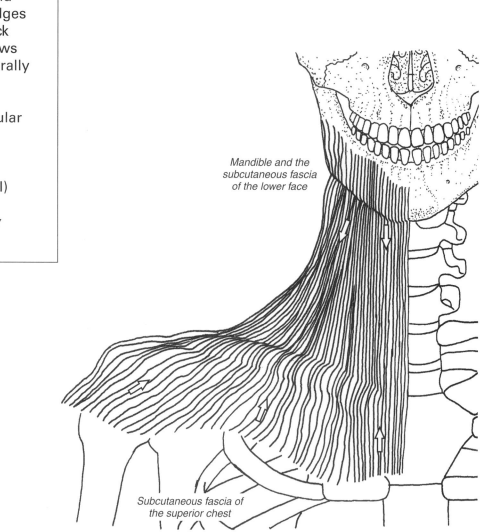

*Mandible and the
subcutaneous fascia
of the lower face*

*Subcutaneous fascia of
the superior chest*

Anterior view of the right platysma

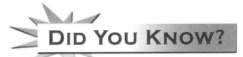

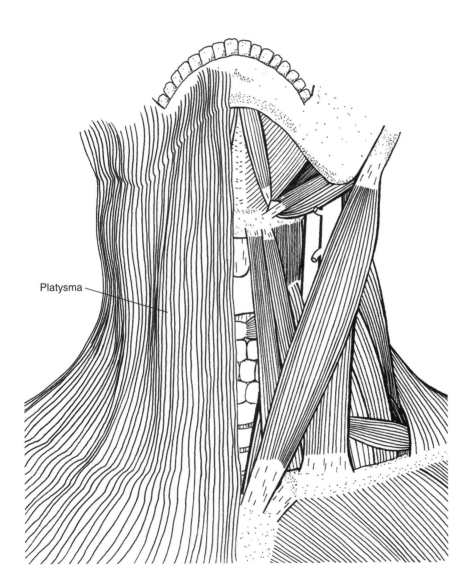

Platysma

Muscles of the Neck

STERNOCLEIDOMASTOID ("SCM")

ster-no-**kli**-do-**mas**-toyd

Actions
Flexion of the neck at
   the spinal joints
Lateral flexion of the
   neck and the head at
   the spinal joints
Contralateral rotation of
   the neck and the head
   at the spinal joints
Extension of the head at
   the atlanto-occipital
   joint
Elevation of the sternum
   and the clavicle

Innervation
Spinal accessory nerve
   (CN XI)

Arterial Supply
The occipital and
   posterior auricular
   arteries

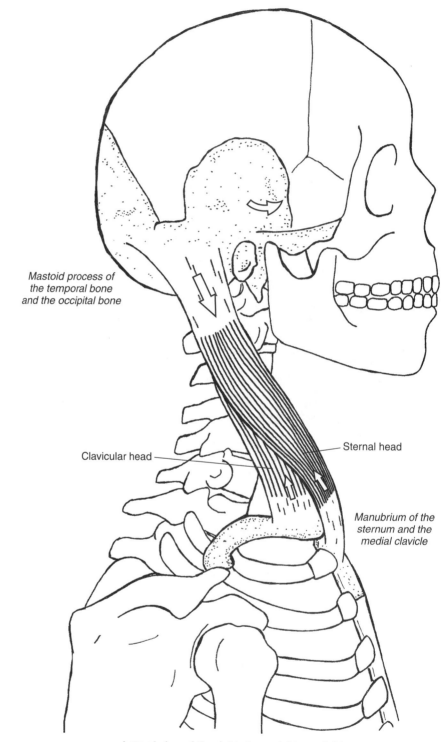

*Mastoid process of
the temporal bone
and the occipital bone*

Clavicular head

Sternal head

*Manubrium of the
sternum and the
medial clavicle*

Lateral view of the right sternocleidomastoid

Muscles of the Neck

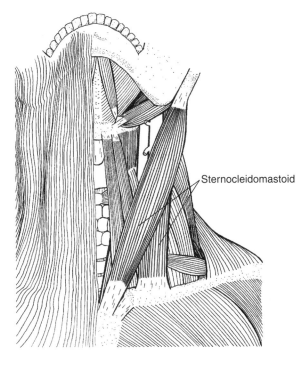

Sternocleidomastoid

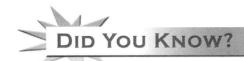

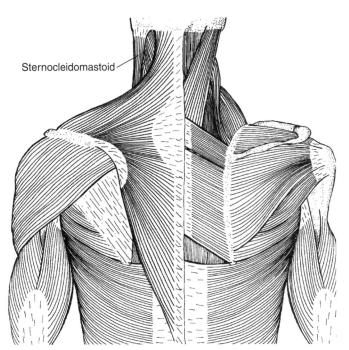

Sternocleidomastoid

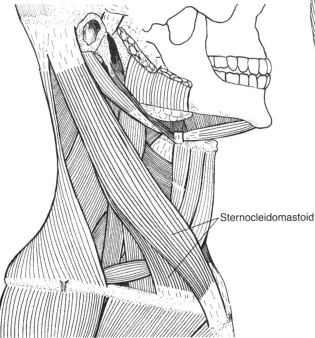

Sternocleidomastoid

Muscles of the Neck

STERNOHYOID

(OF THE HYOID GROUP)

ster-no-**hi**-oyd

Action
Depression of the hyoid

Innervation
The cervical plexus

Arterial Supply
The superior thyroid
  artery

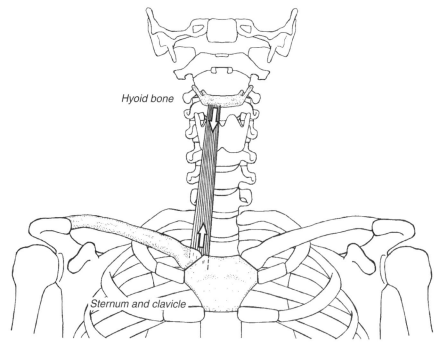

Hyoid bone

Sternum and clavicle

Anterior view of the right sternohyoid

STERNOTHYROID

(OF THE HYOID GROUP)

ster-no-**thi**-royd

Action
Depression of the thyroid
  cartilage

Innervation
The cervical plexus

Arterial Supply
The superior thyroid
  artery

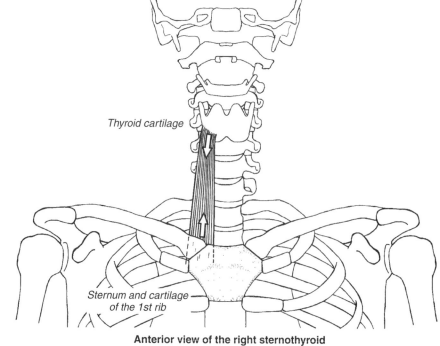

Thyroid cartilage

Sternum and cartilage
of the 1st rib

Anterior view of the right sternothyroid

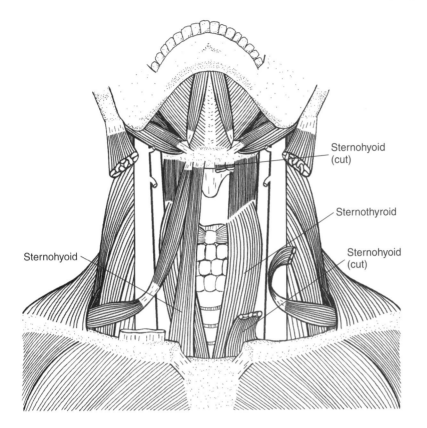

Sternohyoid (cut)

Sternothyroid

Sternohyoid (cut)

Sternohyoid

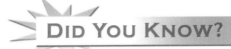

DID YOU KNOW?

The sternohyoid attaches to the posterior surface of both the manubrium of the sternum and the medial clavicle.

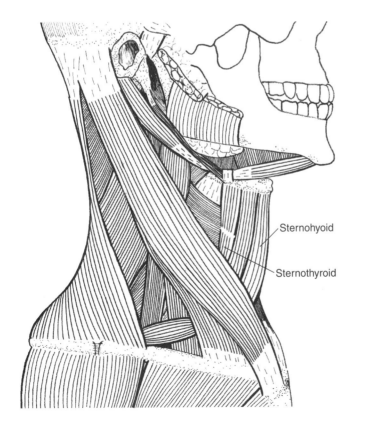

Sternohyoid

Sternothyroid

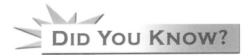

DID YOU KNOW?

The sternothyroid attaches to the posterior surface of both the manubrium of the sternum and the costal cartilage of the 1st rib.

Muscles of the Neck

THYROHYOID
(OF THE HYOID GROUP)

thi-ro-**hi**-oyd

Actions
Depression of the hyoid
Elevation of the thyroid
cartilage

Innervation
The hypoglossal nerve
(CN XII)

Arterial Supply
The superior thyroid
artery

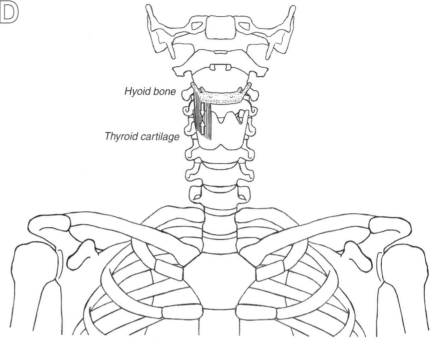

Hyoid bone

Thyroid cartilage

Anterior view of the right thyrohyoid

OMOHYOID
(OF THE HYOID GROUP)

o-mo-**hi**-oyd

Action
Depression of the hyoid

Innervation
The cervical plexus

Arterial Supply
The superior thyroid
artery and the
transverse cervical
artery

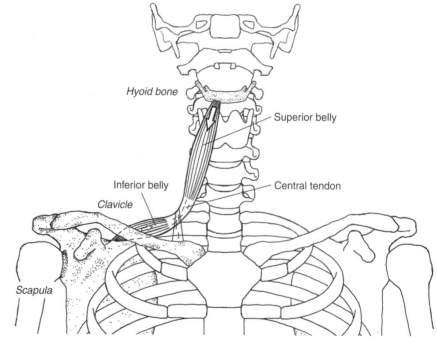

Hyoid bone

Superior belly

Inferior belly

Central tendon

Clavicle

Scapula

Anterior view of the right omohyoid

Muscles of the Neck

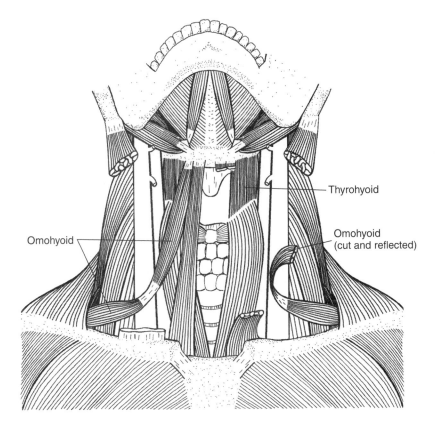

Thyrohyoid

Omohyoid

Omohyoid
(cut and reflected)

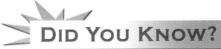

The thyrohyoid can be considered to be an upward continuation of the sternothyroid muscle.

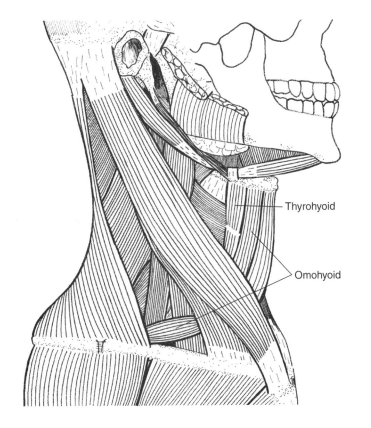

Thyrohyoid

Omohyoid

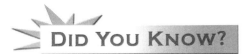

The omohyoid has two bellies separated by a central tendon that attaches to the clavicle.

Muscles of the Neck

DIGASTRIC
(OF THE HYOID GROUP)

di-**gas**-trik

Actions
Elevation of the hyoid
Depression of the
mandible at the
temporomandibular
joint
Retraction of the
mandible at the
temporomandibular
joint

Innervation
The trigeminal (CN V)
and the facial nerve
(CN VII)

Arterial Supply
The occipital, posterior
auricular and facial
arteries

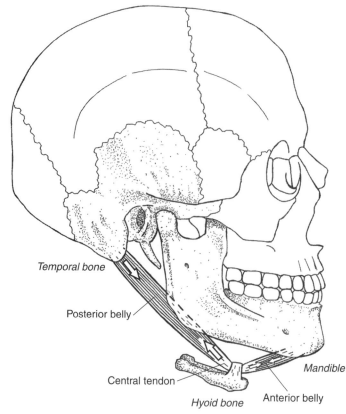

Temporal bone

Posterior belly

Central tendon

Hyoid bone

Mandible

Anterior belly

Lateral view of the right digastric

STYLOHYOID
(OF THE HYOID GROUP)

sti-lo-**hi**-oyd

Action
Elevation of the hyoid

Innervation
The facial nerve (CN VII)

Arterial Supply
The occipital, posterior
auricular and facial
arteries

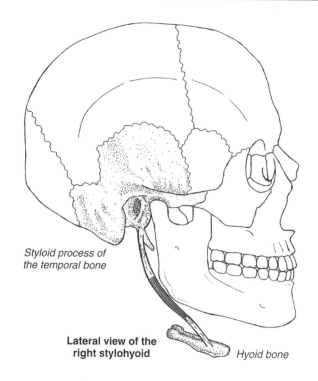

Styloid process of
the temporal bone

**Lateral view of the
right stylohyoid**

Hyoid bone

Muscles of the Neck

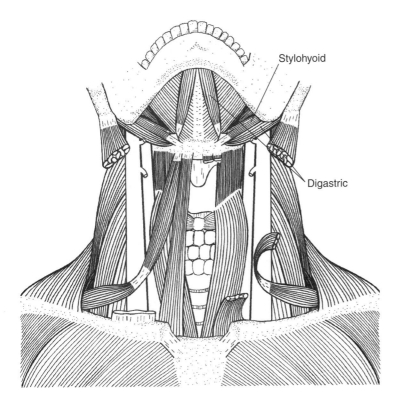

Stylohyoid

Digastric

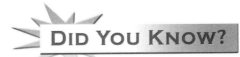

DID YOU KNOW?

The digastric has two bellies that are separated by a central tendon that attaches to the hyoid bone. In fact, the name digastric means "two bellies" in Greek.

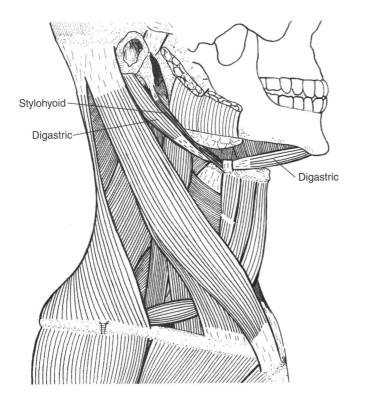

Stylohyoid

Digastric

Digastric

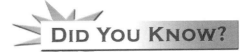

DID YOU KNOW?

The attachment of the stylohyoid onto the hyoid bone is perforated by the central tendon of the digastric.

Muscles of the Neck

MYLOHYOID
(OF THE HYOID GROUP)

my-lo-**hi**-oyd

Actions
Elevation of the hyoid
Depression of the
  mandible at the
  temporomandibular
  joint

Innervation
The trigeminal nerve
  (CN V)

Arterial Supply
The inferior alveolar
  artery

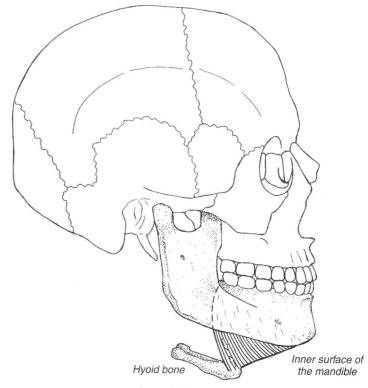

Hyoid bone   *Inner surface of
                       the mandible*

Lateral view of the right mylohyoid

GENIOHYOID
(OF THE HYOID GROUP)

jee-nee-o-**hi**-oyd

Actions
Elevation of the hyoid
Depression of the
  mandible at the
  temporomandibular
  joint

Innervation
The hypoglossal nerve
  (CN XII)

Arterial Supply
The lingual artery

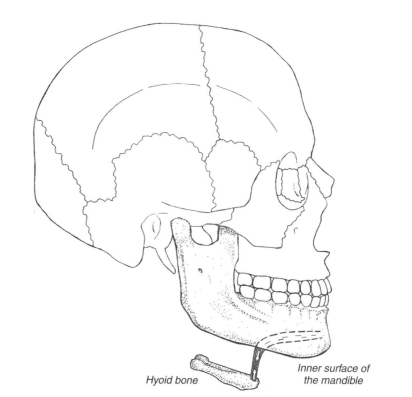

Hyoid bone   *Inner surface of
                       the mandible*

Lateral view of the right geniohyoid

Muscles of the Neck

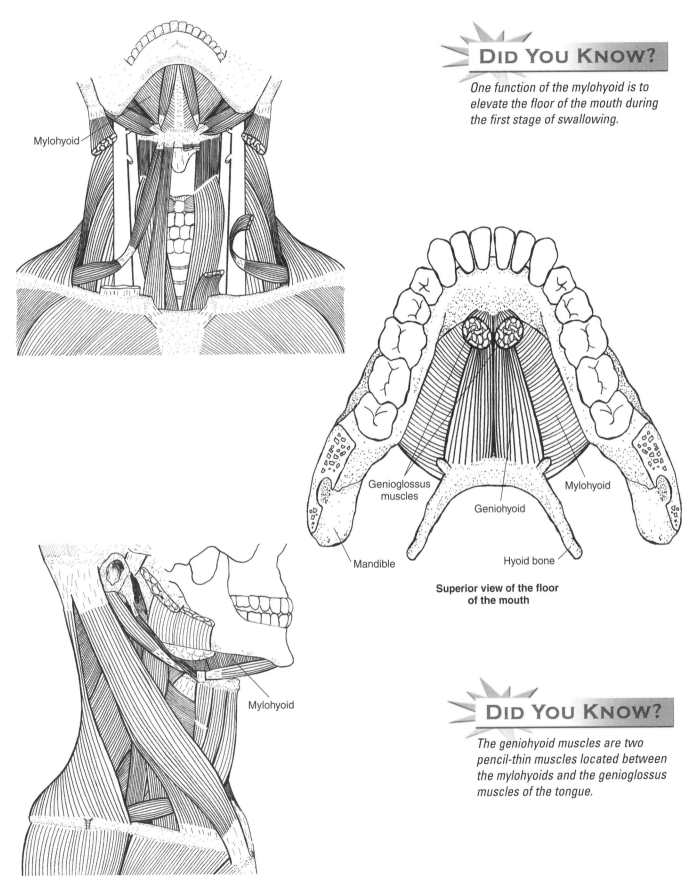

Mylohyoid

DID YOU KNOW?

One function of the mylohyoid is to elevate the floor of the mouth during the first stage of swallowing.

Genioglossus muscles

Geniohyoid

Mylohyoid

Mandible

Hyoid bone

Superior view of the floor of the mouth

Mylohyoid

DID YOU KNOW?

The geniohyoid muscles are two pencil-thin muscles located between the mylohyoids and the genioglossus muscles of the tongue.

Muscles of the Neck

ANTERIOR SCALENE
(OF THE SCALENE GROUP)

an-**tee**-ri-or **skay**-leen

Actions
Flexion of the neck at the
spinal joints
Lateral flexion of the neck
at the spinal joints
Elevation of the 1st rib at
the sternocostal and
costovertebral joints
Contralateral rotation of
the neck at the spinal
joints

Innervation
Cervical spinal nerves

Arterial Supply
The ascending cervical
artery

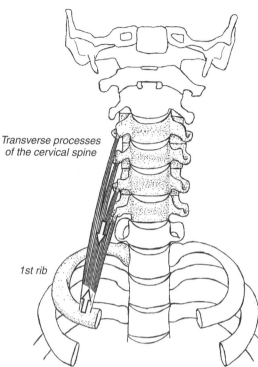

*Transverse processes
of the cervical spine*

1st rib

Anterior view of the right anterior scalene

MIDDLE SCALENE
(OF THE SCALENE GROUP)

mi-dil **skay**-leen

Actions
Lateral flexion of the neck
at the spinal joints
Flexion of the neck at
the spinal joints
Elevation of the 1st rib
at the sternocostal and
costovertebral joints

Innervation
Cervical spinal nerves

Arterial Supply
The transverse cervical
artery

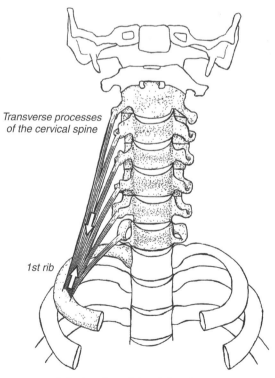

*Transverse processes
of the cervical spine*

1st rib

Anterior view of the right middle scalene

Muscles of the Neck

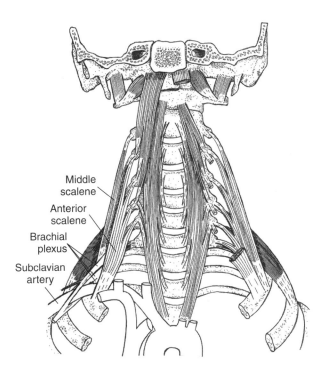

Middle
scalene

Anterior
scalene

Brachial
plexus

Subclavian
artery

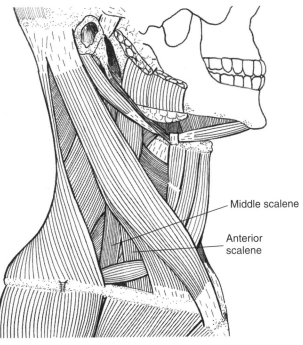

Middle scalene

Anterior
scalene

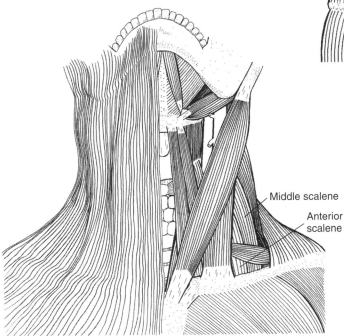

Middle scalene

Anterior
scalene

Muscles of the Neck

POSTERIOR SCALENE

(OF THE SCALENE GROUP)

pos-**tee**-ri-or **skay**-leen

Actions
Lateral flexion of the
   neck at the spinal
   joints
Elevation of the 2nd rib
   at the sternocostal and
   costovertebral joints

Innervation
Cervical spinal nerves

Arterial Supply
The transverse cervical
   artery

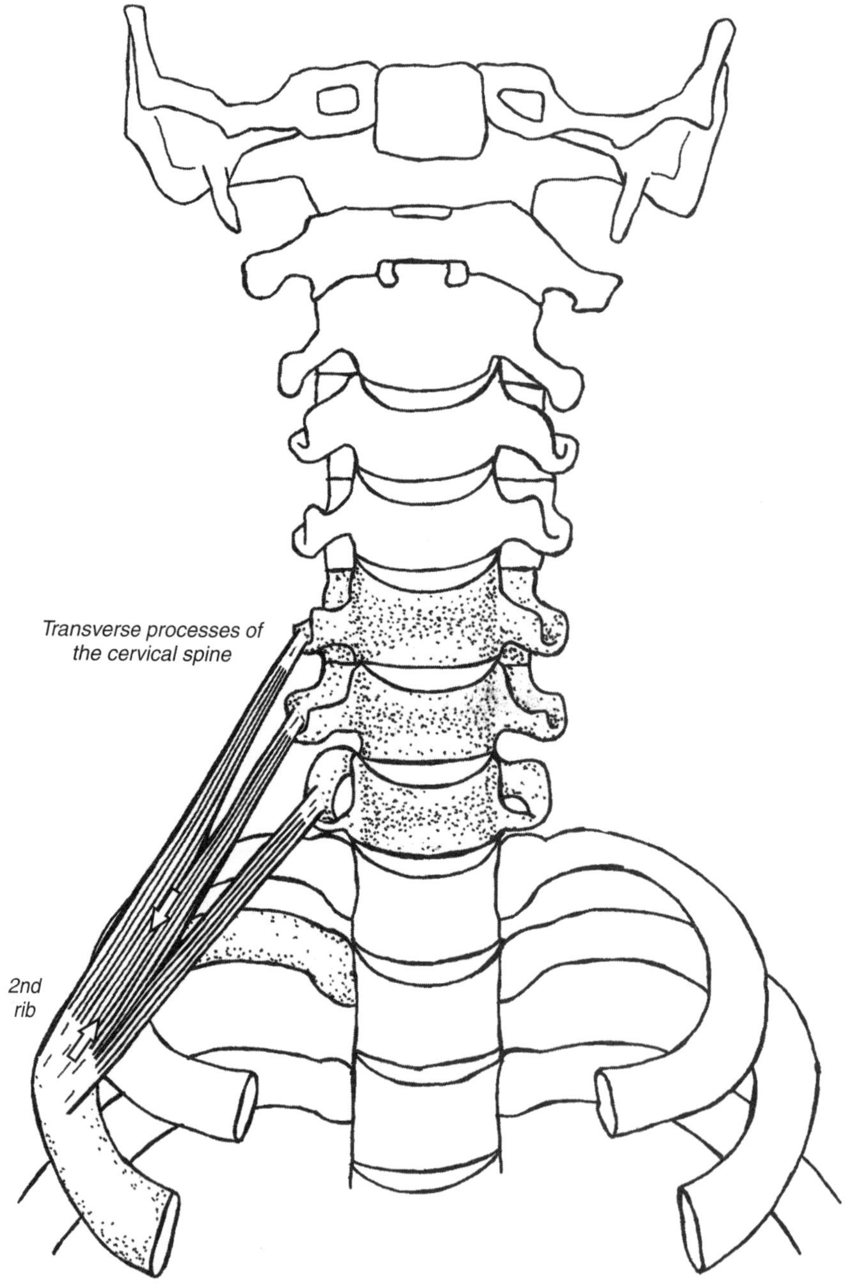

*Transverse processes of
the cervical spine*

*2nd
rib*

Muscles of the Neck

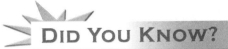

DID YOU KNOW?

The posterior scalene is the smallest and shortest of the three scalenes.

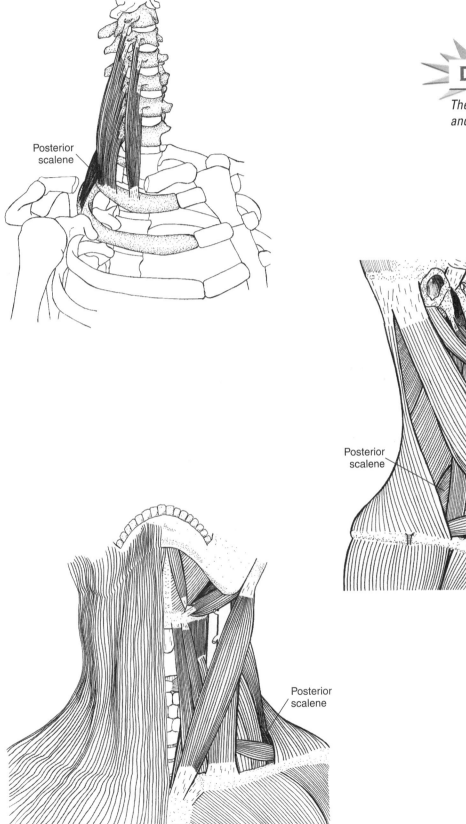

Posterior scalene

Posterior scalene

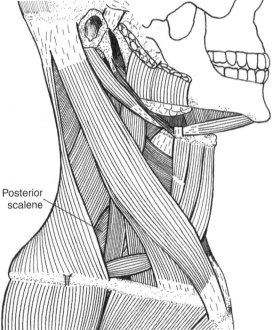

Posterior scalene

Muscles of the Neck

LONGUS COLLI
(OF THE PREVERTEBRAL GROUP)

long-us kol-eye

Actions
Flexion of the neck at the spinal joints
Lateral flexion of the neck at the spinal joints
Contralateral rotation of the neck at the spinal joints

Innervation
Cervical spinal nerves

Arterial Supply
The inferior thyroid artery and the vertebral artery

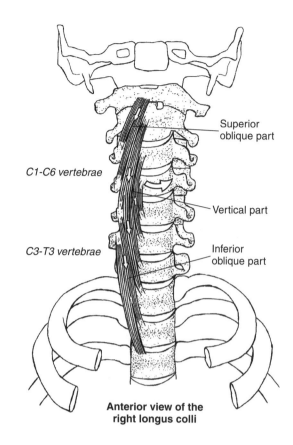

C1-C6 vertebrae

C3-T3 vertebrae

Superior oblique part

Vertical part

Inferior oblique part

Anterior view of the right longus colli

LONGUS CAPITIS
(OF THE PREVERTEBRAL GROUP)

long-us kap-i-tis

Actions
Flexion of the head and the neck at the spinal joints
Lateral flexion of the head and the neck at the spinal joints

Innervation
Cervical spinal nerves

Arterial Supply
The inferior thyroid artery and the vertebral artery

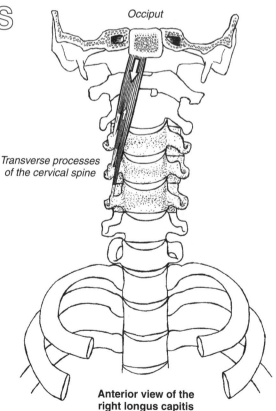

Occiput

Transverse processes of the cervical spine

Anterior view of the right longus capitis

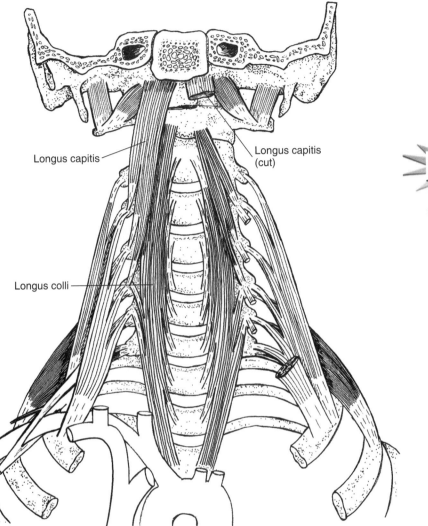

Longus capitis

Longus capitis (cut)

Longus colli

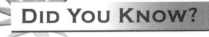

DID YOU KNOW?

The longus colli and longus capitis are very deep in the anterior neck.

Muscles of the Neck

RECTUS CAPITIS ANTERIOR

(OF THE PREVERTEBRAL GROUP)

rek-tus **kap**-i-tis
an-**tee**-ri-or

Action
Flexion of the head at the atlanto-occipital joint

Innervation
Cervical spinal nerves

Arterial Supply
The vertebral artery

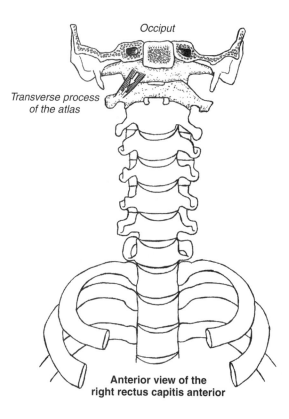

Occiput

Transverse process of the atlas

Anterior view of the right rectus capitis anterior

RECTUS CAPITIS LATERALIS

(OF THE PREVERTEBRAL GROUP)

rek-tus **kap**-i-tis
la-ter-**a**-lis

Action
Lateral flexion of the head at the atlanto-occipital joint

Innervation
Cervical spinal nerves

Arterial Supply
The vertebral artery and the occipital artery

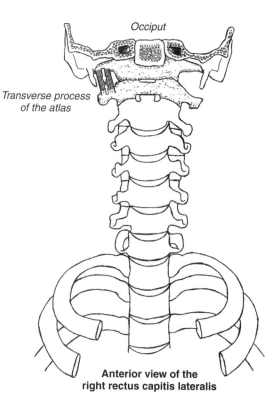

Occiput

Transverse process of the atlas

Anterior view of the right rectus capitis lateralis

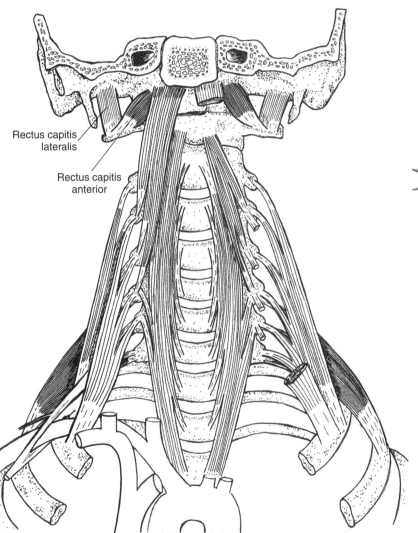

Rectus capitis
lateralis

Rectus capitis
anterior

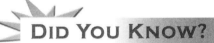

DID YOU KNOW?

The rectus capitis anterior and rectus capitis lateralis are generally considered to be more important as postural stabilization muscles of the head than as movers.

Muscles of the Neck

ANTERIOR VIEW OF THE NECK (SUPERFICIAL)

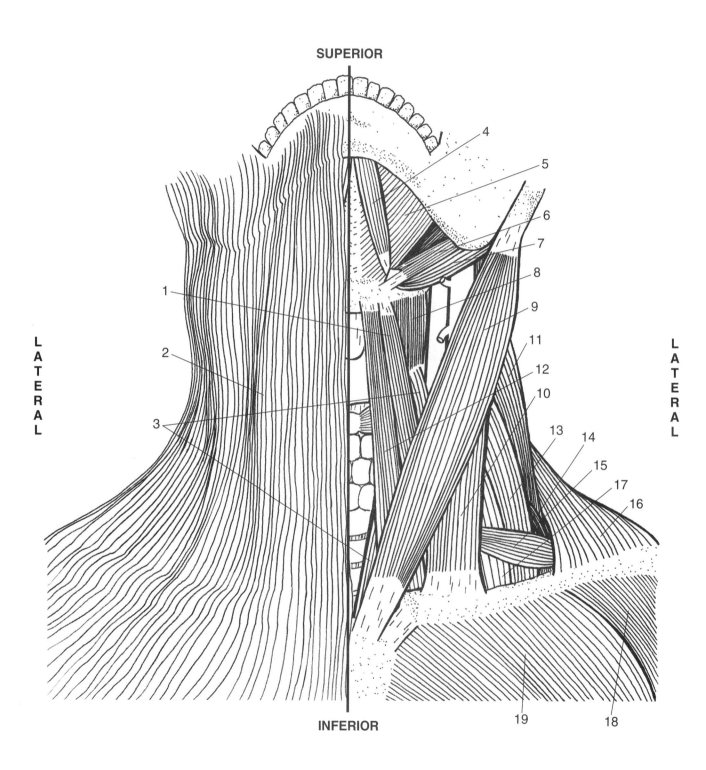

ANTERIOR VIEW OF THE NECK (INTERMEDIATE)

SUPERIOR

LATERAL

LATERAL

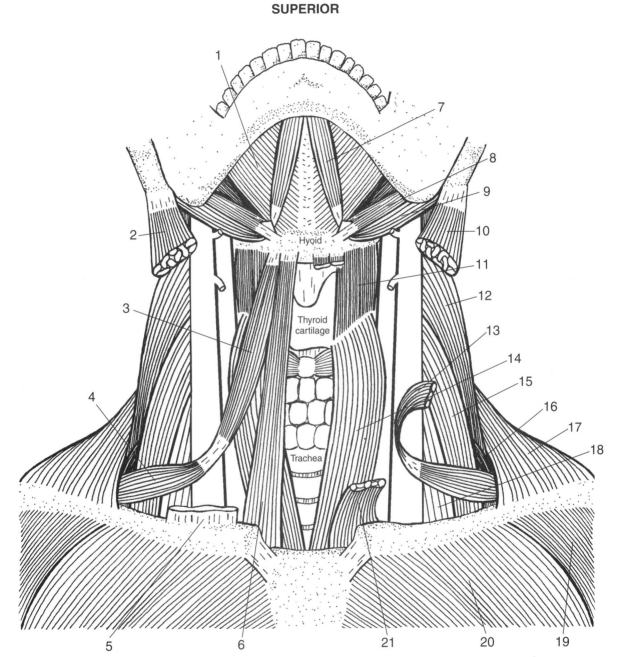

Hyoid

Thyroid
cartilage

Trachea

INFERIOR

Muscles of the Neck

ANTERIOR VIEW OF THE NECK (DEEP)

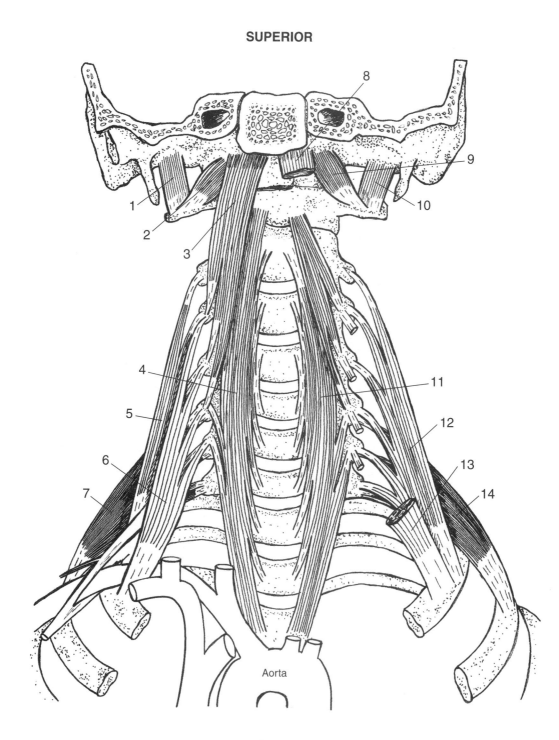

SUPERIOR

LATERAL

LATERAL

Aorta

INFERIOR

LATERAL VIEW OF THE NECK

SUPERIOR

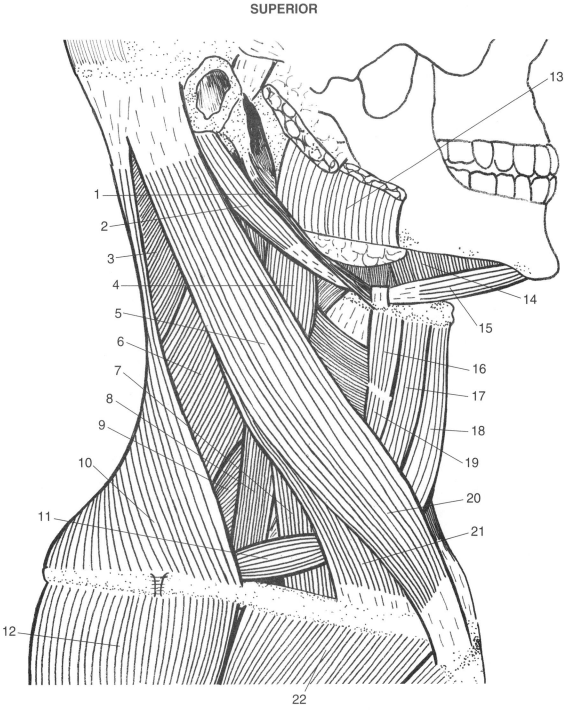

POSTERIOR

ANTERIOR

1
2
3
4
5
6
7
8
9
10
11
12

13
14
15
16
17
18
19
20
21
22

INFERIOR

POSTERIOR VIEW OF THE NECK
(SUPERFICIAL AND INTERMEDIATE)

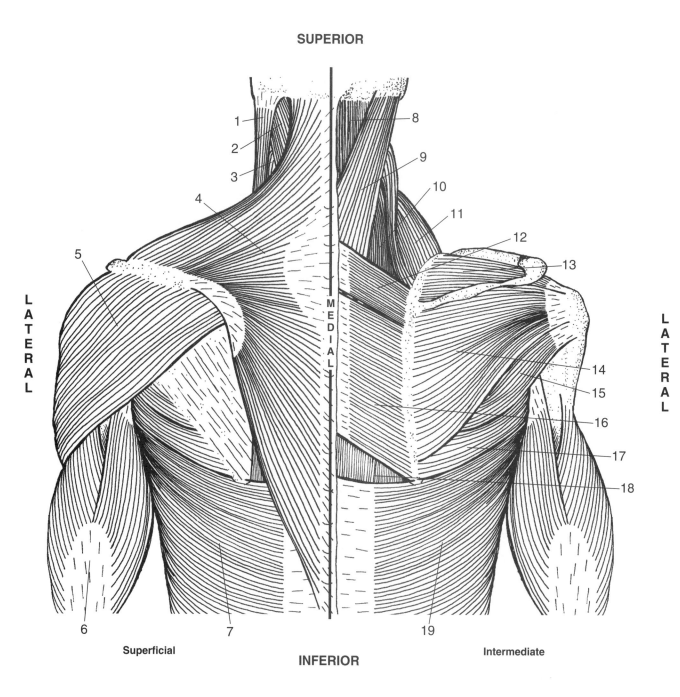

SUPERIOR

LATERAL

MEDIAL

LATERAL

Superficial

Intermediate

INFERIOR

1 2 3 4 5 6 7 8 9 10 11 12 13 14 15 16 17 18 19

POSTERIOR VIEW OF THE NECK
(INTERMEDIATE AND DEEP)

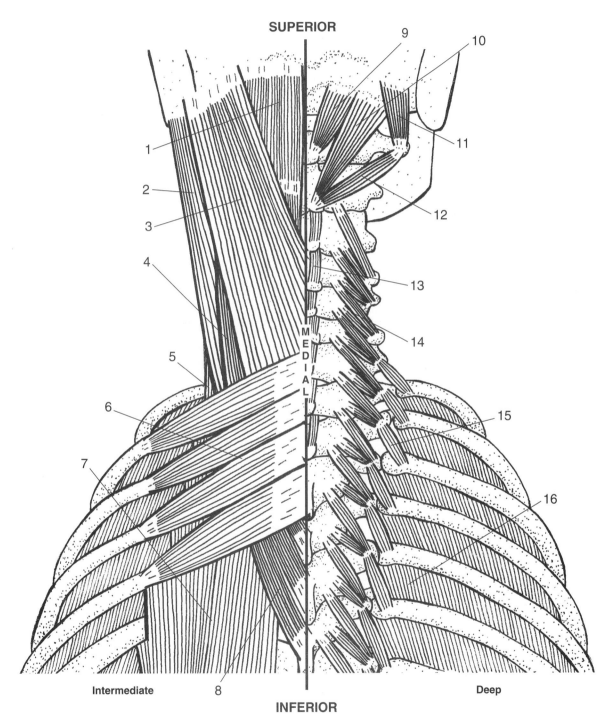

SUPERIOR

LATERAL

MEDIAL

LATERAL

Intermediate

Deep

INFERIOR

Muscles of the Trunk

POSTERIOR VIEW OF THE TRUNK
(SUPERFICIAL AND INTERMEDIATE)

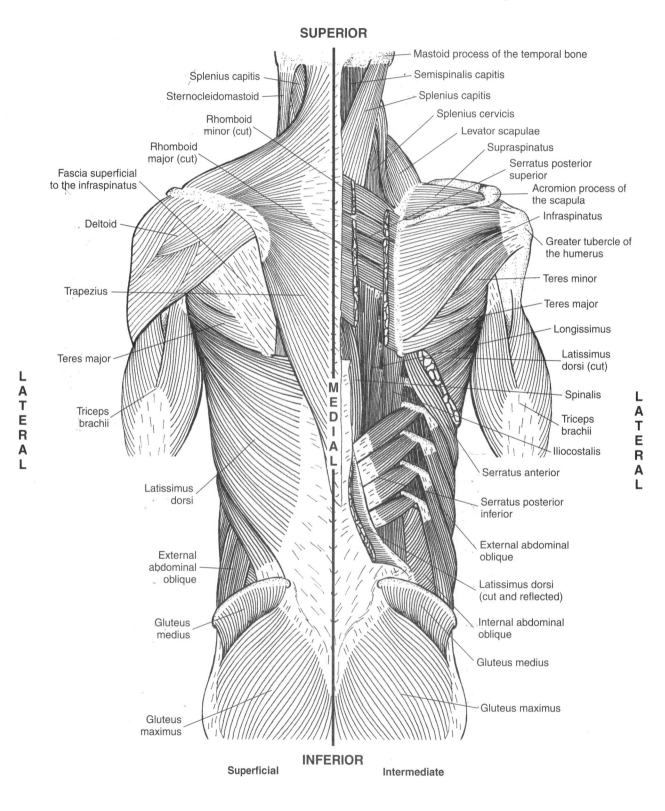

SUPERIOR

Splenius capitis
Sternocleidomastoid
Rhomboid minor (cut)
Rhomboid major (cut)
Fascia superficial to the infraspinatus
Deltoid
Trapezius
Teres major
Triceps brachii
Latissimus dorsi
External abdominal oblique
Gluteus medius
Gluteus maximus

Mastoid process of the temporal bone
Semispinalis capitis
Splenius capitis
Splenius cervicis
Levator scapulae
Supraspinatus
Serratus posterior superior
Acromion process of the scapula
Infraspinatus
Greater tubercle of the humerus
Teres minor
Teres major
Longissimus
Latissimus dorsi (cut)
Spinalis
Triceps brachii
Iliocostalis
Serratus anterior
Serratus posterior inferior
External abdominal oblique
Latissimus dorsi (cut and reflected)
Internal abdominal oblique
Gluteus medius
Gluteus maximus

LATERAL

MEDIAL

LATERAL

INFERIOR

Superficial

Intermediate

POSTERIOR VIEW OF THE TRUNK (DEEP LAYERS)

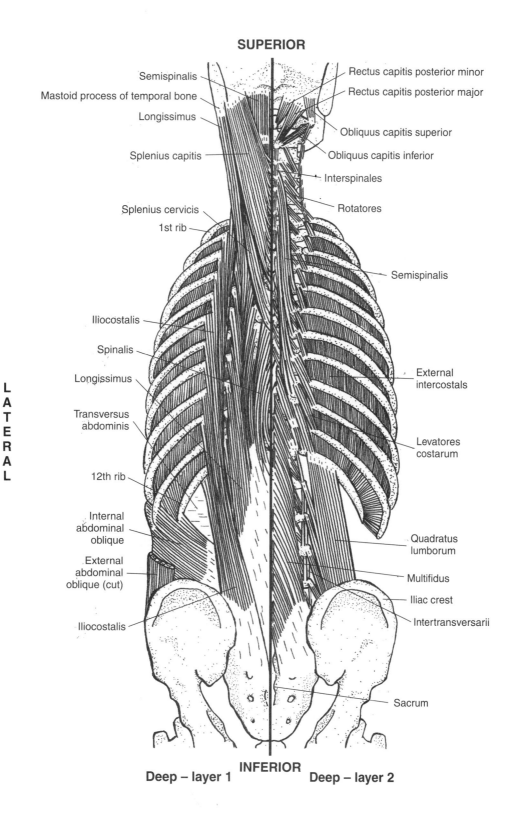

SUPERIOR

Semispinalis

Mastoid process of temporal bone

Longissimus

Splenius capitis

Splenius cervicis

1st rib

Iliocostalis

Spinalis

Longissimus

Transversus abdominis

12th rib

Internal abdominal oblique

External abdominal oblique (cut)

Iliocostalis

Rectus capitis posterior minor

Rectus capitis posterior major

Obliquus capitis superior

Obliquus capitis inferior

Interspinales

Rotatores

Semispinalis

External intercostals

Levatores costarum

Quadratus lumborum

Multifidus

Iliac crest

Intertransversarii

Sacrum

L A T E R A L

L A T E R A L

INFERIOR

Deep – layer 1   Deep – layer 2

Muscles of the Trunk

ANTERIOR VIEW OF THE TRUNK
(SUPERFICIAL AND INTERMEDIATE)

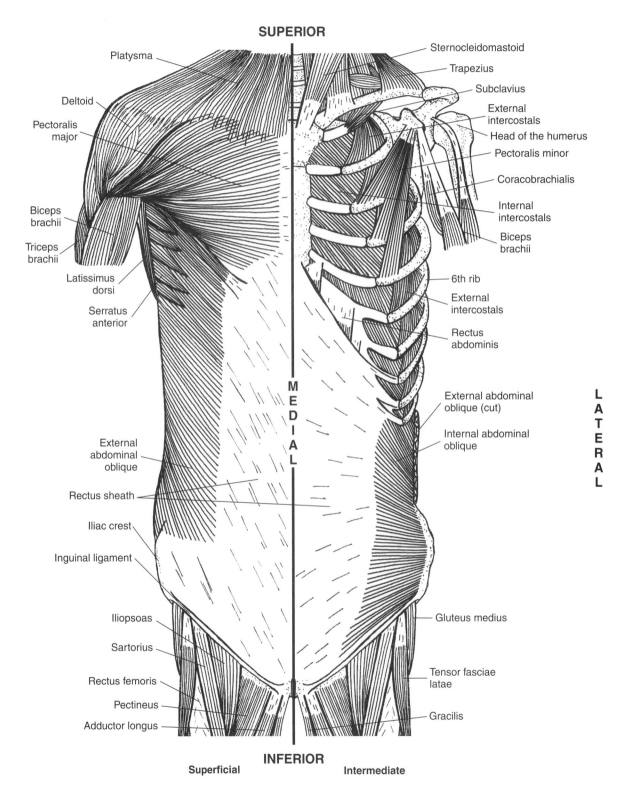

SUPERIOR

Platysma

Sternocleidomastoid

Trapezius

Subclavius

Deltoid

External intercostals

Pectoralis major

Head of the humerus

Pectoralis minor

Coracobrachialis

Biceps brachii

Internal intercostals

Triceps brachii

Biceps brachii

Latissimus dorsi

6th rib

Serratus anterior

External intercostals

Rectus abdominis

LATERAL

MEDIAL

LATERAL

External abdominal oblique (cut)

Internal abdominal oblique

External abdominal oblique

Rectus sheath

Iliac crest

Inguinal ligament

Gluteus medius

Iliopsoas

Sartorius

Tensor fasciae latae

Rectus femoris

Pectineus

Gracilis

Adductor longus

INFERIOR

Superficial

Intermediate

Muscles of the Trunk

ANTERIOR VIEW OF THE TRUNK
(INTERMEDIATE AND DEEP)

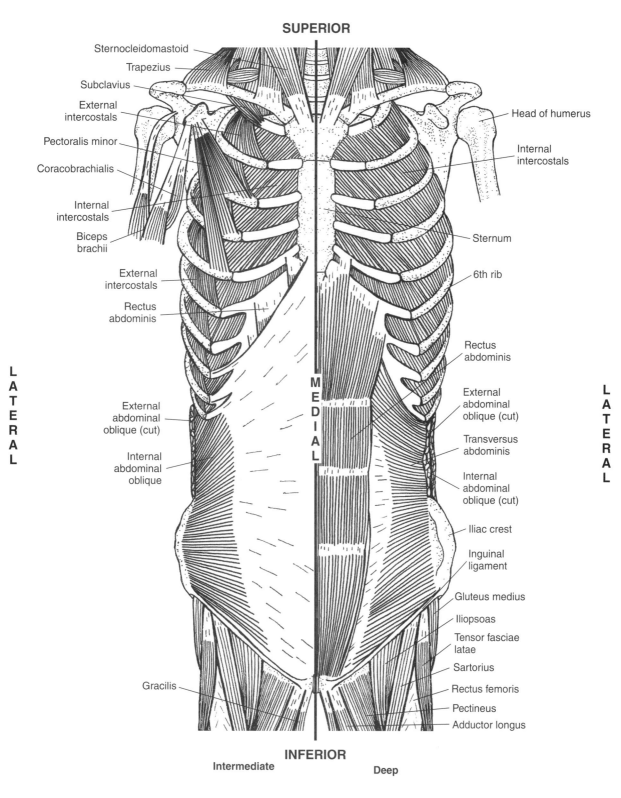

SUPERIOR

Sternocleidomastoid

Trapezius

Subclavius

External
intercostals

Pectoralis minor

Coracobrachialis

Internal
intercostals

Biceps
brachii

External
intercostals

Rectus
abdominis

External
abdominal
oblique (cut)

Internal
abdominal
oblique

Gracilis

Head of humerus

Internal
intercostals

Sternum

6th rib

Rectus
abdominis

External
abdominal
oblique (cut)

Transversus
abdominis

Internal
abdominal
oblique (cut)

Iliac crest

Inguinal
ligament

Gluteus medius

Iliopsoas

Tensor fasciae
latae

Sartorius

Rectus femoris

Pectineus

Adductor longus

LATERAL

MEDIAL

LATERAL

INFERIOR

Intermediate

Deep

Muscles of the Trunk

LATERAL VIEW OF THE TRUNK

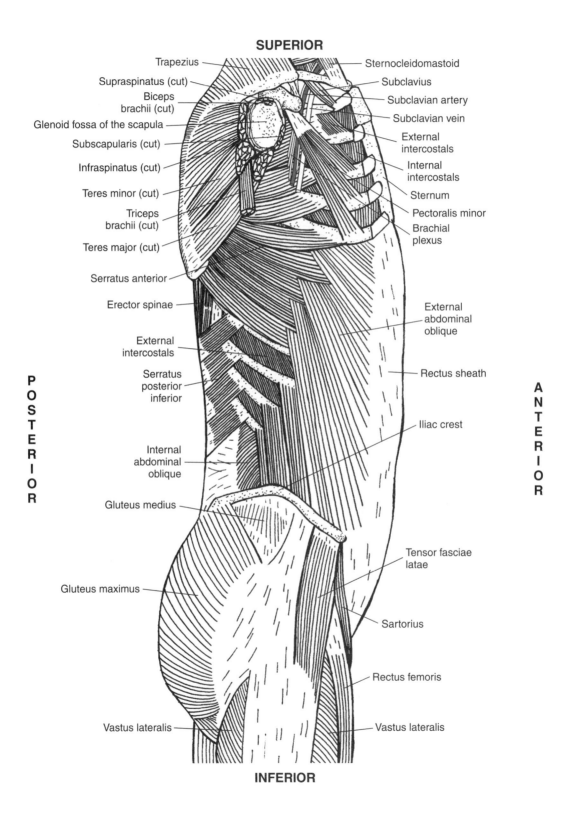

SUPERIOR

Trapezius

Supraspinatus (cut)

Biceps
brachii (cut)

Glenoid fossa of the scapula

Subscapularis (cut)

Infraspinatus (cut)

Teres minor (cut)

Triceps
brachii (cut)

Teres major (cut)

Serratus anterior

Erector spinae

External
intercostals

Serratus
posterior
inferior

Internal
abdominal
oblique

Gluteus medius

Gluteus maximus

Vastus lateralis

Sternocleidomastoid

Subclavius

Subclavian artery

Subclavian vein

External
intercostals

Internal
intercostals

Sternum

Pectoralis minor

Brachial
plexus

External
abdominal
oblique

Rectus sheath

Iliac crest

Tensor fasciae
latae

Sartorius

Rectus femoris

Vastus lateralis

POSTERIOR

ANTERIOR

INFERIOR

CROSS SECTION VIEWS OF THE TRUNK

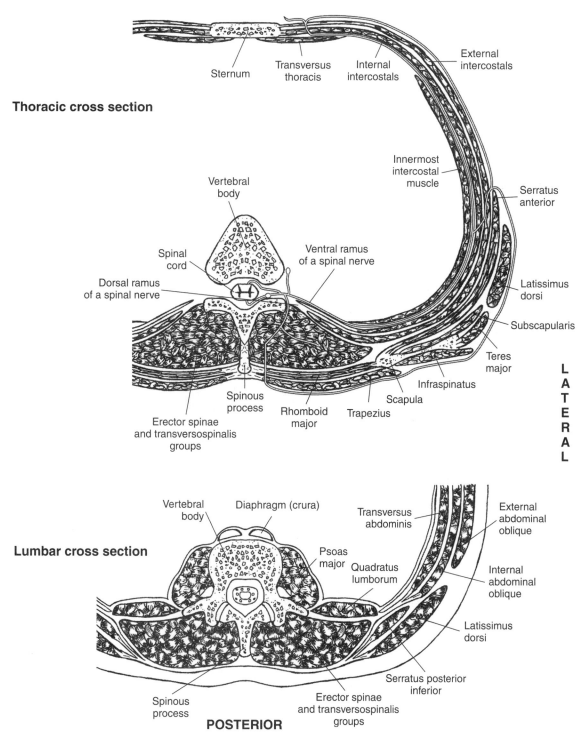

ANTERIOR

Thoracic cross section

Sternum

Transversus thoracis

Internal intercostals

External intercostals

Innermost intercostal muscle

Serratus anterior

Vertebral body

Ventral ramus of a spinal nerve

Spinal cord

Dorsal ramus of a spinal nerve

Latissimus dorsi

Subscapularis

Teres major

Infraspinatus

Scapula

Trapezius

Spinous process

Rhomboid major

Erector spinae and transversospinalis groups

LATERAL

Lumbar cross section

Vertebral body

Diaphragm (crura)

Transversus abdominis

External abdominal oblique

Psoas major

Quadratus lumborum

Internal abdominal oblique

Latissimus dorsi

Serratus posterior inferior

Spinous process

Erector spinae and transversospinalis groups

POSTERIOR

Muscles of the Trunk

LATISSIMUS DORSI (THE "LAT")

la-**tis**-i-mus **door**-si

Actions
Medial rotation of the arm at the shoulder joint

Adduction of the arm at the shoulder joint

Extension of the arm at the shoulder joint

Anterior tilt of the pelvis at the lumbosacral joint

Depression of the scapula at the scapulocostal joint

Lateral deviation of the trunk at the scapulocostal joint

Elevation of the trunk at the scapulocostal joint

Contralateral rotation of the trunk at the scapulocostal joint

Elevation of the pelvis at the lumbosacral joint

Innervation
The thoracodorsal nerve

Arterial Supply
The thoracodorsal artery and the dorsal branches of the posterior intercostal arteries

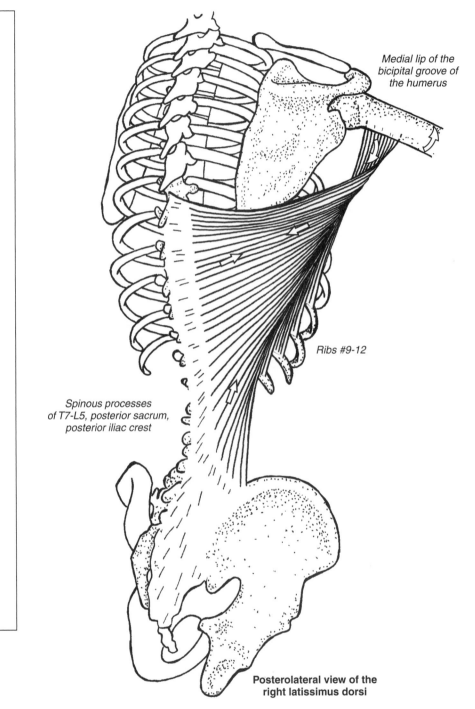

Medial lip of the bicipital groove of the humerus

Ribs #9-12

Spinous processes of T7-L5, posterior sacrum, posterior iliac crest

Posterolateral view of the right latissimus dorsi

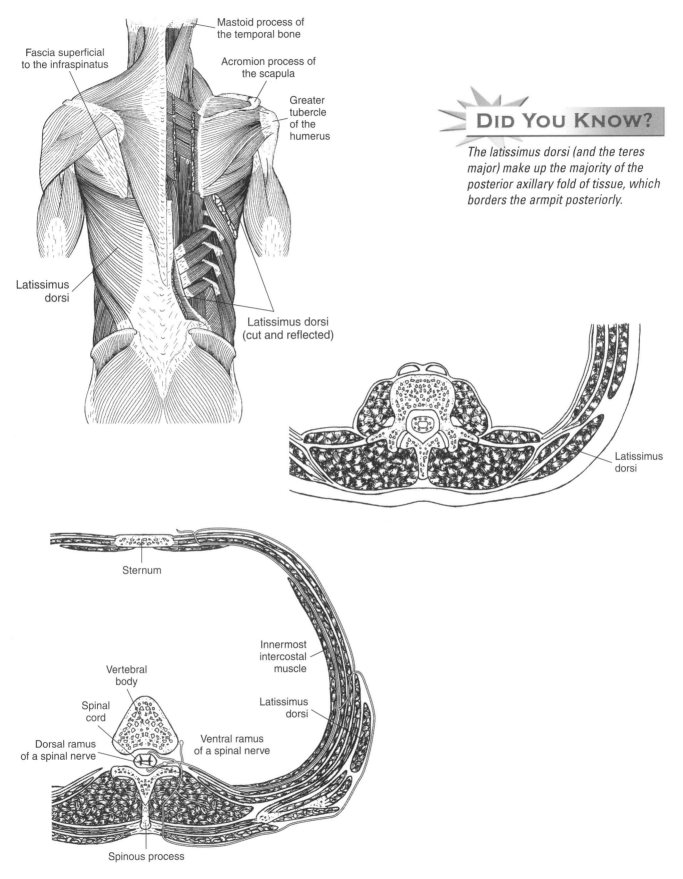

Mastoid process of the temporal bone

Fascia superficial to the infraspinatus

Acromion process of the scapula

Greater tubercle of the humerus

Latissimus dorsi

Latissimus dorsi (cut and reflected)

DID YOU KNOW?

The latissimus dorsi (and the teres major) make up the majority of the posterior axillary fold of tissue, which borders the armpit posteriorly.

Latissimus dorsi

Sternum

Innermost intercostal muscle

Vertebral body

Spinal cord

Latissimus dorsi

Dorsal ramus of a spinal nerve

Ventral ramus of a spinal nerve

Spinous process

Muscles of the Trunk

RHOMBOIDS MAJOR AND MINOR

rom-boyd **may**-jor, **my**-nor

Actions
Retraction (adduction) of the scapula at the scapulocostal joint
Elevation of the scapula at the scapulocostal joint
Downward rotation of the scapula at the scapulocostal joint
Contralateral rotation of the trunk at the spinal joints

Innervation
The dorsal scapular nerve

Arterial Supply
The dorsal scapular artery

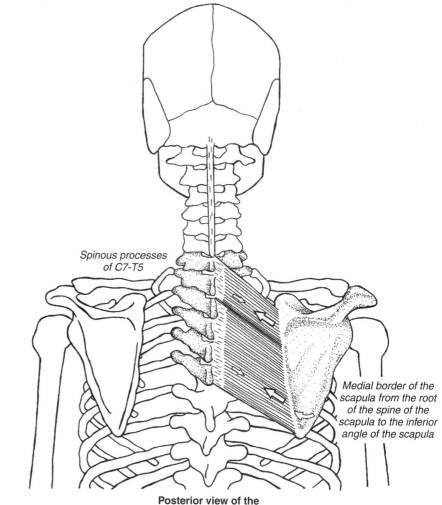

Spinous processes of C7-T5

Medial border of the scapula from the root of the spine of the scapula to the inferior angle of the scapula

Posterior view of the right rhomboids major and minor

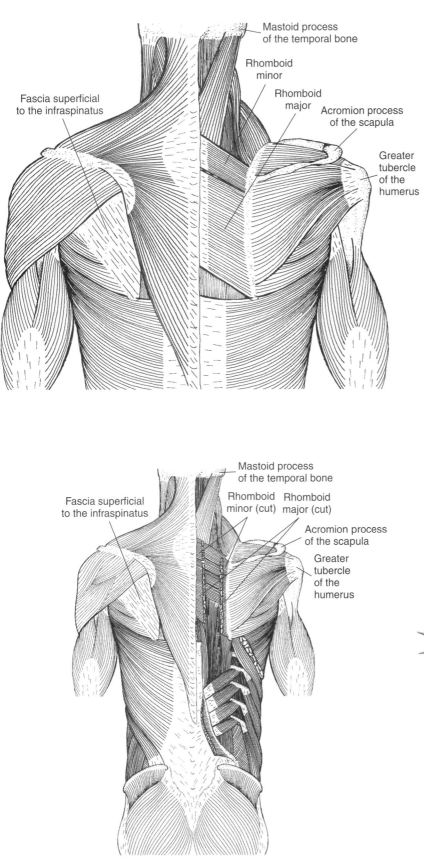

Mastoid process
of the temporal bone

Rhomboid
minor

Rhomboid
major

Acromion process
of the scapula

Greater
tubercle
of the
humerus

Fascia superficial
to the infraspinatus

Mastoid process
of the temporal bone

Rhomboid   Rhomboid
minor (cut)   major (cut)

Acromion process
of the scapula

Greater
tubercle
of the
humerus

Fascia superficial
to the infraspinatus

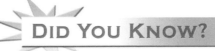

DID YOU KNOW?

The rhomboids are sometimes known as the 'Christmas tree' muscles. When you look at them bilaterally with the spine between them, they look like a Christmas tree.

Muscles of the Trunk

SERRATUS ANTERIOR

ser-**a**-tus an-**tee**-ri-or

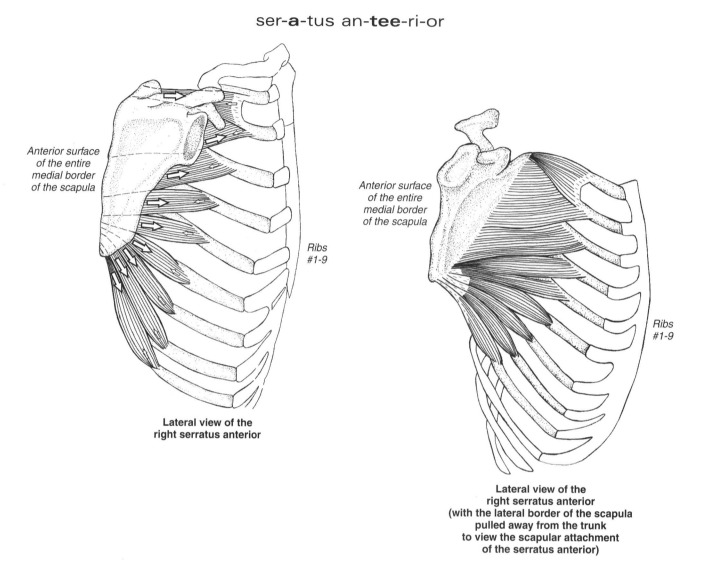

Anterior surface of the entire medial border of the scapula

Ribs #1-9

Lateral view of the right serratus anterior

Anterior surface of the entire medial border of the scapula

Ribs #1-9

Lateral view of the right serratus anterior (with the lateral border of the scapula pulled away from the trunk to view the scapular attachment of the serratus anterior)

Actions	**Innervation**	**Arterial Supply**
Protraction (abduction) of the scapula at the scapulocostal joint Upward rotation of the scapula at the scapulocostal joint Elevation of the scapula at the scapulocostal joint Depression of the scapula at the scapulocostal joint	The long thoracic nerve	The dorsal scapular artery and the lateral thoracic artery

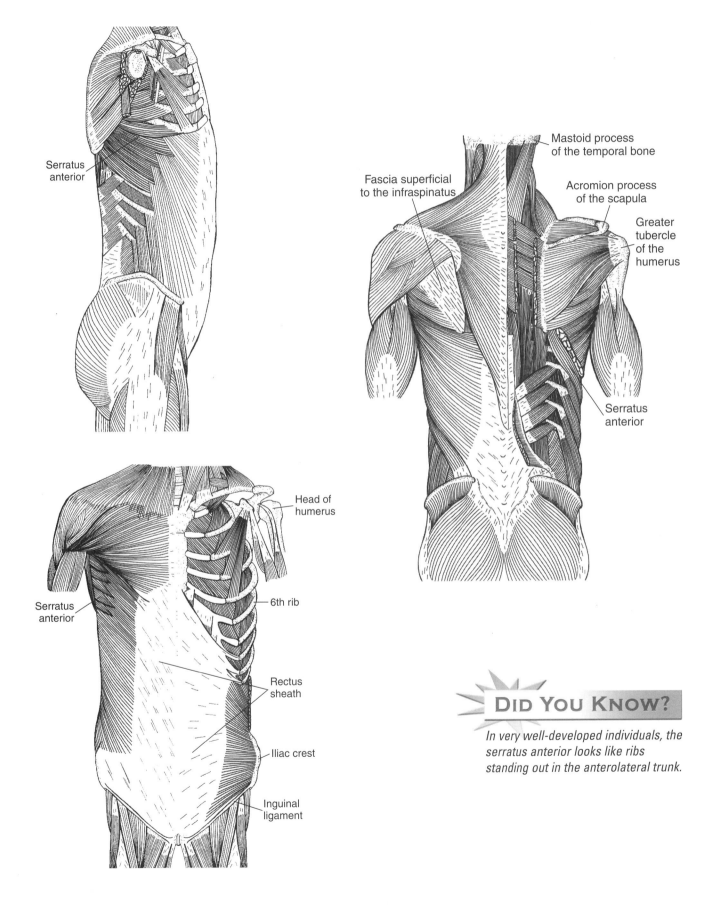

Serratus
anterior

Mastoid process
of the temporal bone

Fascia superficial
to the infraspinatus

Acromion process
of the scapula

Greater
tubercle
of the
humerus

Serratus
anterior

Head of
humerus

Serratus
anterior

6th rib

Rectus
sheath

Iliac crest

Inguinal
ligament

DID YOU KNOW?

In very well-developed individuals, the serratus anterior looks like ribs standing out in the anterolateral trunk.

Muscles of the Trunk

SERRATUS POSTERIOR SUPERIOR

ser-**a**-tus pos-**tee**-ri-or
sue-**pee**-ri-or

Action
Elevation of ribs #2-5 at the sternocostal and costovertebral joints

Innervation
Intercostal nerves

Arterial Supply
The dorsal branches of the posterior intercostal arteries

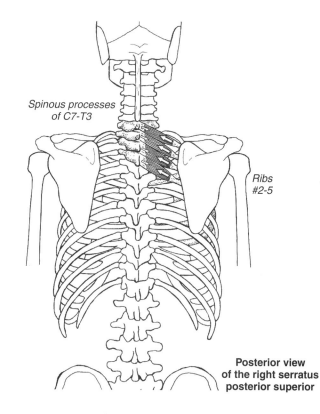

Spinous processes of C7-T3

Ribs #2-5

Posterior view of the right serratus posterior superior

SERRATUS POSTERIOR INFERIOR

ser-**a**-tus pos-**tee**-ri-or
in-**fee**-ri-or

Actions
Depression of ribs #9-12 at the sternocostal and costovertebral joints

Innervation
Subcostal nerve and intercostal nerves

Arterial Supply
The dorsal branches of the posterior intercostal arteries

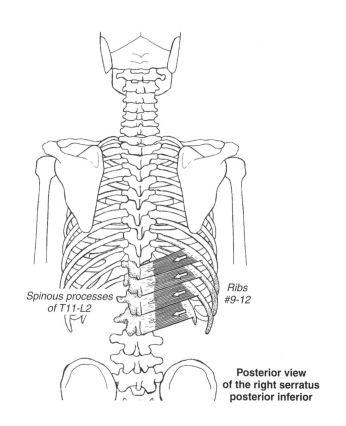

Spinous processes of T11-L2

Ribs #9-12

Posterior view of the right serratus posterior inferior

Muscles of the Trunk

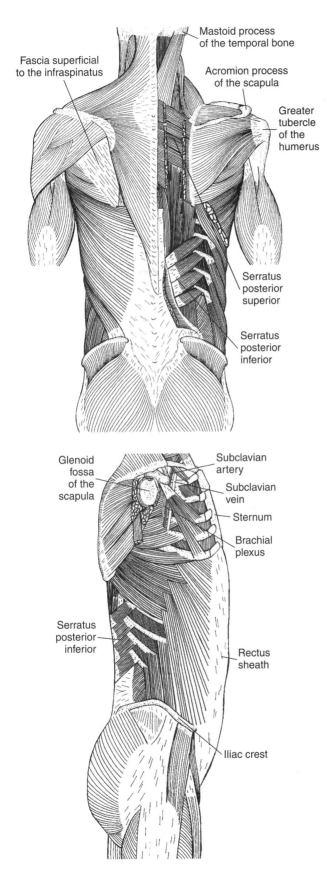

Mastoid process
of the temporal bone

Fascia superficial
to the infraspinatus

Acromion process
of the scapula

Greater
tubercle
of the
humerus

Serratus
posterior
superior

Serratus
posterior
inferior

Glenoid
fossa
of the
scapula

Subclavian
artery

Subclavian
vein

Sternum

Brachial
plexus

Serratus
posterior
inferior

Rectus
sheath

Iliac crest

DID YOU KNOW?

By their action of moving the ribs, the serratus posterior superior and inferior muscles are primarily important as muscles of respiration.

Muscles of the Trunk

THE ERECTOR SPINAE GROUP

ee-**rek**-tor **spee**-nee

Actions

Extension of the trunk and the neck and the head at the spinal joints

Lateral flexion of the trunk and the neck and the head at the spinal joints

Ipsilateral rotation of the trunk and the neck and the head at the spinal joints

Anterior tilt of the pelvis at the lumbosacral joint

Elevation of the pelvis at the lumbosacral joint

Contralateral rotation of the pelvis at the lumbosacral joint

Innervation

Spinal nerves

Arterial Supply

The dorsal branches of the posterior inter-costal and lumbar arteries

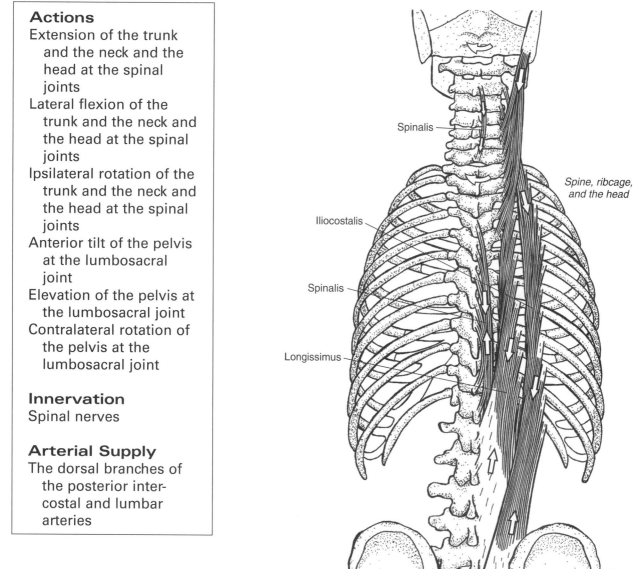

Spinalis

Iliocostalis

Spinalis

Longissimus

Spine, ribcage, and the head

Pelvis

Posterior view of the right erector spinae group

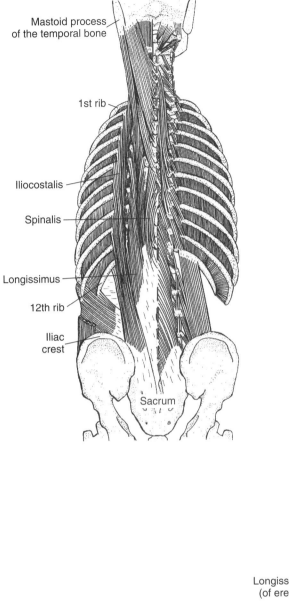

Mastoid process
of the temporal bone

1st rib

Iliocostalis

Spinalis

Longissimus

12th rib

Iliac
crest

Sacrum

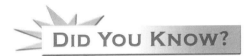

DID YOU KNOW?

The erector spinae group, as its name implies, makes the spine erect, i.e., it does extension of the spine.

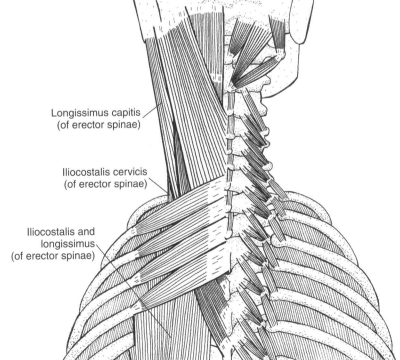

Longissimus capitis
(of erector spinae)

Iliocostalis cervicis
(of erector spinae)

Iliocostalis and
longissimus
(of erector spinae)

Muscles of the Trunk

Actions

Extension of the trunk and the neck at the spinal joints

Lateral flexion of the trunk and the neck at the spinal joints

Ipsilateral rotation of the trunk and the neck at the spinal joints

Anterior tilt of the pelvis at the lumbosacral joint

Elevation of the pelvis at the lumbosacral joint

Contralateral rotation of the pelvis at the lumbosacral joint

Innervation

Spinal nerves

Arterial Supply

The dorsal branches of the posterior intercostal and lumbar arteries

ILIOCOSTALIS
(OF THE ERECTOR SPINAE GROUP)

il-ee-o-kos-**ta**-lis

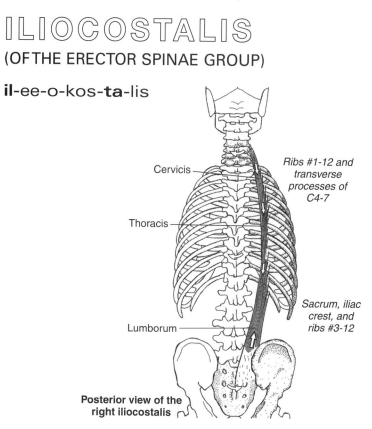

Cervicis

Thoracis

Lumborum

Ribs #1-12 and transverse processes of C4-7

Sacrum, iliac crest, and ribs #3-12

Posterior view of the right iliocostalis

Actions

Extension of the trunk and the neck and the head at the spinal joints

Lateral flexion of the trunk and the neck and the head at the spinal joints

Ipsilateral rotation of the trunk and the neck and the head at the spinal joints

Anterior tilt of the pelvis at the lumbosacral joint

Elevation of the pelvis at the lumbosacral joint

Contralateral rotation of the pelvis at the lumbosacral joint

Innervation

Spinal nerves

Arterial Supply

The dorsal branches of the posterior intercostal and lumbar arteries

LONGISSIMUS
(OF THE ERECTOR SPINAE GROUP)

lon-**jis**-i-mus

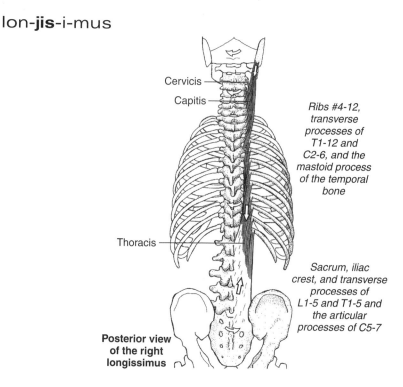

Cervicis

Capitis

Thoracis

Ribs #4-12, transverse processes of T1-12 and C2-6, and the mastoid process of the temporal bone

Sacrum, iliac crest, and transverse processes of L1-5 and T1-5 and the articular processes of C5-7

Posterior view of the right longissimus

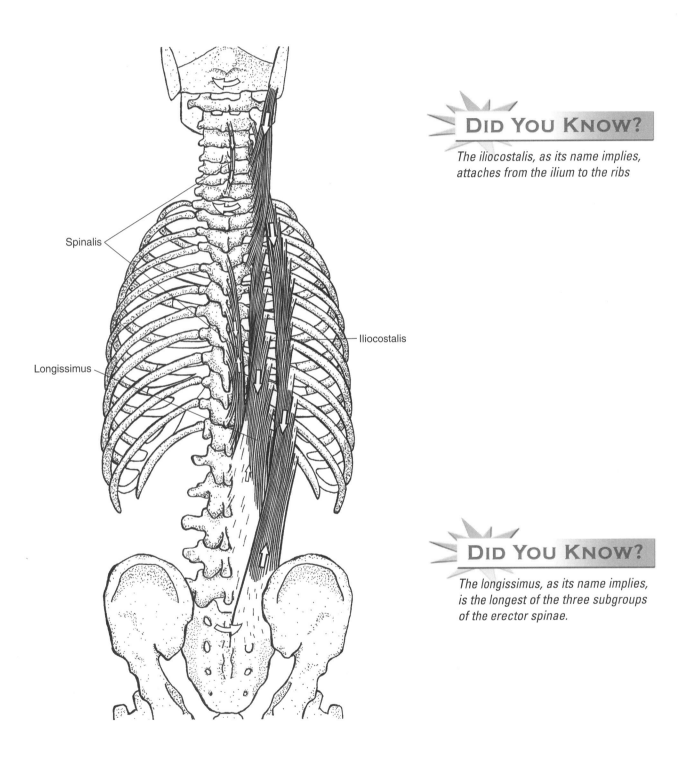

Spinalis

Longissimus

Iliocostalis

Muscles of the Trunk

SPINALIS
(OF THE ERECTOR SPINAE GROUP)

spy-**na**-lis

Actions
Extension of the trunk and the neck and the head at the spinal joints

Lateral flexion of the trunk and the neck and the head at the spinal joints

Ipsilateral rotation of the trunk and the neck and the head at the spinal joints

Innervation
Spinal nerves

Arterial Supply
The dorsal branches of the posterior intercostal and lumbar arteries

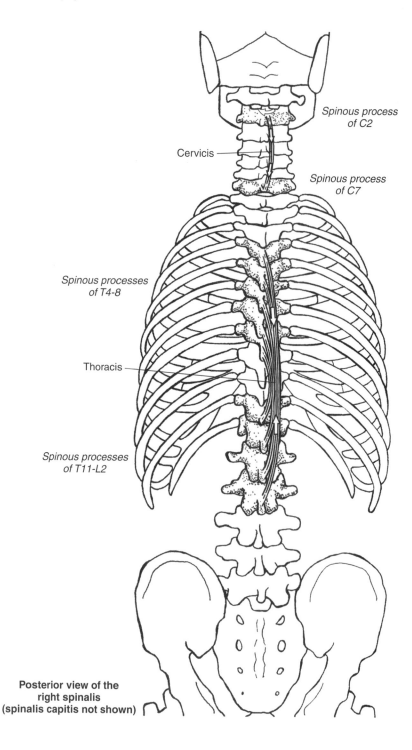

Spinous process of C2

Cervicis

Spinous process of C7

Spinous processes of T4-8

Thoracis

Spinous processes of T11-L2

Posterior view of the right spinalis (spinalis capitis not shown)

Muscles of the Trunk

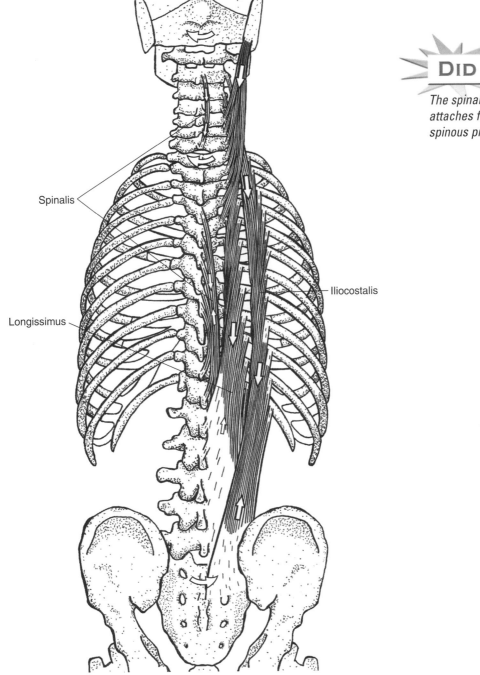

Spinalis

Longissimus

Iliocostalis

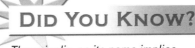

DID YOU KNOW?

The spinalis, as its name implies, attaches from spinous processes to spinous processes.

Muscles of the Trunk

THE TRANSVERSOSPINALIS GROUP

trans-**ver**-so-spy-**na**-lis

Actions
Extension of the trunk
and the neck and the
head at the spinal
joints
Lateral flexion of the
trunk and the neck and
the head at the spinal
joints
Contralateral rotation of
the trunk and the neck
at the spinal joints
Anterior tilt of the pelvis
at the lumbosacral
joint
Elevation of the pelvis at
the lumbosacral joint
Ipsilateral rotation
of the pelvis at the
lumbosacral joint

Innervation
Spinal nerves

Arterial Supply
The occipital artery and
the dorsal branches of
the posterior inter-
costal and lumbar
arteries

Semispinalis

Rotatores

Spine and
the head

Multifidus

Pelvis

**Posterior view of the
transversospinalis group
(semispinalis and multifidus on the right)
(rotatores on the left)**

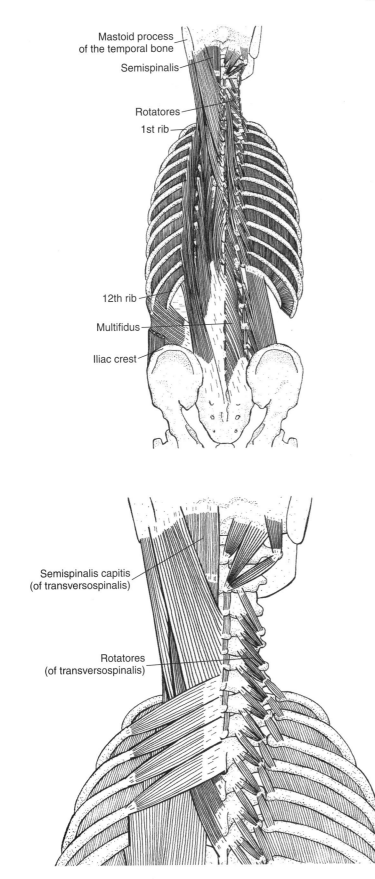

Mastoid process
of the temporal bone

Semispinalis

Rotatores

1st rib

12th rib

Multifidus

Iliac crest

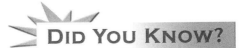

DID YOU KNOW?

The transversospinalis group, as its name implies, attaches from transverse processes to spinous processes.

Semispinalis capitis
(of transversospinalis)

Rotatores
(of transversospinalis)

Muscles of the Trunk

Actions

Extension of the trunk
and the neck and the
head at the spinal
joints

Lateral flexion of the
trunk and the neck and
the head at the spinal
joints

Contralateral rotation of
the trunk and the neck
at the spinal joints

Innervation

Spinal nerves

Arterial Supply

The occipital artery and
the dorsal branches
of the posterior
intercostal arteries

SEMISPINALIS

(OF THE TRANSVERSOSPINALIS GROUP)

sem-ee-spy-**na**-lis

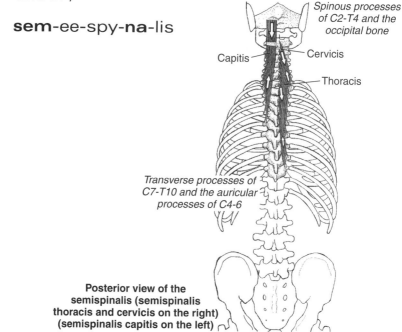

Spinous processes
of C2-T4 and the
occipital bone

Capitis   Cervicis

Thoracis

Transverse processes of
C7-T10 and the auricular
processes of C4-6

**Posterior view of the
semispinalis (semispinalis
thoracis and cervicis on the right)
(semispinalis capitis on the left)**

Actions

Extension of the trunk
and the neck at the
spinal joints

Lateral flexion of the
trunk and the neck at
the spinal joints

Contralateral rotation of
the trunk and the neck
at the spinal joints

Anterior tilt of the pelvis
at the lumbosacral joint

Elevation of the pelvis at
the lumbosacral joint

Ipsilateral rotation of the
pelvis at the lumbo-
sacral joint

Innervation

Spinal nerves

Arterial Supply

The dorsal branches
of the posterior
intercostal and
lumbar arteries

MULTIFIDUS

(OF THE TRANSVERSOSPINALIS GROUP)

mul-**tif**-id-us

Spinous processes
of vertebrae 2-4
segmental levels
superior to the
inferior attachment

Posterior sacrum,
posterior superior
iliac spine (PSIS),
posterior sacro-iliac
ligament and L5-C4
vertebrae

**Posterior view of the
right multifidus**

Muscles of the Trunk

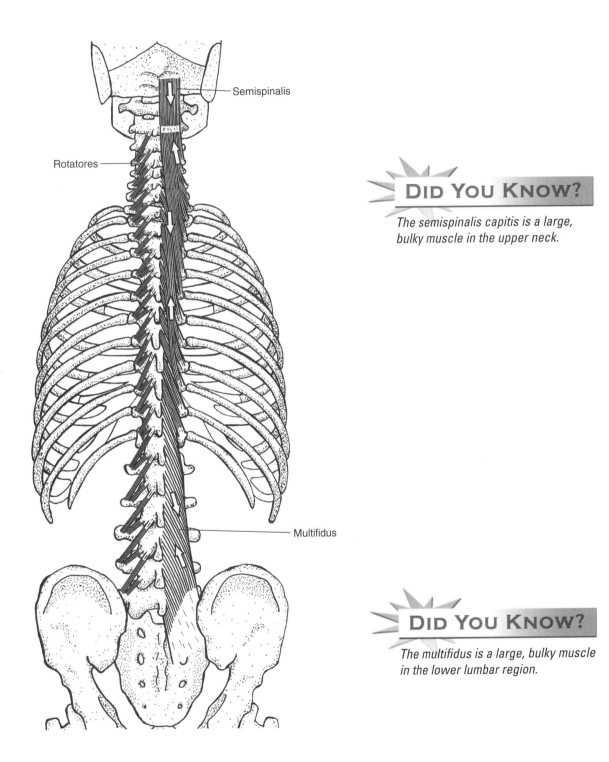

Semispinalis

Rotatores

Multifidus

DID YOU KNOW?

The semispinalis capitis is a large, bulky muscle in the upper neck.

DID YOU KNOW?

The multifidus is a large, bulky muscle in the lower lumbar region.

Muscles of the Trunk

ROTATORES
(OF THE TRANSVERSOSPINALIS GROUP)

ro-ta-**to**-reez

Actions
Contralateral rotation of
the trunk and the neck
at the spinal joints
Extension of the trunk
and the neck at the
spinal joints

Innervation
Spinal nerves

Arterial Supply
The dorsal branches of
the posterior inter-
costal and lumbar
arteries

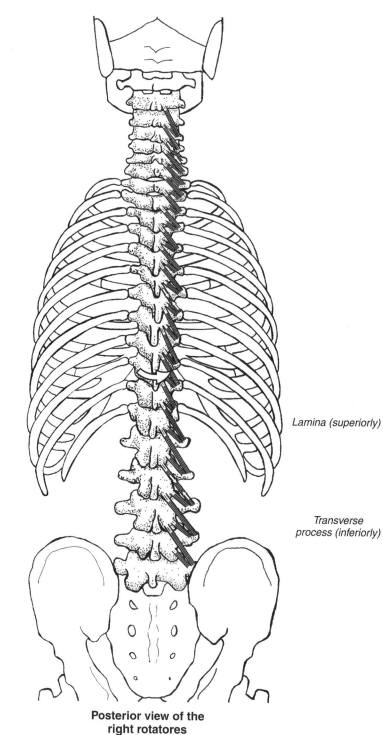

Lamina (superiorly)

*Transverse
process (inferiorly)*

**Posterior view of the
right rotatores**

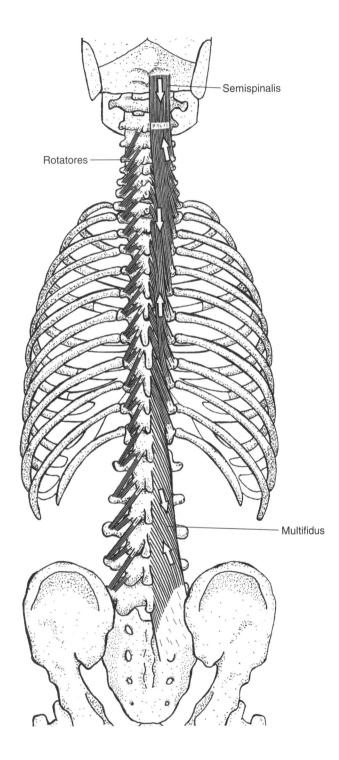

Semispinalis

Rotatores

Multifidus

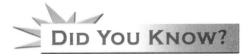

DID YOU KNOW?

The rotatores, as their name implies, are best at rotation (contralaterally) of the spine.

Muscles of the Trunk

QUADRATUS LUMBORUM

kwod-**ray**-tus lum-**bor**-um

Actions
Elevation of the pelvis at
the lumbosacral joint
Anterior tilt of the pelvis
at the lumbosacral joint
Lateral flexion of the
trunk at the spinal
joints
Extension of the trunk at
the spinal joints
Depression of the 12th
rib at the costoverte-
bral joints

Innervation
Lumbar plexus

Arterial Supply
Branches of the subcostal
and lumbar arteries

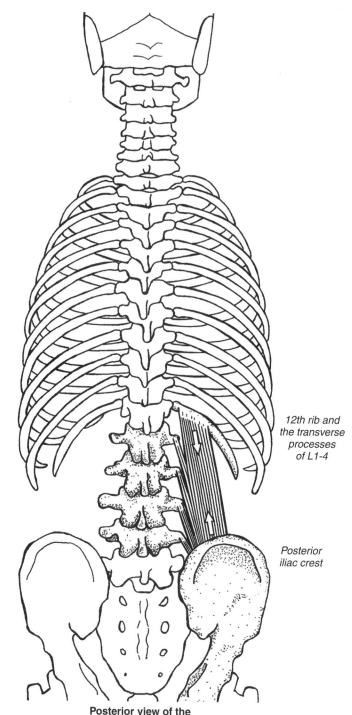

*12th rib and
the transverse
processes
of L1-4*

*Posterior
iliac crest*

**Posterior view of the
right quadratus lumborum**

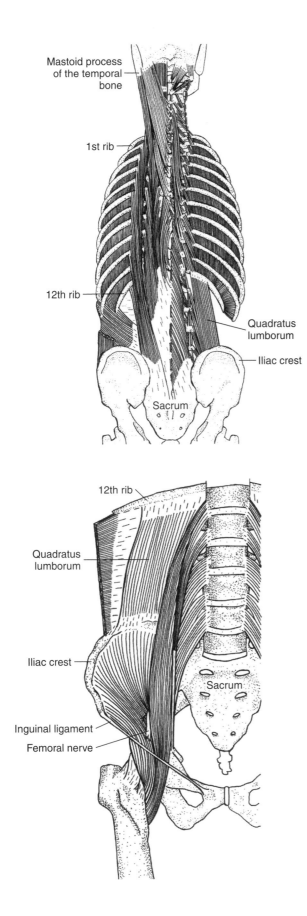

Mastoid process of the temporal bone

1st rib

12th rib

Quadratus lumborum

Iliac crest

Sacrum

12th rib

Quadratus lumborum

Iliac crest

Inguinal ligament

Femoral nerve

Sacrum

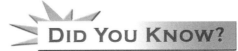

DID YOU KNOW?

When palpating the quadratus lumborum, it must be accessed from the side.

Muscles of the Trunk

INTERSPINALES

in-ter-spy-**na**-leez

Action
Extension of the neck and the trunk at the spinal joints

Innervation
Spinal nerves

Arterial Supply
The dorsal branches of the posterior intercostal arteries

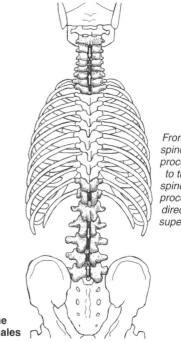

From a spinous process to the spinous process directly superior

Posterior view of the right and left interspinales

INTERTRANSVERSARII

in-ter-trans-ver-**sa**-ri-eye

Action
Lateral flexion of the neck and the trunk at the spinal joints

Innervation
Spinal nerves

Arterial Supply
The dorsal branches of the posterior inter-costal arteries

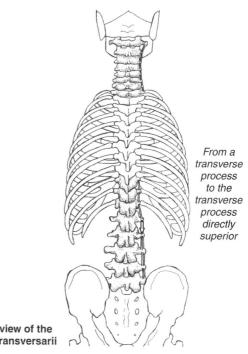

From a transverse process to the transverse process directly superior

Posterior view of the right intertransversarii

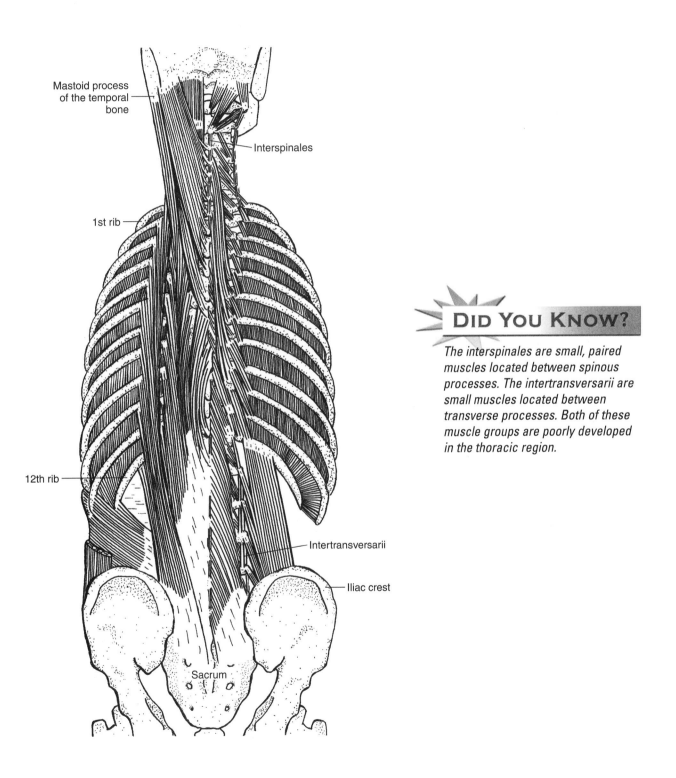

Mastoid process
of the temporal
bone

Interspinales

1st rib

12th rib

Intertransversarii

Iliac crest

Sacrum

DID YOU KNOW?

The interspinales are small, paired muscles located between spinous processes. The intertransversarii are small muscles located between transverse processes. Both of these muscle groups are poorly developed in the thoracic region.

Muscles of the Trunk

Actions
Elevation of the ribs at the sternocostal and costovertebral joints

Extension of the trunk at the spinal joints

Lateral flexion of the trunk at the spinal joints

Contralateral rotation of the trunk at the spinal joints

Innervation
Spinal nerves

Arterial Supply
The dorsal branches of the posterior intercostal arteries

LEVATORES COSTARUM

le-va-**to**-rez (singular: le-**vay**-tor) kos-**tar**-um

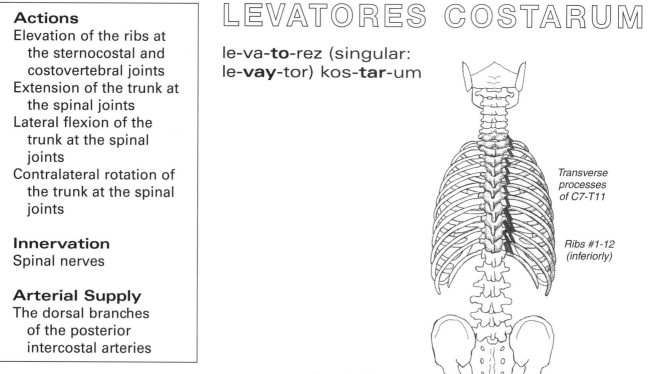

Transverse processes of C7-T11

Ribs #1-12 (inferiorly)

Posterior view of the right levatores costarum

SUBCOSTALES

sub-kos-**tal**-eez

Action
Depression of ribs #8-10 at the sternocostal and costovertebral joints

Innervation
Intercostal nerves

Arterial Supply
The dorsal branches of the posterior inter-costal arteries

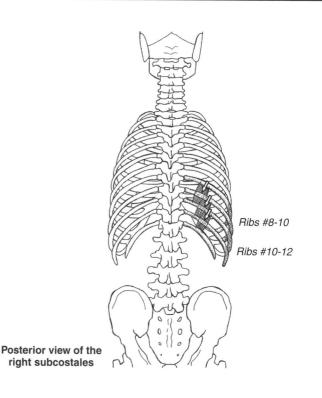

Ribs #8-10

Ribs #10-12

Posterior view of the right subcostales

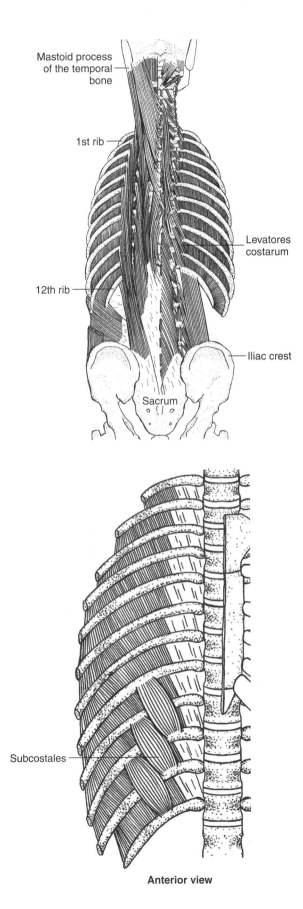

Mastoid process
of the temporal
bone

1st rib

Levatores
costarum

12th rib

Iliac crest

Sacrum

Subcostales

Anterior view

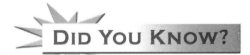

DID YOU KNOW?

As their name implies, the levatores costarum elevate the ribs.

DID YOU KNOW?

There are usually three subcostales muscles and they are located deep to the ribcage.

Muscles of the Trunk

PECTORALIS MAJOR

pek-to-ra-lis **may**-jor

Actions
Adduction of the arm at
the shoulder joint
Medial rotation of the
arm at the shoulder
joint
Flexion of the arm at the
shoulder joint
(clavicular head)
Extension of the arm at
the shoulder joint
(sternocostal head)
Abduction of the arm at
the shoulder joint
(clavicular head,
above 90°)
Depression of the scapula
at the scapulocostal
joint
Elevation of the trunk at
the scapulocostal joint
Lateral deviation of
the trunk at the
scapulocostal joint
Ipsilateral rotation of
the trunk at the
scapulocostal joint

Innervation
The medial and lateral
pectoral nerves

Arterial Supply
The pectoral branches of
the thoracoacromial
trunk

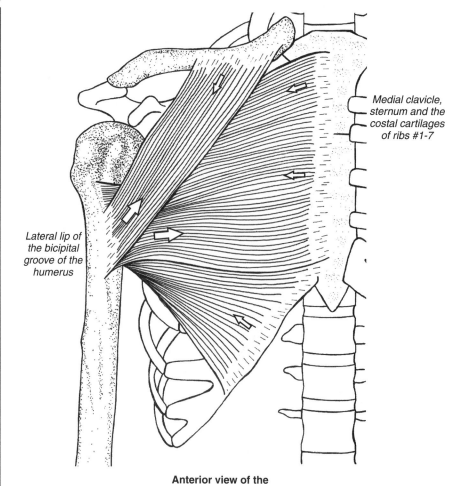

Medial clavicle, sternum and the costal cartilages of ribs #1-7

Lateral lip of the bicipital groove of the humerus

**Anterior view of the
right pectoralis major**

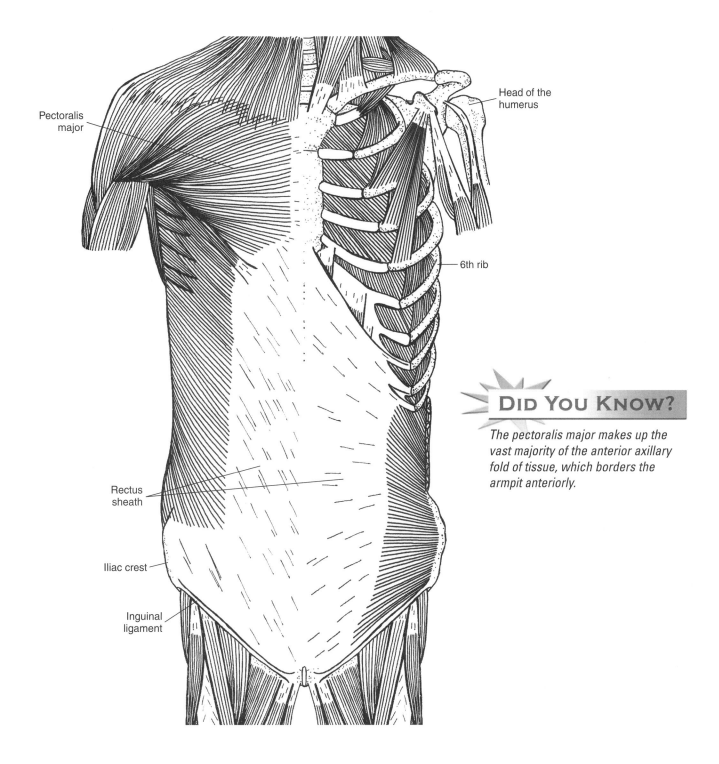

Pectoralis
major

Head of the
humerus

6th rib

Rectus
sheath

Iliac crest

Inguinal
ligament

DID YOU KNOW?

The pectoralis major makes up the
vast majority of the anterior axillary
fold of tissue, which borders the
armpit anteriorly.

Muscles of the Trunk

PECTORALIS MINOR

pek-to-**ra**-lis **my**-nor

Actions
Protraction (abduction) of the scapula at the scapulocostal joint
Depression of the scapula at the scapulocostal joint
Elevation of ribs #3-5 at the sternocostal and costovertebral joints
Downward rotation of the scapula at the scapulocostal joint

Innervation
The medial and lateral pectoral nerves

Arterial Supply
The pectoral branches of the thoracoacromial trunk

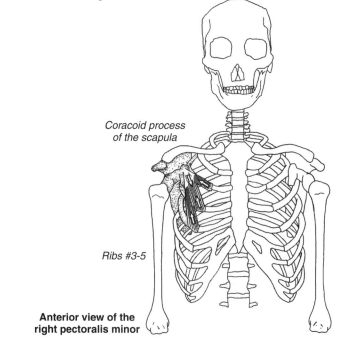

Coracoid process of the scapula

Ribs #3-5

Anterior view of the right pectoralis minor

SUBCLAVIUS

sub-**klay**-vee-us

Actions
Depression of the clavicle at the sternoclavicular joint
Elevation of the 1st rib at the sternocostal and costovertebral joints
Protraction of the clavicle at the sternoclavicular joint
Downward rotation of the clavicle at the sterno-clavicular joint

Innervation
A nerve from the brachial plexus

Arterial Supply
The clavicular branch of the thoracoacromial trunk and the supra-scapular artery

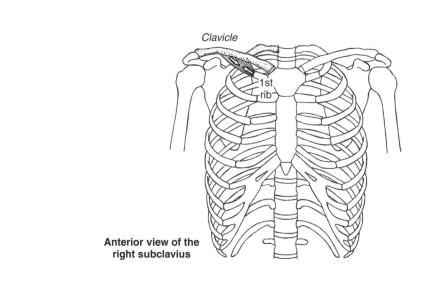

Clavicle

1st rib

Anterior view of the right subclavius

Muscles of the Trunk

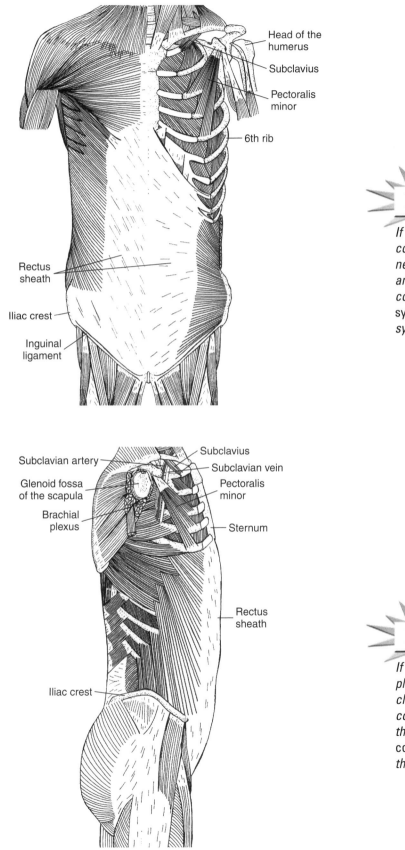

Head of the humerus

Subclavius

Pectoralis minor

6th rib

Rectus sheath

Iliac crest

Inguinal ligament

Subclavian artery

Glenoid fossa of the scapula

Brachial plexus

Iliac crest

Subclavius

Subclavian vein

Pectoralis minor

Sternum

Rectus sheath

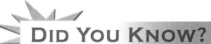

DID YOU KNOW?

If the pectoralis minor is tight, it may compress the brachial plexus of nerves and/or the subclavian artery and vein against the ribcage. This condition is called pectoralis minor syndrome, *a type of thoracic outlet syndrome.*

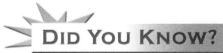

DID YOU KNOW?

If the subclavius is tight, the brachial plexus of nerves and/or the subclavian artery and vein can be compressed between the 1st rib and the clavicle; this condition is called costoclavicular syndrome, *a type of thoracic outlet syndrome.*

Muscles of the Trunk

EXTERNAL INTERCOSTALS

eks-turn-al in-ter-**kos**-tals

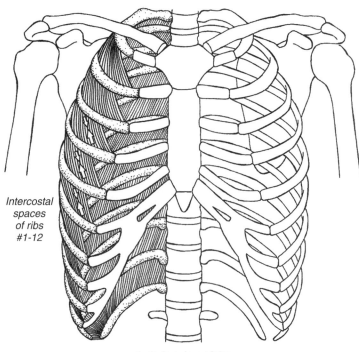

Intercostal spaces of ribs #1-12

**Anterior view of the
right external intercostals**

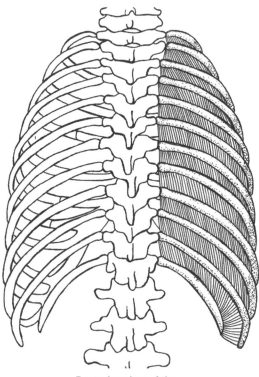

**Posterior view of the
right external intercostals**

Actions	**Innervation**	**Arterial Supply**
Elevation of ribs #2-12 at the sternocostal and costoclavicular joints Depression of ribs #1-11 at the sternocostal and costoclavicular joints	Intercostal nerves	Anterior intercostal arteries and the posterior inter-costal arteries

Muscles of the Trunk

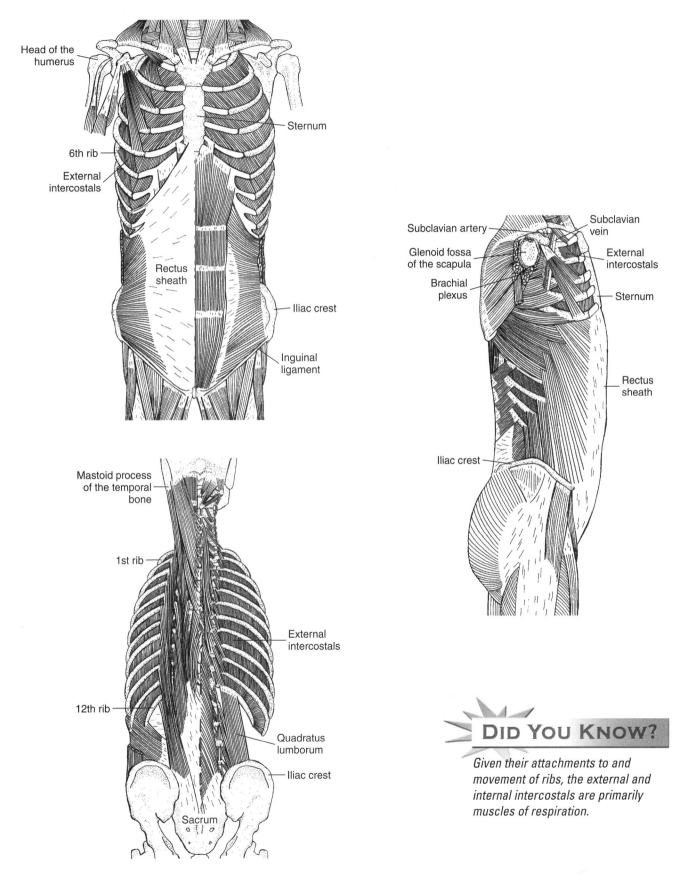

Head of the
humerus

Sternum

6th rib

External
intercostals

Rectus
sheath

Iliac crest

Inguinal
ligament

Subclavian artery
Subclavian
vein

Glenoid fossa
of the scapula

External
intercostals

Brachial
plexus

Sternum

Rectus
sheath

Iliac crest

Mastoid process
of the temporal
bone

1st rib

External
intercostals

12th rib

Quadratus
lumborum

Iliac crest

Sacrum

DID YOU KNOW?

Given their attachments to and movement of ribs, the external and internal intercostals are primarily muscles of respiration.

Muscles of the Trunk

INTERNAL INTERCOSTALS

in-turn-al in-ter-kos-tals

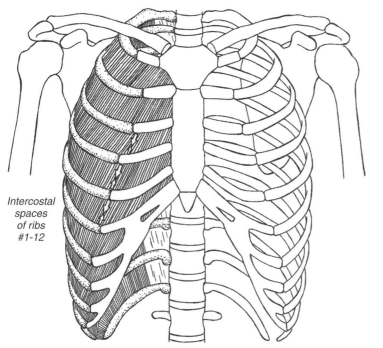

Intercostal spaces of ribs #1-12

Anterior view of the right internal intercostals

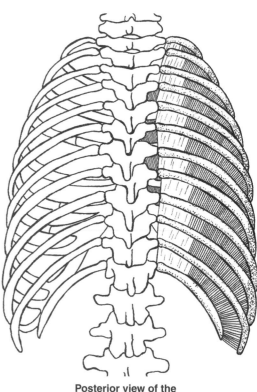

Posterior view of the right internal intercostals

Actions	Innervation	Arterial Supply
Depression of ribs #1-11 at the sternocostal and costoclavicular joints Elevation of ribs #2-12 at the sternocostal and costoclavicular joints	Intercostal nerves	Anterior intercostal arteries and the posterior intercostal arteries

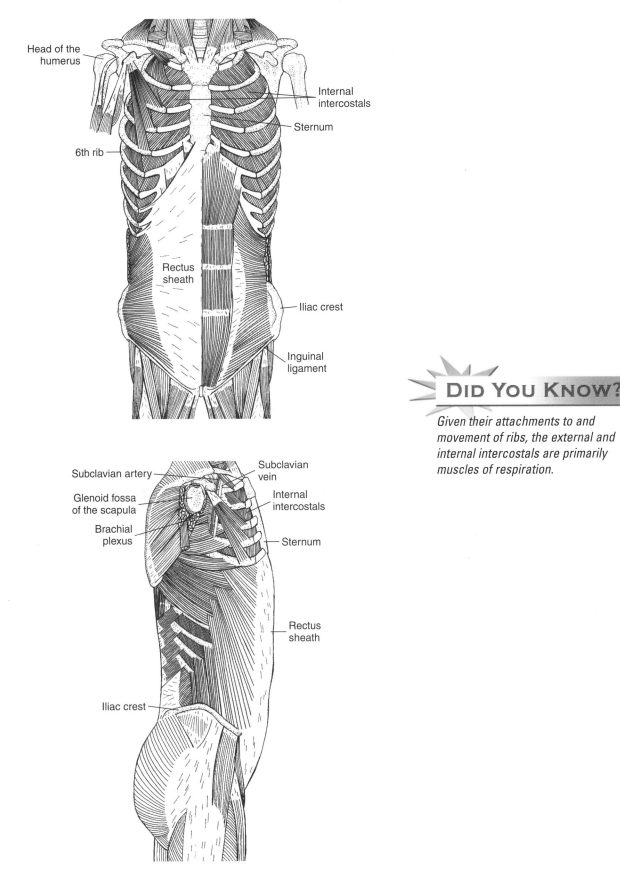

Head of the
humerus

Internal
intercostals

Sternum

6th rib

Rectus
sheath

Iliac crest

Inguinal
ligament

Subclavian artery

Subclavian
vein

Glenoid fossa
of the scapula

Internal
intercostals

Brachial
plexus

Sternum

Rectus
sheath

Iliac crest

DID YOU KNOW?

*Given their attachments to and
movement of ribs, the external and
internal intercostals are primarily
muscles of respiration.*

Muscles of the Trunk

RECTUS ABDOMINIS

rek-tus ab-**dom**-i-nis

Actions
Flexion of the trunk at the
spinal joints
Posterior tilt of the pelvis
at the lumbosacral joint
Lateral flexion of the
trunk at the spinal
joints
Compression of the
abdominal contents

Innervation
Intercostal nerves

Arterial Supply
The superior epigastric
artery and the inferior
epigastric artery

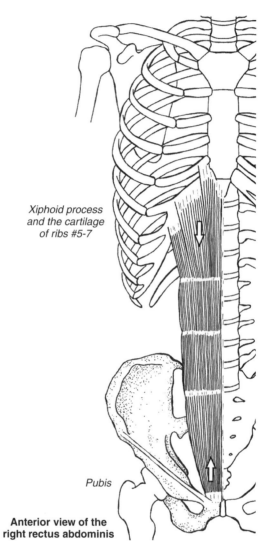

*Xiphoid process
and the cartilage
of ribs #5-7*

Pubis

**Anterior view of the
right rectus abdominis**

Muscles of the Trunk

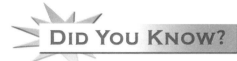

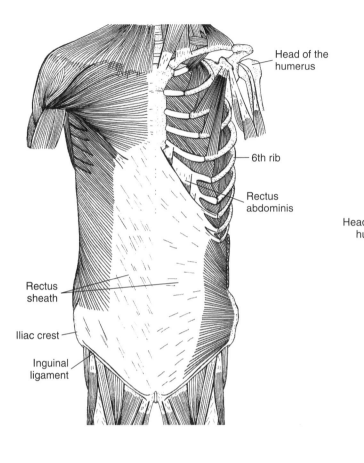

Head of the
humerus

6th rib

Rectus
abdominis

Rectus
sheath

Iliac crest

Inguinal
ligament

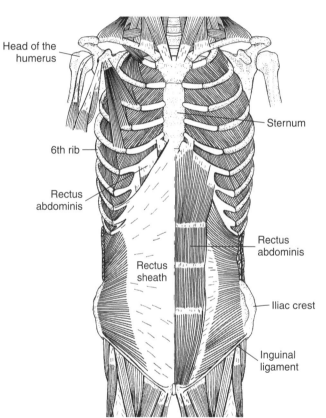

Head of the
humerus

Sternum

6th rib

Rectus
abdominis

Rectus
sheath

Rectus
abdominis

Iliac crest

Inguinal
ligament

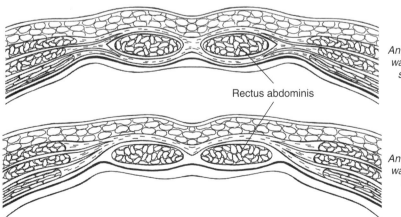

Rectus abdominis

*Anterior abdominal
wall cross section
superior to the
arcuate line*

*Anterior abdominal
wall cross section
inferior to the
arcuate line*

Muscles of the Trunk

Actions
Flexion of the trunk at the
  spinal joints
Lateral flexion of the trunk
  at the spinal joints
Contralateral rotation of the
  trunk at the spinal joints
Posterior tilt of the pelvis at
  the lumbosacral joint
Ipsilateral rotation of the
  pelvis at the lumbosacral
  joint
Compression of the
  abdominal contents

Innervation
Intercostal nerves

Arterial Supply
The subcostal and posterior
  intercostal arteries and
  the deep circumflex iliac
  artery

EXTERNAL ABDOMINAL OBLIQUE

eks-turn-al
ab-**dom**-in-al
o-**bleek**

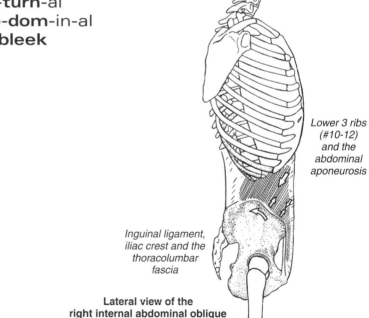

Lower 8 ribs
(ribs #5-12)

Anterior iliac
crest, pubic
bone, and the
abdominal
aponeurosis

**Lateral view of the
right external abdominal oblique**

Actions
Flexion of the trunk at the
  spinal joints
Lateral flexion of the trunk
  at the spinal joints
Ipsilateral rotation of the
  trunk at the spinal joints
Posterior tilt of the pelvis at
  the lumbosacral joint
Contralateral rotation of the
  pelvis at the lumbosacral
  joint
Compression of the
  abdominal contents

Innervation
Intercostal nerves

Arterial Supply
The subcostal and posterior
  intercostal arteries and
  the deep circumflex iliac
  artery

INTERNAL ABDOMINAL OBLIQUE

in-**turn**-al
ab-**dom**-in-al
o-**bleek**

Lower 3 ribs
(#10-12)
and the
abdominal
aponeurosis

Inguinal ligament,
iliac crest and the
thoracolumbar
fascia

**Lateral view of the
right internal abdominal oblique**

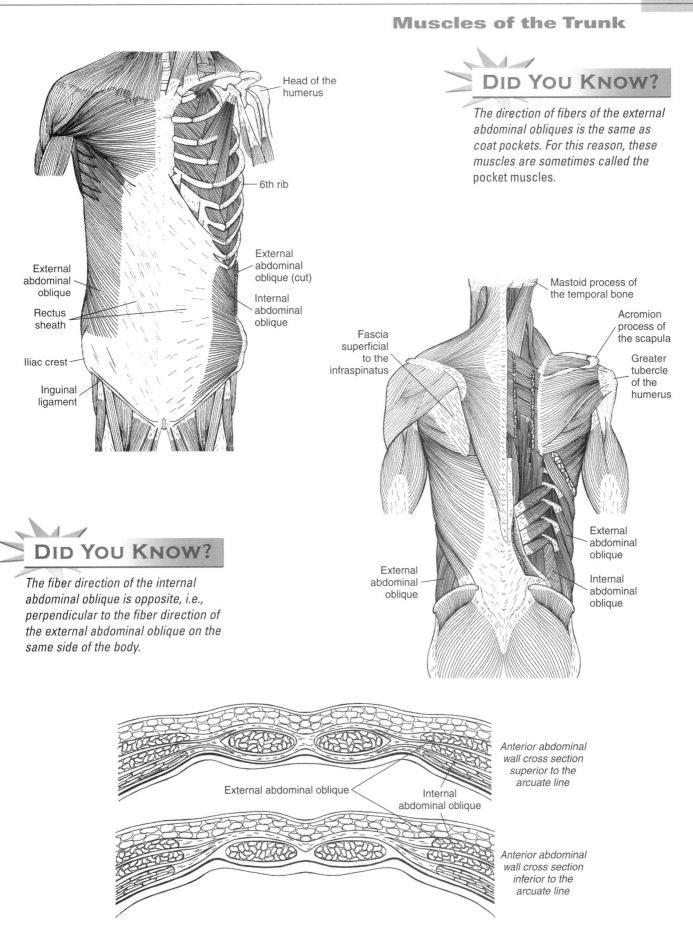

Head of the humerus

6th rib

External abdominal oblique (cut)

Internal abdominal oblique

External abdominal oblique

Rectus sheath

Iliac crest

Inguinal ligament

DID YOU KNOW?

The direction of fibers of the external abdominal obliques is the same as coat pockets. For this reason, these muscles are sometimes called the pocket muscles.

Mastoid process of the temporal bone

Acromion process of the scapula

Greater tubercle of the humerus

Fascia superficial to the infraspinatus

External abdominal oblique

Internal abdominal oblique

External abdominal oblique

DID YOU KNOW?

The fiber direction of the internal abdominal oblique is opposite, i.e., perpendicular to the fiber direction of the external abdominal oblique on the same side of the body.

External abdominal oblique

Internal abdominal oblique

Anterior abdominal wall cross section superior to the arcuate line

Anterior abdominal wall cross section inferior to the arcuate line

Muscles of the Trunk

TRANSVERSUS ABDOMINIS

trans-**ver**-sus ab-**dom**-i-nis

Action
Compression of the
  abdominal contents

Innervation
Intercostal nerves

Arterial Supply
The subcostal and
  posterior intercostal
  arteries and the deep
  circumflex iliac artery

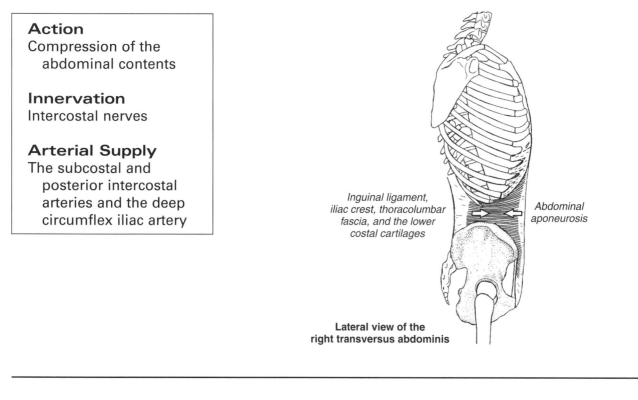

*Inguinal ligament,
iliac crest, thoracolumbar
fascia, and the lower
costal cartilages*

*Abdominal
aponeurosis*

**Lateral view of the
right transversus abdominis**

TRANSVERSUS THORACIS

trans-**ver**-sus thor-**as**-is

Action
Depression of ribs #2-6
  at the sternocostal and
  costovertebral joints

Innervation
Intercostal nerves

Arterial Supply
The anterior intercostal
  arteries

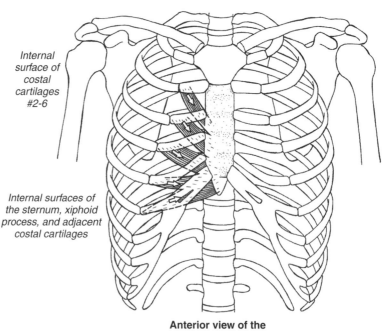

*Internal
surface of
costal
cartilages
#2-6*

*Internal surfaces of
the sternum, xiphoid
process, and adjacent
costal cartilages*

**Anterior view of the
right transversus thoracis**

Muscles of the Trunk

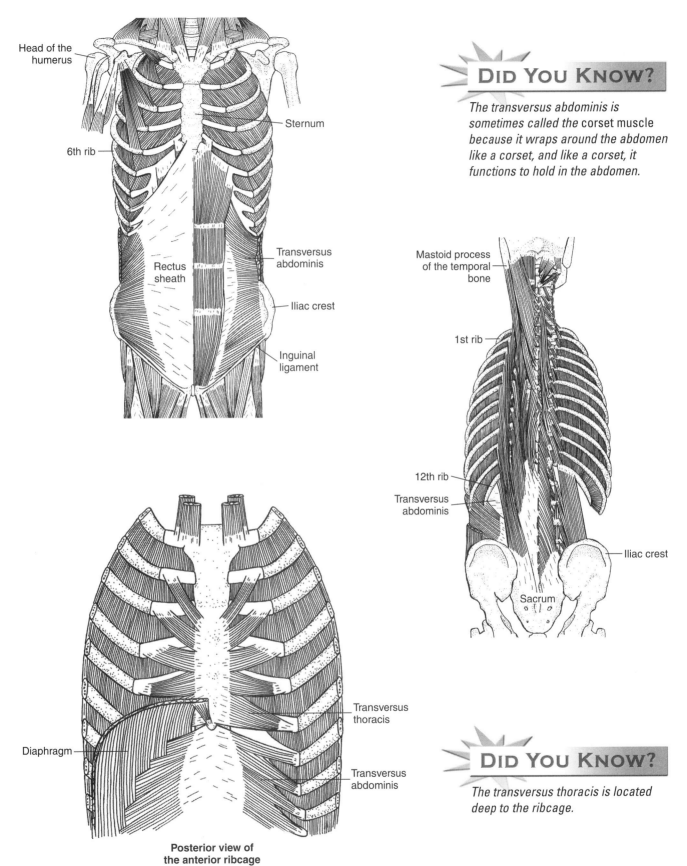

Head of the humerus

Sternum

6th rib

Rectus sheath

Transversus abdominis

Iliac crest

Inguinal ligament

DID YOU KNOW?

The transversus abdominis is sometimes called the corset muscle because it wraps around the abdomen like a corset, and like a corset, it functions to hold in the abdomen.

Mastoid process of the temporal bone

1st rib

12th rib

Transversus abdominis

Iliac crest

Sacrum

Transversus thoracis

Diaphragm

Transversus abdominis

Posterior view of the anterior ribcage

DID YOU KNOW?

The transversus thoracis is located deep to the ribcage.

Muscles of the Trunk

DIAPHRAGM

di-a-fram

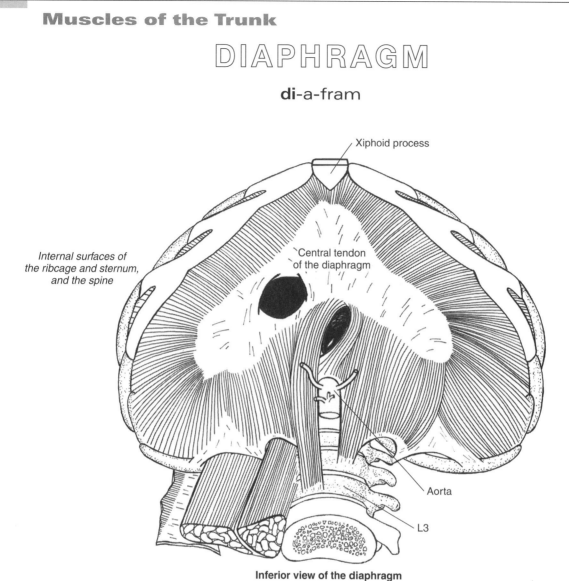

Xiphoid process

*Internal surfaces of
the ribcage and sternum,
and the spine*

Central tendon
of the diaphragm

Aorta

L3

Inferior view of the diaphragm

Action	**Innervation**	**Arterial Supply**
Increases the volume of the thoracic cavity	The phrenic nerve	Branches of the aorta and the internal thoracic artery

Muscles of the Trunk

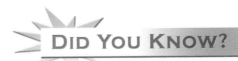

DID YOU KNOW?

The diaphragm is an unusual muscle in that it is under both conscious and unconscious control by the nervous system.

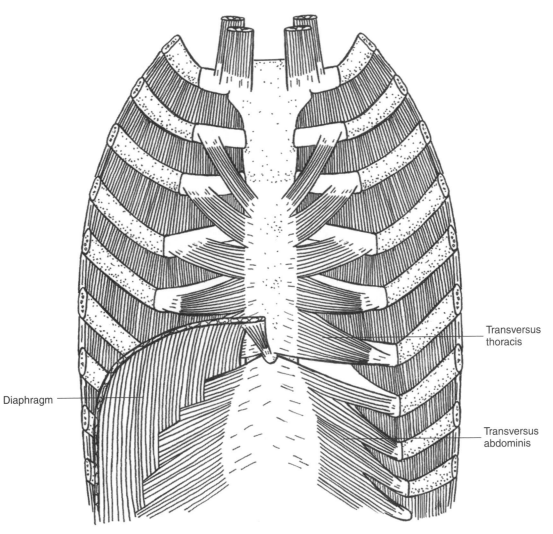

Transversus thoracis

Diaphragm

Transversus abdominis

Posterior view

Muscles of the Trunk

POSTERIOR VIEW OF THE TRUNK
(SUPERFICIAL AND INTERMEDIATE)

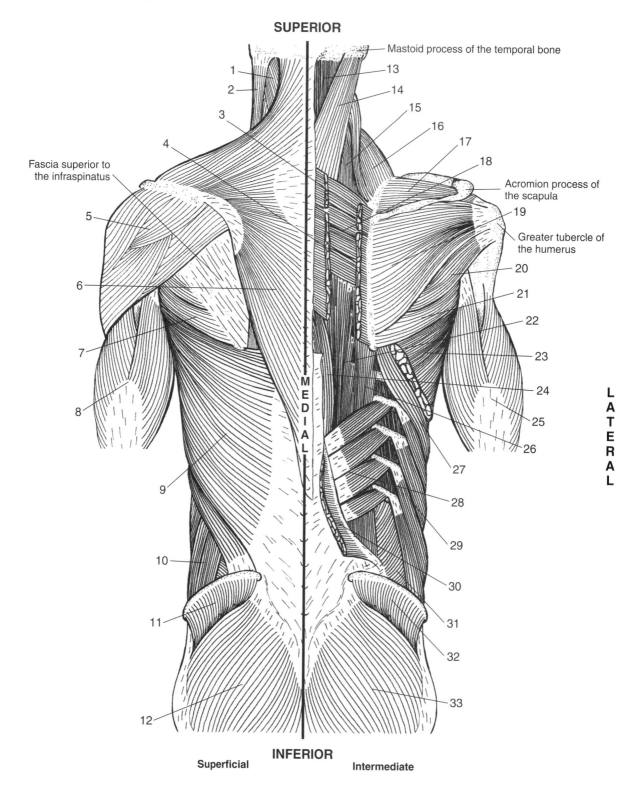

SUPERIOR

Mastoid process of the temporal bone

Fascia superior to
the infraspinatus

Acromion process of
the scapula

Greater tubercle of
the humerus

LATERAL

MEDIAL

LATERAL

INFERIOR

Superficial   Intermediate

POSTERIOR VIEW OF THE TRUNK (DEEP LAYERS)

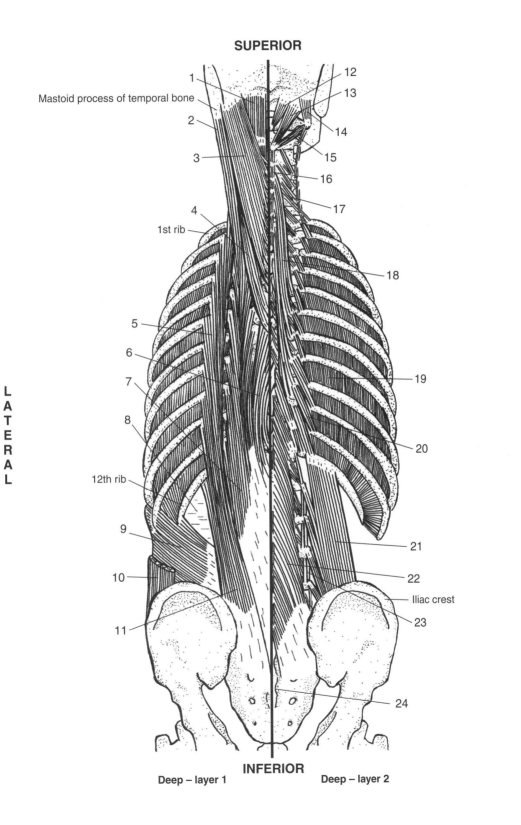

SUPERIOR

1

Mastoid process of temporal bone

2

3

4

1st rib

5

6

7

8

12th rib

9

10

11

12

13

14

15

16

17

18

19

20

21

22

Iliac crest

23

24

LATERAL

LATERAL

INFERIOR

Deep – layer 1   Deep – layer 2

Muscles of the Trunk

ANTERIOR VIEW OF THE TRUNK
(SUPERFICIAL AND INTERMEDIATE)

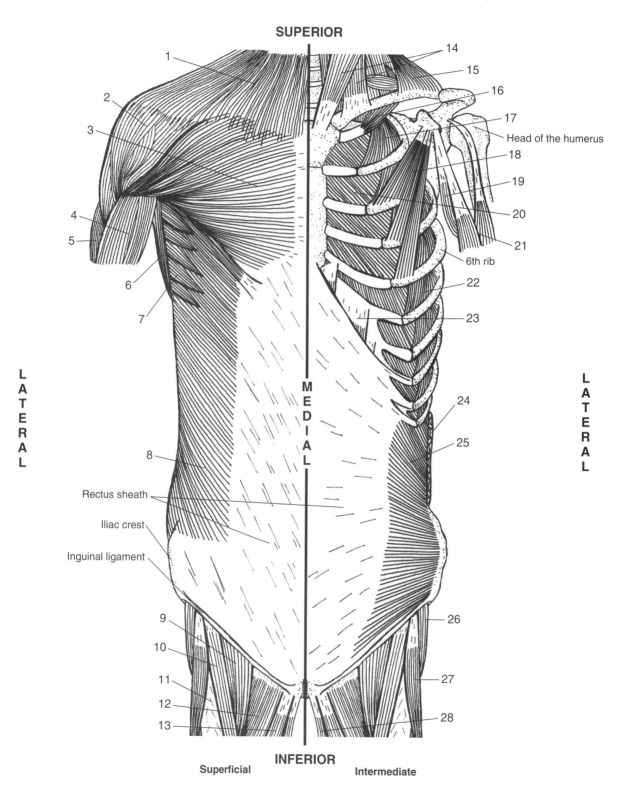

SUPERIOR

1

2

3

4

5

6

7

8

14

15

16

17

Head of the humerus

18

19

20

21

6th rib

22

23

24

25

Rectus sheath

Iliac crest

Inguinal ligament

9

10

11

12

13

26

27

28

LATERAL

MEDIAL

LATERAL

INFERIOR

Superficial

Intermediate

ANTERIOR VIEW OF THE TRUNK
(INTERMEDIATE AND DEEP)

SUPERIOR

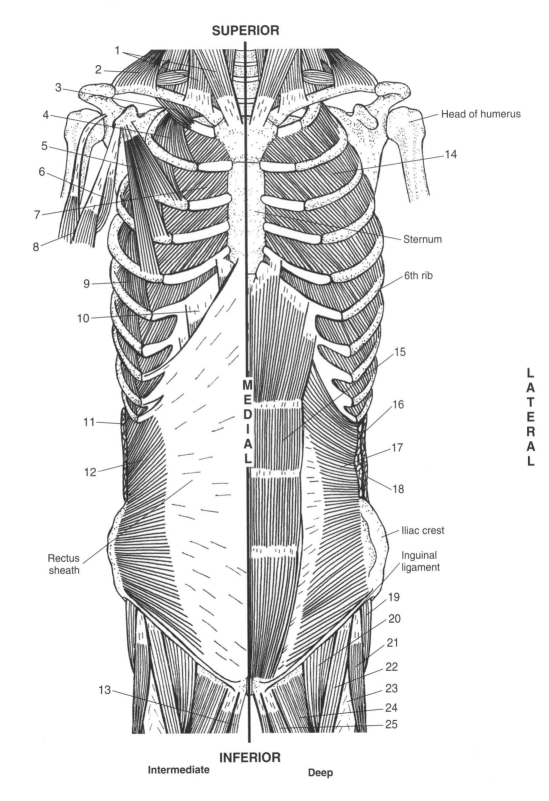

Head of humerus

14

Sternum

6th rib

LATERAL

MEDIAL

LATERAL

15

16

17

18

Iliac crest

Inguinal
ligament

Rectus
sheath

19
20
21
22
23
24
25

13

INFERIOR

Intermediate   Deep

Muscles of the Trunk

LATERAL VIEW OF THE TRUNK

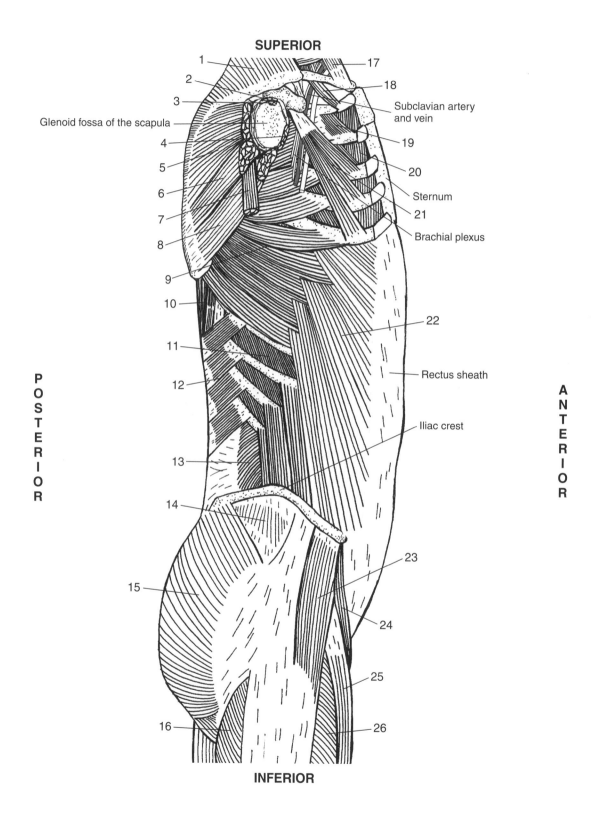

SUPERIOR

1

2

3

Glenoid fossa of the scapula

4

5

6

7

8

9

10

11

12

13

14

15

16

17

18

Subclavian artery
and vein

19

20

Sternum

21

Brachial plexus

22

Rectus sheath

Iliac crest

23

24

25

26

POSTERIOR

ANTERIOR

INFERIOR

CROSS SECTION VIEWS OF THE TRUNK

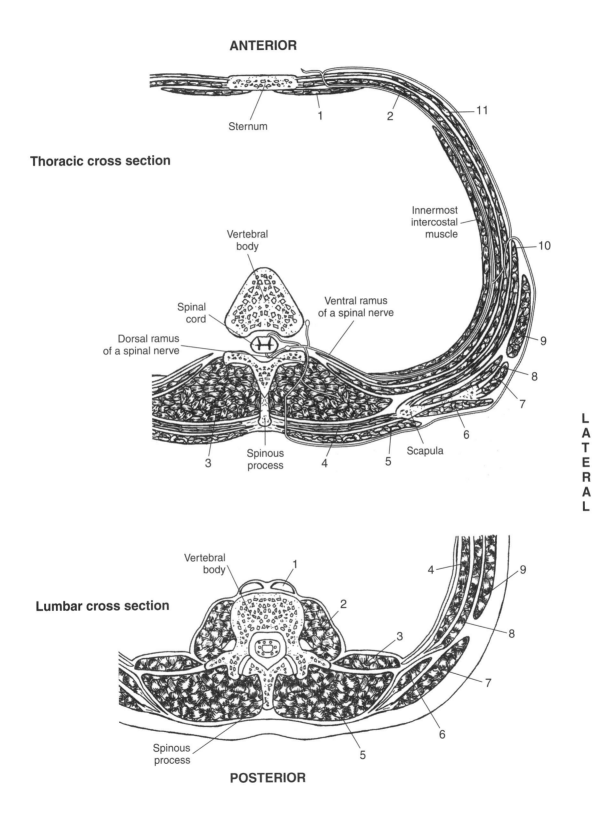

ANTERIOR

Thoracic cross section

Sternum

1

2

11

Innermost intercostal muscle

10

Vertebral body

Spinal cord

Ventral ramus of a spinal nerve

9

Dorsal ramus of a spinal nerve

8

7

3

Spinous process

4

5

Scapula

6

LATERAL

Lumbar cross section

Vertebral body

1

2

4

9

3

8

7

5

6

Spinous process

POSTERIOR

Muscles of the Pelvis

ANTERIOR VIEW OF THE RIGHT PELVIS

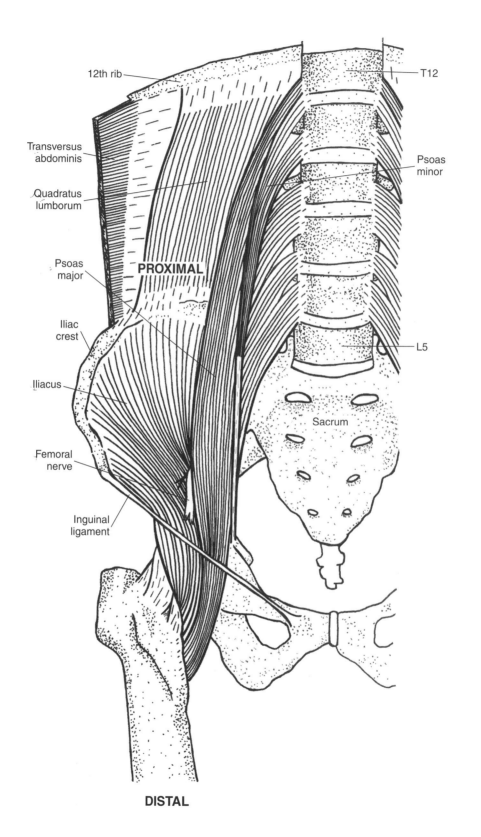

12th rib

T12

Transversus
abdominis

Psoas
minor

Quadratus
lumborum

Psoas
major

PROXIMAL

Iliac
crest

L5

Iliacus

Sacrum

Femoral
nerve

Inguinal
ligament

L
A
T
E
R
A
L

M
E
D
I
A
L

DISTAL

LATERAL VIEW OF THE RIGHT PELVIS

PROXIMAL

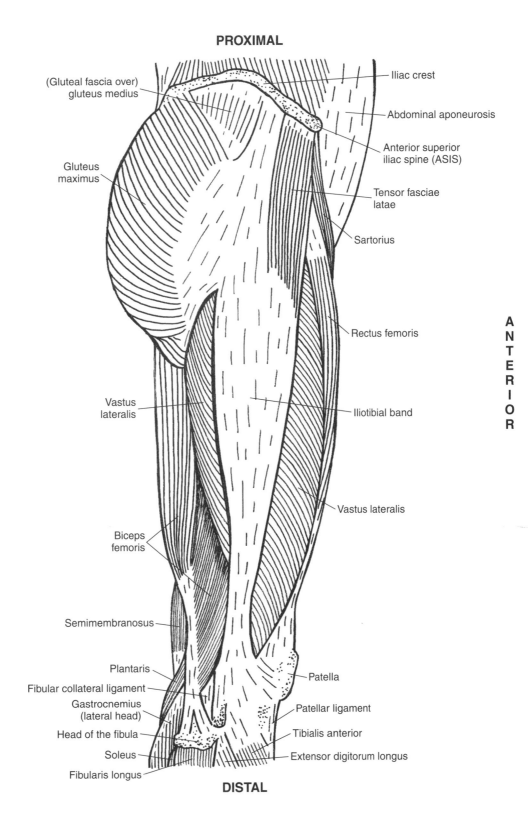

(Gluteal fascia over) gluteus medius

Gluteus maximus

Iliac crest

Abdominal aponeurosis

Anterior superior iliac spine (ASIS)

Tensor fasciae latae

Sartorius

Rectus femoris

Vastus lateralis

Iliotibial band

Vastus lateralis

Biceps femoris

Semimembranosus

Plantaris

Fibular collateral ligament

Gastrocnemius (lateral head)

Head of the fibula

Soleus

Fibularis longus

Patella

Patellar ligament

Tibialis anterior

Extensor digitorum longus

POSTERIOR

ANTERIOR

DISTAL

Muscles of the Pelvis

POSTERIOR VIEW OF THE RIGHT PELVIS (SUPERFICIAL)

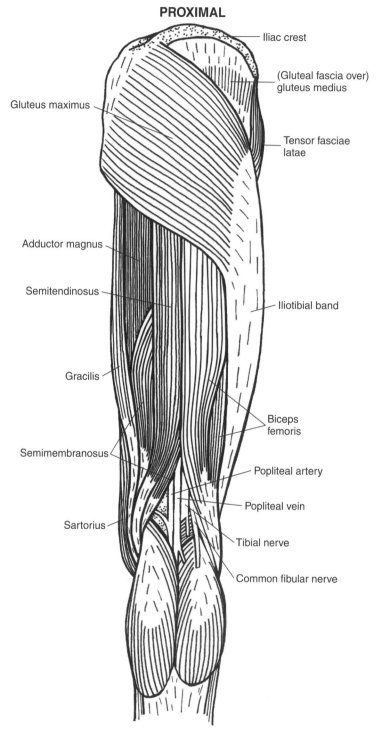

PROXIMAL

Iliac crest

(Gluteal fascia over) gluteus medius

Gluteus maximus

Tensor fasciae latae

Adductor magnus

Semitendinosus

Iliotibial band

Gracilis

M E D I A L

L A T E R A L

Biceps femoris

Semimembranosus

Popliteal artery

Popliteal vein

Sartorius

Tibial nerve

Common fibular nerve

DISTAL

POSTERIOR VIEW OF THE RIGHT PELVIS (DEEP)

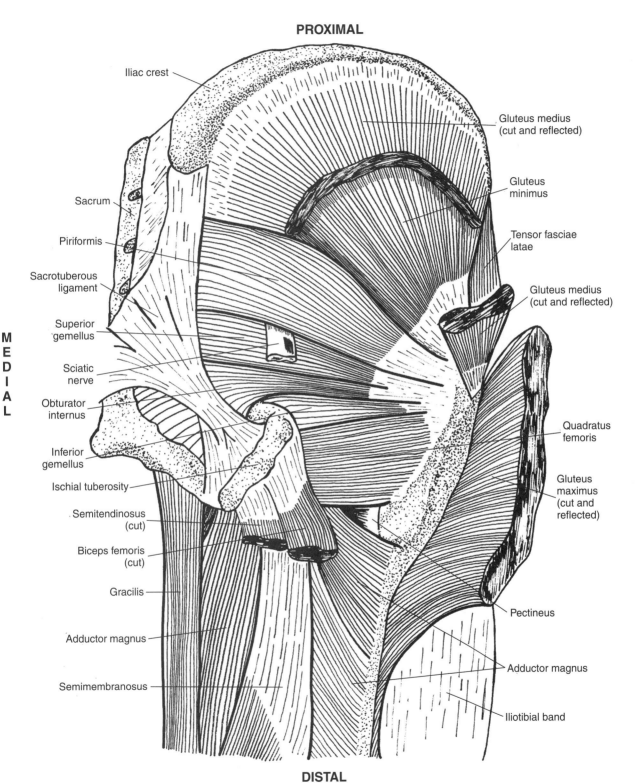

PROXIMAL

Iliac crest

Sacrum

Piriformis

Sacrotuberous ligament

Superior gemellus

Sciatic nerve

Obturator internus

Inferior gemellus

Ischial tuberosity

Semitendinosus (cut)

Biceps femoris (cut)

Gracilis

Adductor magnus

Semimembranosus

MEDIAL

LATERAL

Gluteus medius (cut and reflected)

Gluteus minimus

Tensor fasciae latae

Gluteus medius (cut and reflected)

Quadratus femoris

Gluteus maximus (cut and reflected)

Pectineus

Adductor magnus

Iliotibial band

DISTAL

Muscles of the Pelvis

PSOAS MAJOR
(OF THE ILIOPSOAS)

so-as **may**-jor

Actions
Flexion of the thigh at the hip joint
Lateral rotation of the thigh at the hip joint
Flexion of the trunk at the spinal joints
Lateral flexion of the trunk at the spinal joints
Anterior tilt of the pelvis at the hip joint
Contralateral rotation of the trunk at the spinal joints
Contralateral rotation of the pelvis at the hip joint

Innervation
Lumbar plexus

Arterial Supply
The lumbar arteries

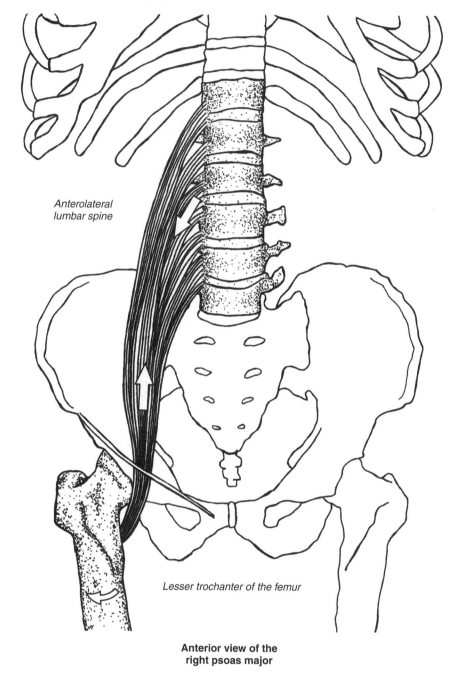

Anterolateral lumbar spine

Lesser trochanter of the femur

Anterior view of the right psoas major

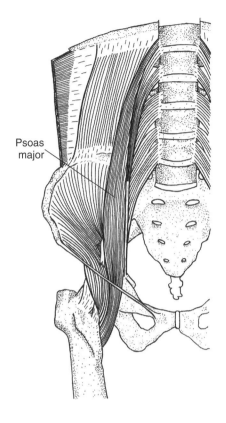

Psoas
major

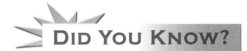

DID YOU KNOW?

The reason that old-fashioned sit-ups have been replaced by abdominal curl-ups or crunches is to avoid creating an overly strengthened and perhaps overly tight psoas major.

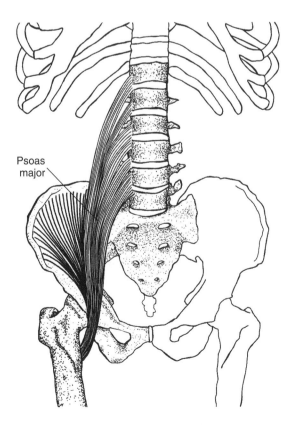

Psoas
major

Muscles of the Pelvis

ILIACUS
(OF THE ILIOPSOAS)

i-lee-**ak**-us

Actions
Flexion of the thigh at
the hip joint
Lateral rotation of the
thigh at the hip joint
Anterior tilt of the pelvis
at the hip joint
Contralateral rotation of
the pelvis at the hip
joint

Innervation
The femoral nerve

Arterial Supply
The iliolumbar artery

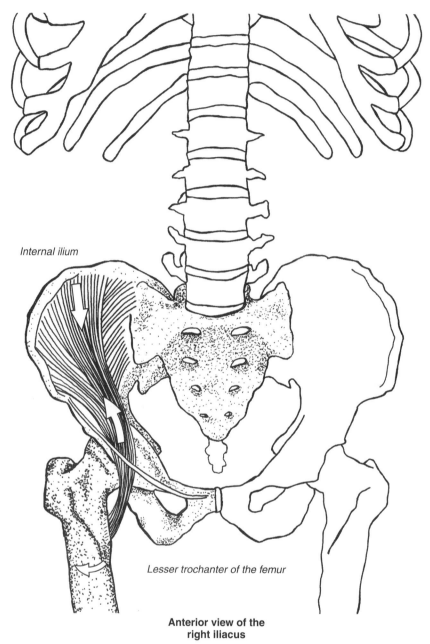

Internal ilium

Lesser trochanter of the femur

**Anterior view of the
right iliacus**

Muscles of the Pelvis

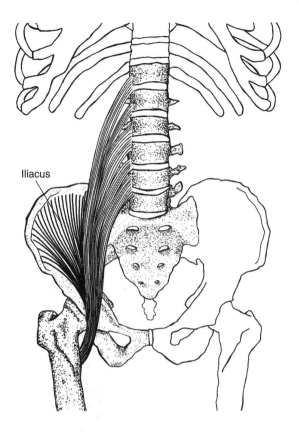

Iliacus

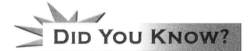

DID YOU KNOW?

The distal tendon of the iliacus joins into the distal tendon of the psoas major; together, these two muscles are often called the iliopsoas muscle.

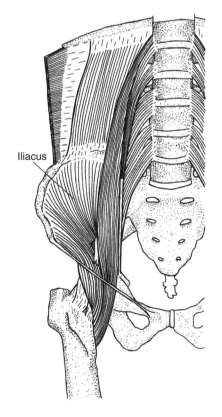

Iliacus

Muscles of the Pelvis

PSOAS MINOR

so-as **my**-nor

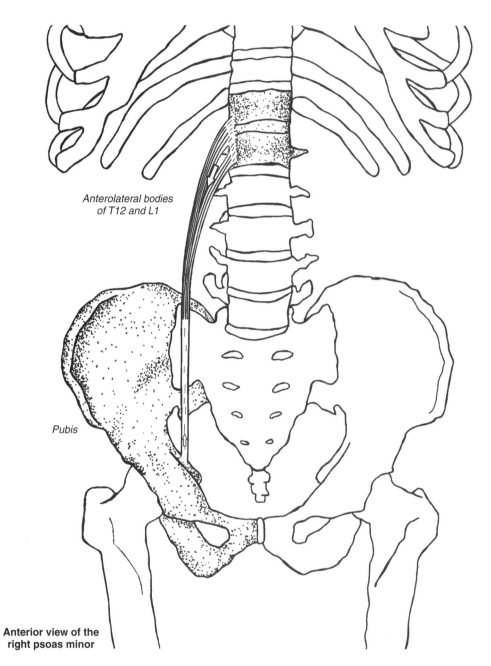

*Anterolateral bodies
of T12 and L1*

Pubis

**Anterior view of the
right psoas minor**

Actions	Innervation	Arterial Supply
Flexion of the trunk at the spinal joints	L1 spinal nerve	Lumbar arteries
Posterior tilt of the pelvis at the lumbosacral joint		

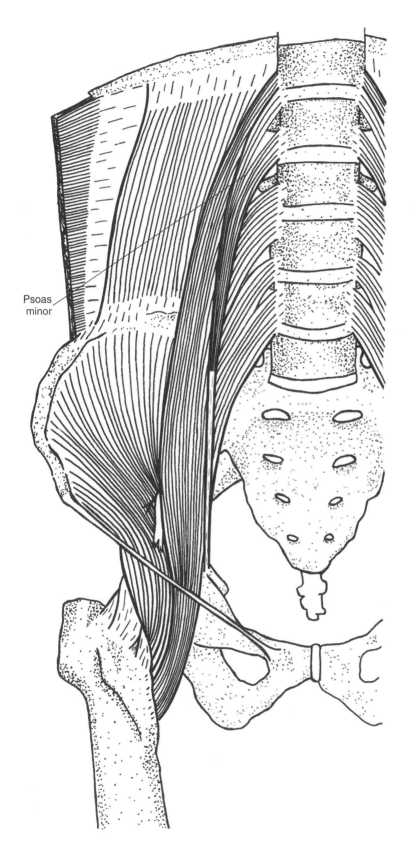

Psoas
minor

Muscles of the Pelvis

GLUTEUS MAXIMUS

gloo-tee-us **max**-i-mus

Actions
Extension of the thigh at
the hip joint
Lateral rotation of the
thigh at the hip joint
Abduction of the thigh at
the hip joint (upper ⅓)
Adduction of the thigh at
the hip joint (lower ⅔)
Posterior tilt of the pelvis
at the hip joint
Contralateral rotation of
the pelvis at the hip
joint
Extension of the leg at
the knee joint

Innervation
The inferior gluteal
nerve (L5, S1, 2)

Arterial Supply
The superior gluteal
artery and the inferior
gluteal artery

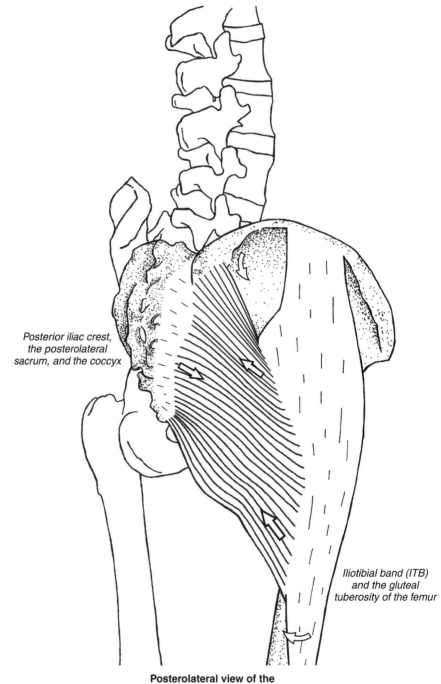

Posterior iliac crest,
the posterolateral
sacrum, and the coccyx

Iliotibial band (ITB)
and the gluteal
tuberosity of the femur

**Posterolateral view of the
right gluteus maximus**

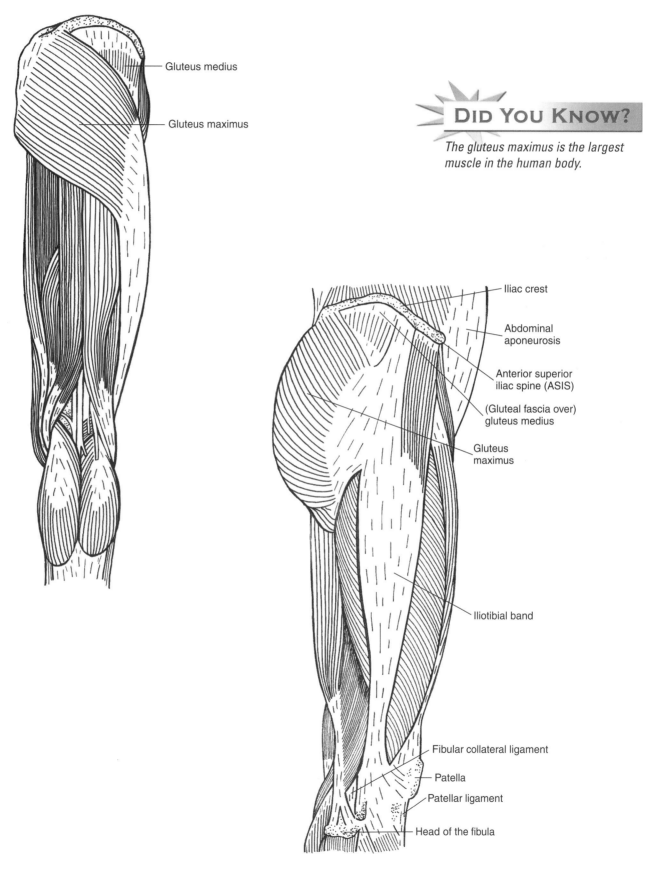

Gluteus medius

Gluteus maximus

DID YOU KNOW?

The gluteus maximus is the largest muscle in the human body.

Iliac crest

Abdominal aponeurosis

Anterior superior iliac spine (ASIS)

(Gluteal fascia over) gluteus medius

Gluteus maximus

Iliotibial band

Fibular collateral ligament

Patella

Patellar ligament

Head of the fibula

Muscles of the Pelvis

GLUTEUS MEDIUS

gloo-tee-us **meed**-ee-us

Actions
Abduction of the thigh at the hip joint (entire muscle)

Flexion of the thigh at the hip joint (anterior fibers)

Medial rotation of the thigh at the hip joint (anterior fibers)

Extension of the thigh at the hip joint (posterior fibers)

Lateral rotation of the thigh at the hip joint (posterior fibers)

Posterior tilt of the pelvis at the hip joint (posterior fibers)

Anterior tilt of the pelvis at the hip joint (anterior fibers)

Depression (lateral tilt) of the pelvis at the hip joint (entire muscle)

Ipsilateral rotation of the pelvis at the hip joint (anterior fibers)

Contralateral rotation of the pelvis at the hip joint (posterior fibers)

Innervation
The superior gluteal nerve

Arterial Supply
The superior gluteal artery

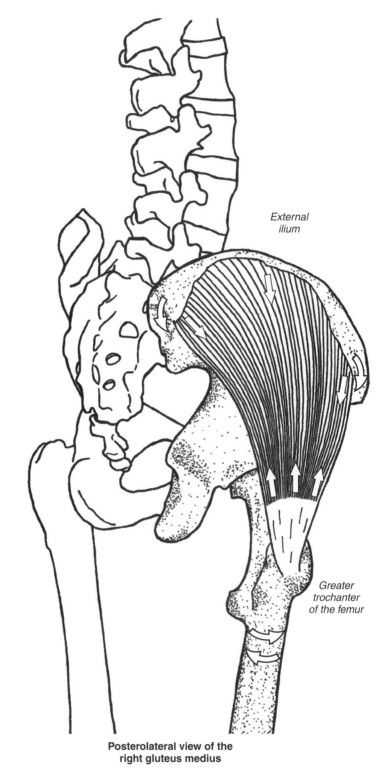

External ilium

Greater trochanter of the femur

Posterolateral view of the right gluteus medius

Muscles of the Pelvis

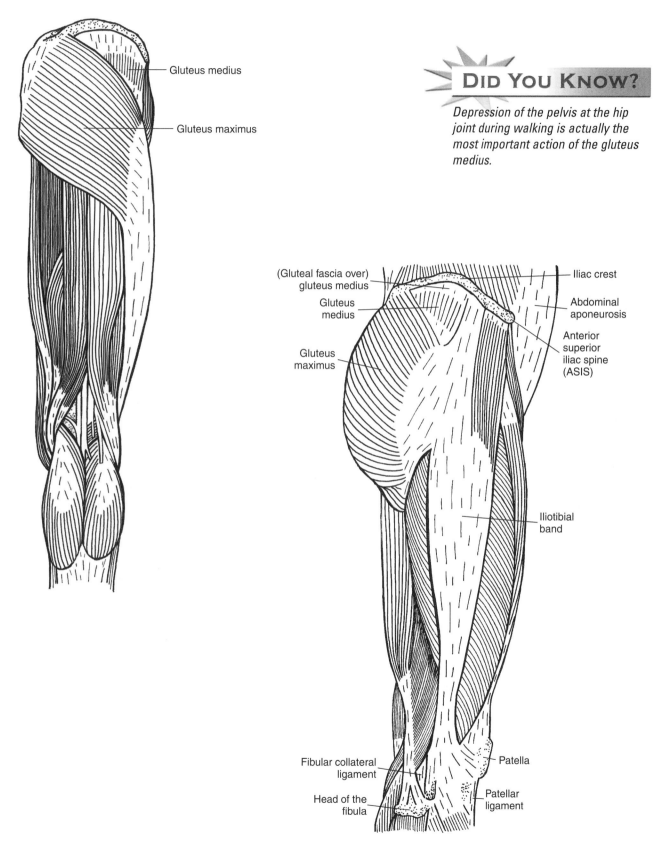

Gluteus medius

Gluteus maximus

DID YOU KNOW?

Depression of the pelvis at the hip joint during walking is actually the most important action of the gluteus medius.

(Gluteal fascia over) gluteus medius

Iliac crest

Gluteus medius

Abdominal aponeurosis

Gluteus maximus

Anterior superior iliac spine (ASIS)

Iliotibial band

Fibular collateral ligament

Patella

Head of the fibula

Patellar ligament

Muscles of the Pelvis

GLUTEUS MINIMUS

gloo-tee-us **min**-i-mus

Actions
Abduction of the thigh at the hip joint (entire muscle)

Flexion of the thigh at the hip joint (anterior fibers)

Medial rotation of the thigh at the hip joint (anterior fibers)

Extension of the thigh at the hip joint (posterior fibers)

Lateral rotation of the thigh at the hip joint (posterior fibers)

Posterior tilt of the pelvis at the hip joint (posterior fibers)

Anterior tilt of the pelvis at the hip joint (anterior fibers)

Depression (lateral tilt) of the pelvis at the hip joint (entire muscle)

Ipsilateral rotation of the pelvis at the hip joint (anterior fibers)

Contralateral rotation of the pelvis at the hip joint (posterior fibers)

Innervation
The superior gluteal nerve

Arterial Supply
The superior gluteal artery

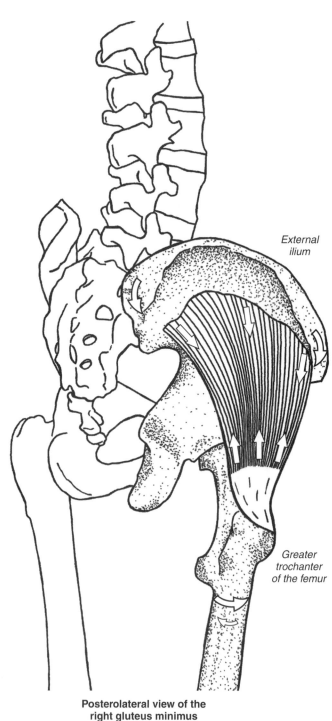

External ilium

Greater trochanter of the femur

Posterolateral view of the right gluteus minimus

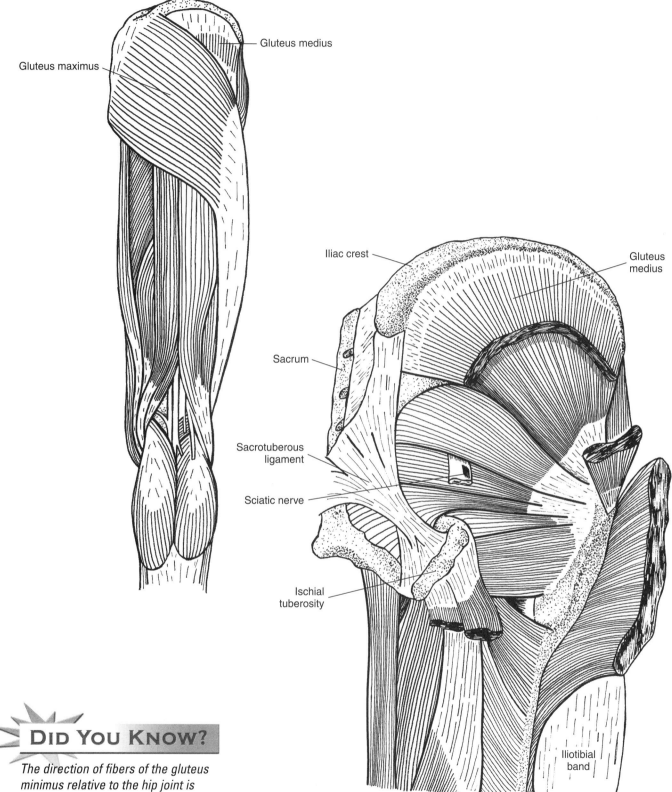

Gluteus medius

Gluteus maximus

Iliac crest

Gluteus medius

Sacrum

Sacrotuberous ligament

Sciatic nerve

Ischial tuberosity

Iliotibial band

DID YOU KNOW?

The direction of fibers of the gluteus minimus relative to the hip joint is identical to the more superficial gluteus medius; therefore, these two muscles have the same actions.

Muscles of the Pelvis

PIRIFORMIS
(OF THE DEEP LATERAL ROTATORS OF THE THIGH)

pi-ri-**for**-mis

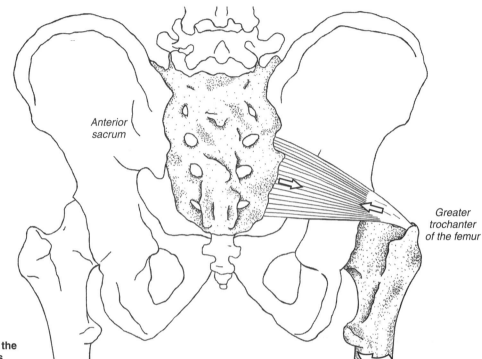

Anterior sacrum

Greater trochanter of the femur

Posterior view of the right piriformis
(sacrotuberous ligament not shown)

Actions
Lateral rotation of the
  thigh at the hip joint
Abduction of the thigh at
  the hip joint (if the
  thigh is flexed)
Medial rotation of the
  thigh at the hip joint
  (if the thigh is flexed)
Contralateral rotation of
  the pelvis at the hip
  joint

Innervation
Nerve to piriformis
  (of the lumbosacral
  plexus)

Arterial Supply
The superior and inferior
  gluteal arteries

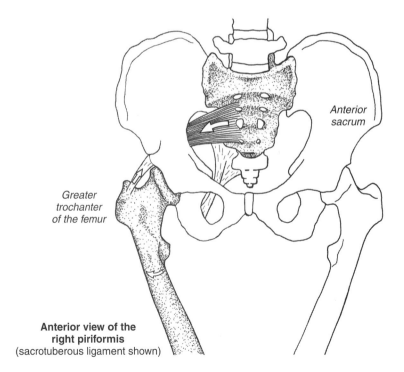

Anterior sacrum

Greater trochanter of the femur

Anterior view of the right piriformis
(sacrotuberous ligament shown)

Muscles of the Pelvis

Piriformis

Sciatic
nerve

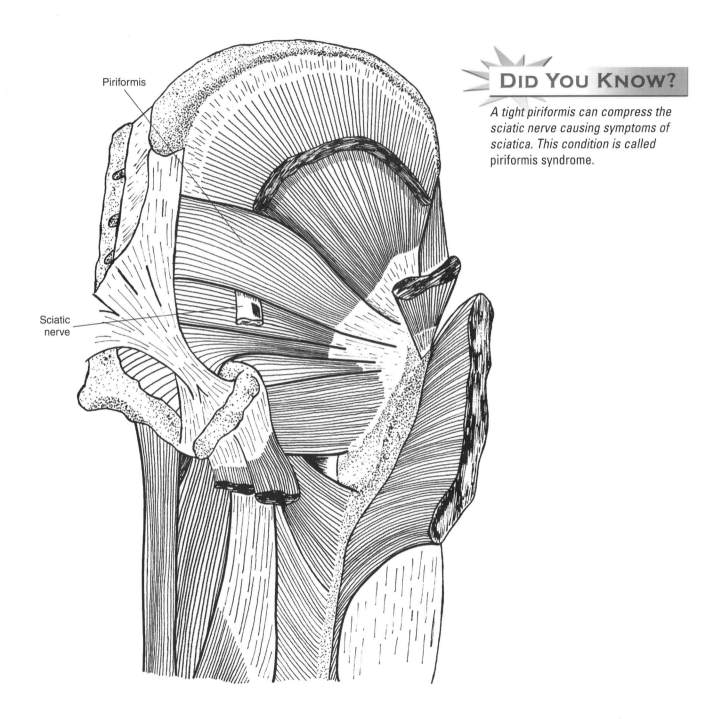

DID YOU KNOW?

A tight piriformis can compress the sciatic nerve causing symptoms of sciatica. This condition is called piriformis syndrome.

Muscles of the Pelvis

SUPERIOR GEMELLUS
(OF THE DEEP LATERAL ROTATORS OF THE THIGH)

su-**pee**-ree-or jee-**mel**-us

Actions
Lateral rotation of the
thigh at the hip joint
Abduction of the thigh at
the hip joint (if the
thigh is flexed)
Contralateral rotation of
the pelvis at the hip
joint

Innervation
Nerve to obturator
internus (of the
lumbosacral plexus)

Arterial Supply
The inferior gluteal
artery

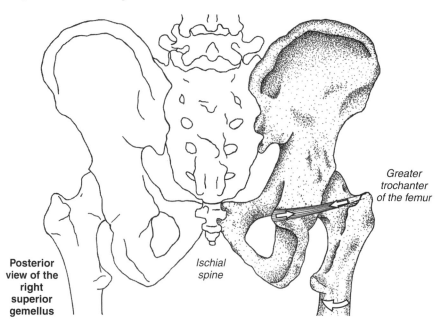

Greater trochanter of the femur

**Posterior
view of the
right
superior
gemellus**

Ischial spine

OBTURATOR INTERNUS
(OF THE DEEP LATERAL ROTATORS OF THE THIGH)

ob-too-**ray**-tor in-**ter**-nus

Actions
Lateral rotation of the
thigh at the hip joint
Abduction of the thigh at
the hip joint (if the
thigh is flexed)
Contralateral rotation of
the pelvis at the hip
joint

Innervation
Nerve to obturator
internus (of the
lumbosacral plexus)

Arterial Supply
The superior and inferior
gluteal arteries

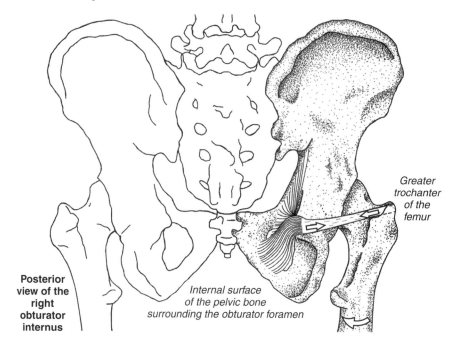

Greater trochanter of the femur

**Posterior
view of the
right
obturator
internus**

*Internal surface
of the pelvic bone
surrounding the obturator foramen*

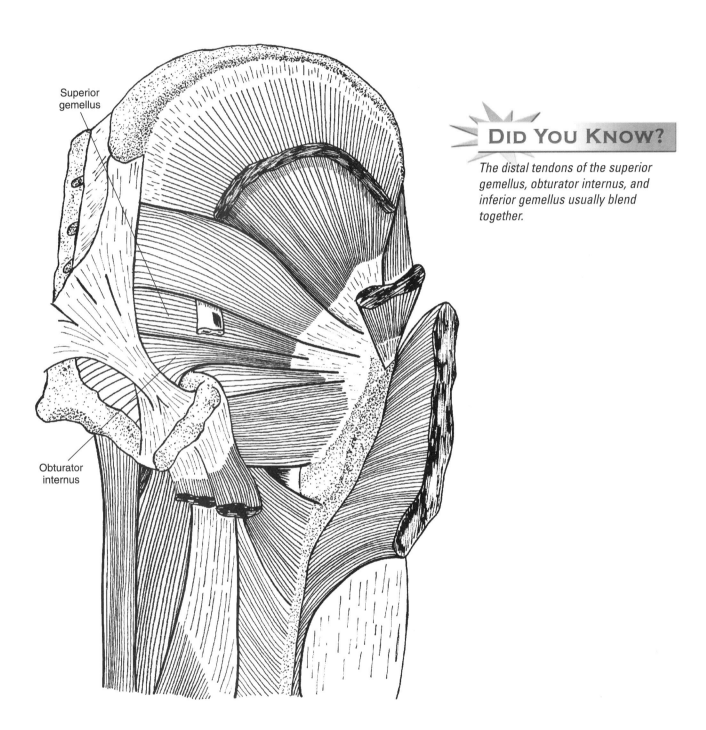

Superior gemellus

Obturator internus

DID YOU KNOW?

The distal tendons of the superior gemellus, obturator internus, and inferior gemellus usually blend together.

Muscles of the Pelvis

INFERIOR GEMELLUS
(OF THE DEEP LATERAL ROTATORS OF THE THIGH)

in-**fee**-ree-or jee-**mel**-us

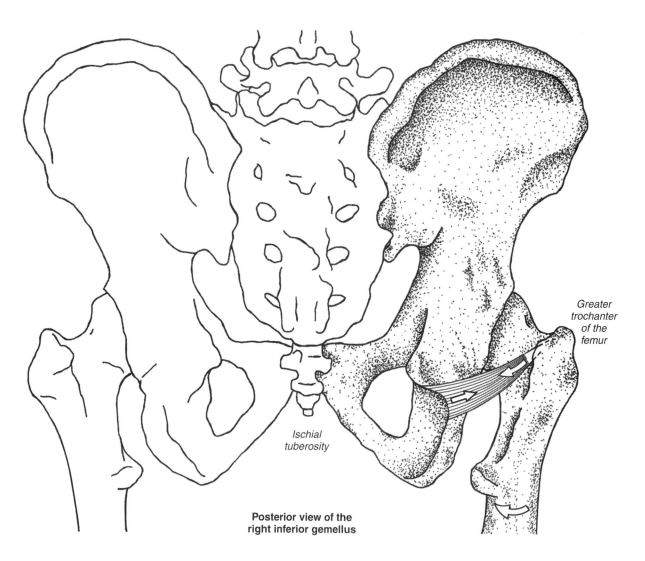

Greater
trochanter
of the
femur

Ischial
tuberosity

**Posterior view of the
right inferior gemellus**

Actions	**Innervation**	**Arterial Supply**
Lateral rotation of the thigh at the hip joint Abduction of the thigh at the hip joint (if the thigh is flexed) Contralateral rotation of the pelvis at the hip joint	Nerve to quadratus femoris (of the lumbosacral plexus)	The inferior gluteal artery

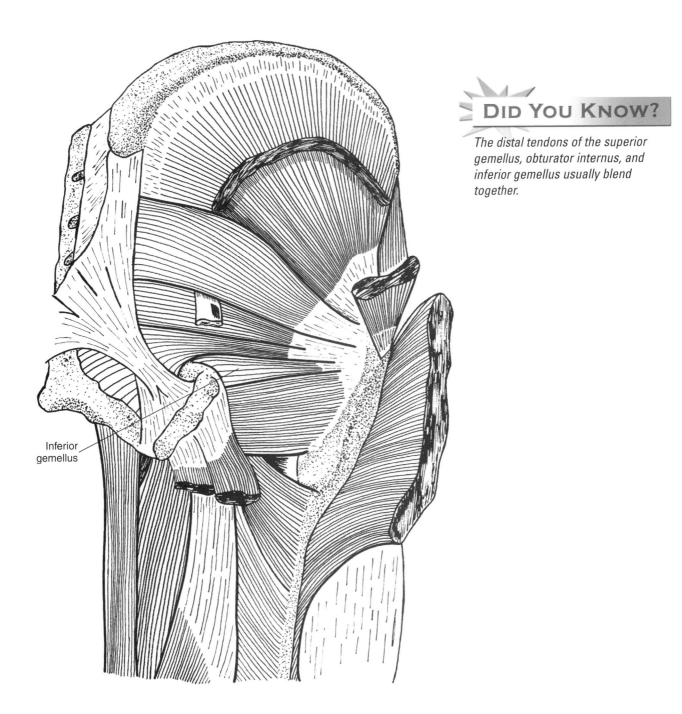

Inferior
gemellus

Muscles of the Pelvis

OBTURATOR EXTERNUS

(OF THE DEEP LATERAL ROTATORS OF THE THIGH)

ob-too-**ray**-tor ex-**ter**-nus

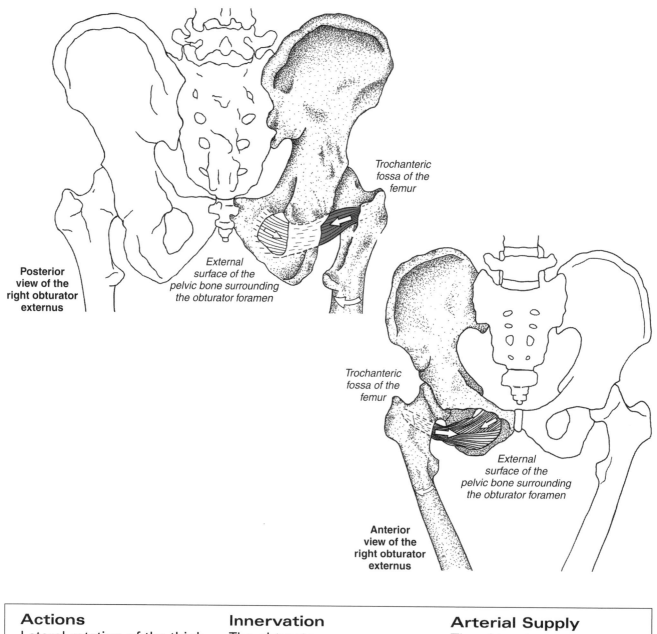

Trochanteric
fossa of the
femur

Posterior
view of the
right obturator
externus

External
surface of the
pelvic bone surrounding
the obturator foramen

Trochanteric
fossa of the
femur

External
surface of the
pelvic bone surrounding
the obturator foramen

Anterior
view of the
right obturator
externus

Actions	Innervation	Arterial Supply
Lateral rotation of the thigh at the hip joint	The obturator nerve	The obturator artery
Contralateral rotation of the pelvis at the hip joint		

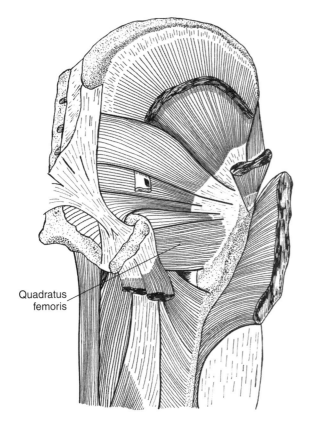

Quadratus
femoris

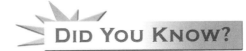

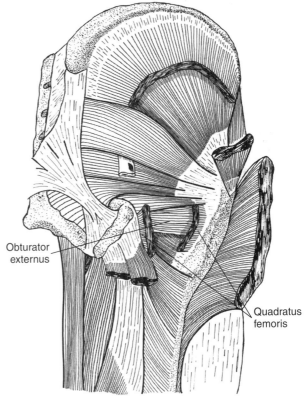

Obturator
externus

Quadratus
femoris

Muscles of the Pelvis

QUADRATUS FEMORIS
(OF THE DEEP LATERAL ROTATORS OF THE THIGH)

kwod-**rate**-us **fem**-o-ris

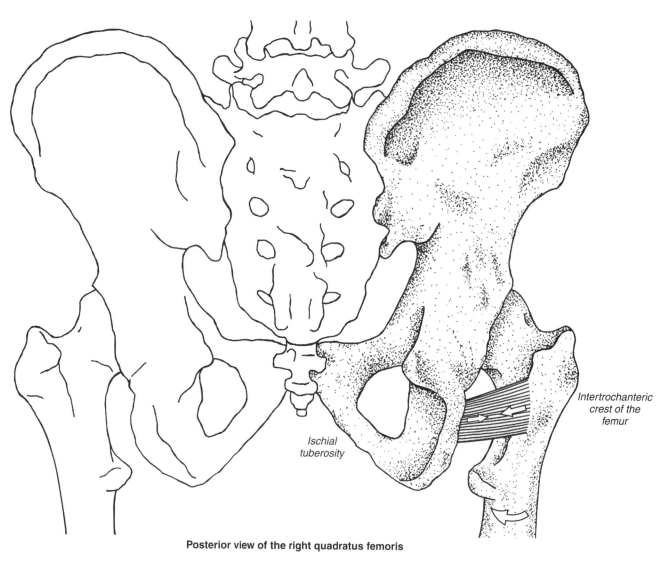

Intertrochanteric crest of the femur

Ischial tuberosity

Posterior view of the right quadratus femoris

Actions	**Innervation**	**Arterial Supply**
Lateral rotation of the thigh at the hip joint Adduction of the thigh at the hip joint Contralateral rotation of the pelvis at the hip joint	Nerve to quadratus femoris (of the lumbosacral plexus)	The inferior gluteal artery

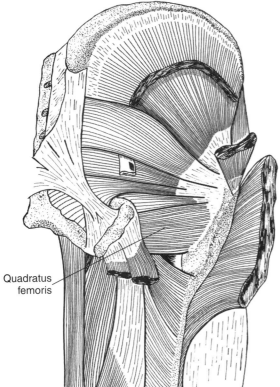

Quadratus
femoris

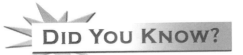

DID YOU KNOW?

The quadratus femoris attaches sufficiently distal on the femur to be able to do adduction of the thigh at the hip joint.

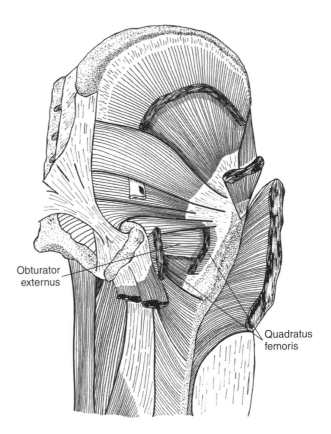

Obturator
externus

Quadratus
femoris

Muscles of the Pelvis

ANTERIOR VIEW OF THE RIGHT PELVIS

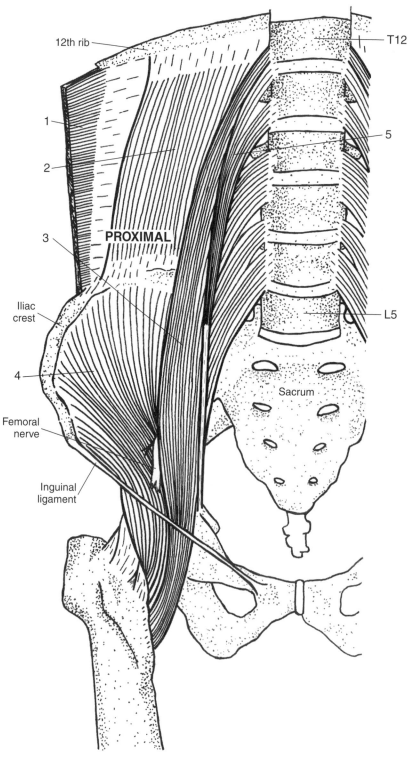

12th rib

T12

1

5

2

PROXIMAL

3

Iliac
crest

L5

4

Sacrum

Femoral
nerve

Inguinal
ligament

LATERAL

MEDIAL

DISTAL

LATERAL VIEW OF THE RIGHT PELVIS

PROXIMAL

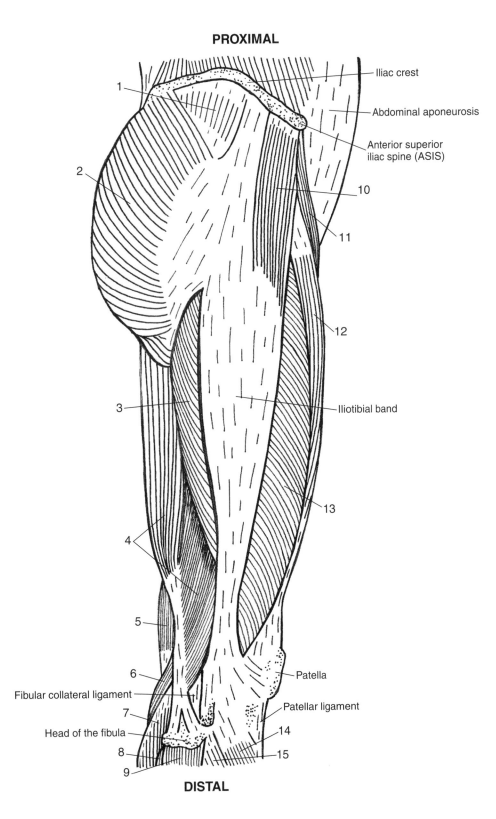

Iliac crest

Abdominal aponeurosis

Anterior superior
iliac spine (ASIS)

10

11

12

POSTERIOR

ANTERIOR

Iliotibial band

13

Patella

Fibular collateral ligament

Patellar ligament

Head of the fibula

14

15

DISTAL

Muscles of the Pelvis

POSTERIOR VIEW OF THE RIGHT PELVIS (SUPERFICIAL)

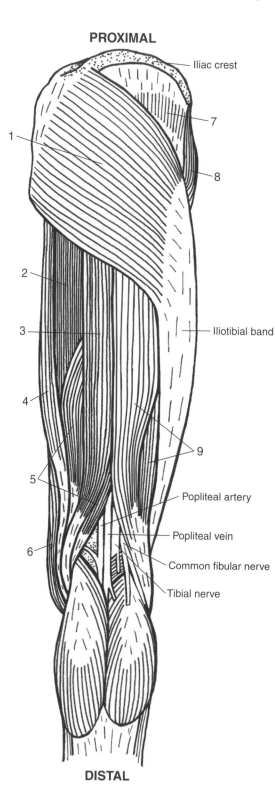

PROXIMAL

Iliac crest

7

1

8

2

M E D I A L

L A T E R A L

3

Iliotibial band

4

9

5

Popliteal artery

6

Popliteal vein

Common fibular nerve

Tibial nerve

DISTAL

POSTERIOR VIEW OF THE RIGHT PELVIS (DEEP)

PROXIMAL

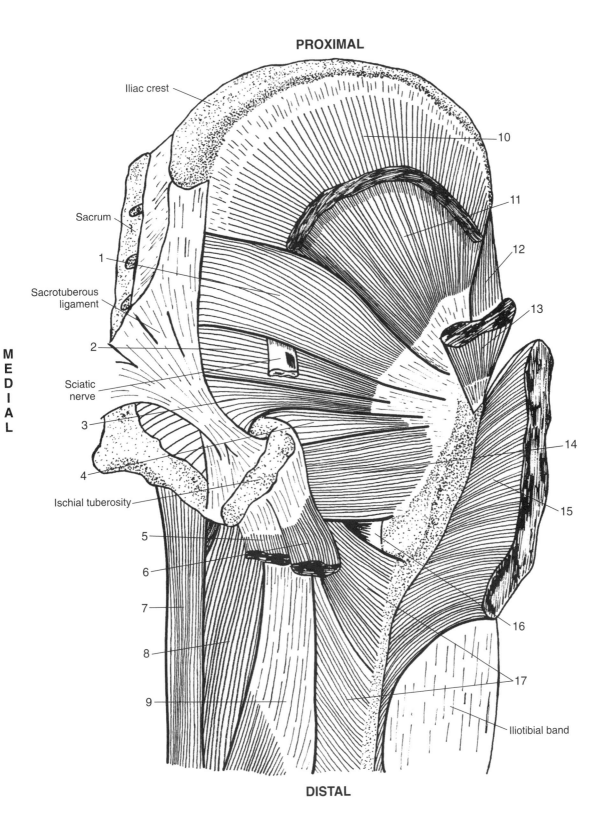

Iliac crest

Sacrum

Sacrotuberous
ligament

Sciatic
nerve

Ischial tuberosity

MEDIAL

LATERAL

10

11

12

13

14

15

16

17

1

2

3

4

5

6

7

8

9

Iliotibial band

DISTAL

ANTERIOR VIEW OF THE RIGHT THIGH (SUPERFICIAL)

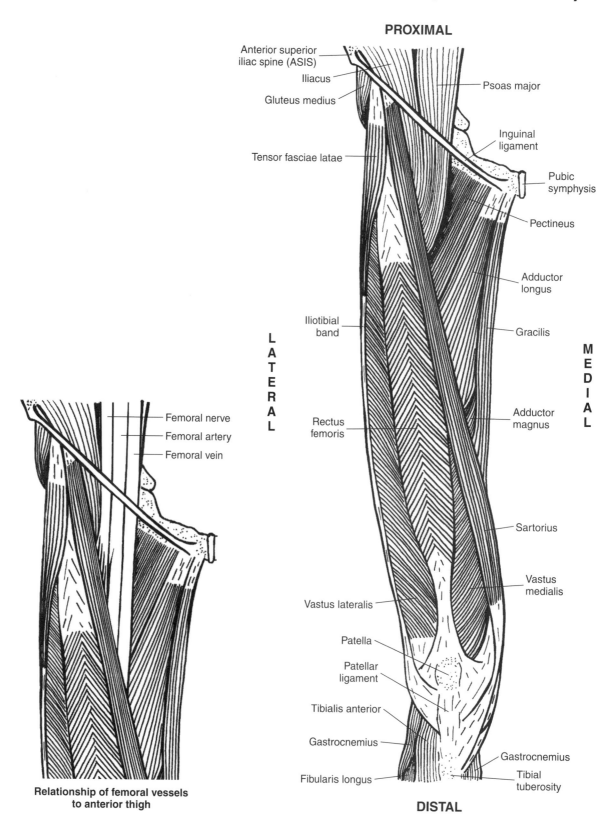

PROXIMAL

Anterior superior
iliac spine (ASIS)

Iliacus

Gluteus medius

Tensor fasciae latae

Psoas major

Inguinal
ligament

Pubic
symphysis

Pectineus

Adductor
longus

Gracilis

Iliotibial
band

Rectus
femoris

Adductor
magnus

LATERAL

MEDIAL

Sartorius

Vastus
medialis

Vastus lateralis

Patella

Patellar
ligament

Tibialis anterior

Gastrocnemius

Gastrocnemius

Fibularis longus

Tibial
tuberosity

DISTAL

Femoral nerve

Femoral artery

Femoral vein

**Relationship of femoral vessels
to anterior thigh**

ANTERIOR VIEW OF THE RIGHT THIGH (DEEP)

PROXIMAL

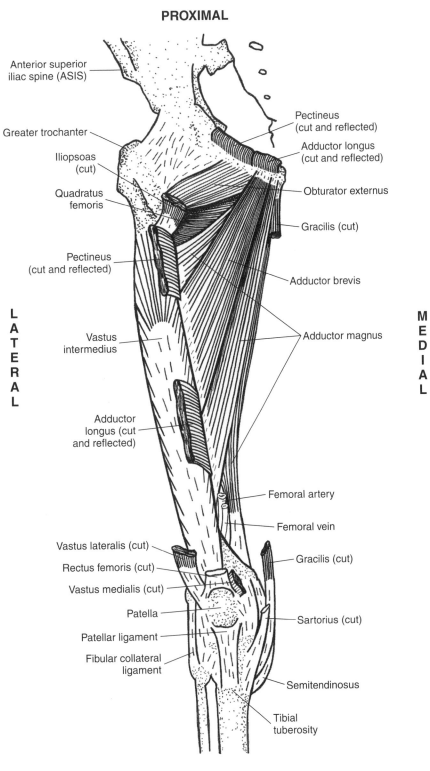

Anterior superior
iliac spine (ASIS)

Greater trochanter

Iliopsoas
(cut)

Quadratus
femoris

Pectineus
(cut and reflected)

Vastus
intermedius

Adductor
longus (cut
and reflected)

Vastus lateralis (cut)

Rectus femoris (cut)

Vastus medialis (cut)

Patella

Patellar ligament

Fibular collateral
ligament

Pectineus
(cut and reflected)

Adductor longus
(cut and reflected)

Obturator externus

Gracilis (cut)

Adductor brevis

Adductor magnus

Femoral artery

Femoral vein

Gracilis (cut)

Sartorius (cut)

Semitendinosus

Tibial
tuberosity

LATERAL

MEDIAL

DISTAL

Muscles of the Thigh

POSTERIOR VIEW OF THE RIGHT THIGH (SUPERFICIAL)

PROXIMAL

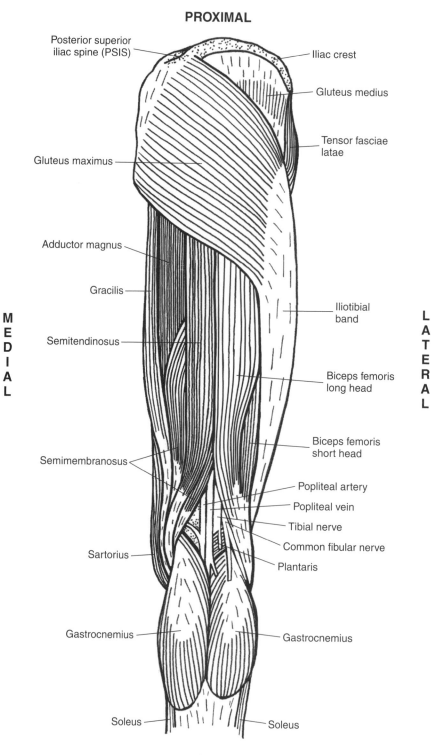

Posterior superior iliac spine (PSIS)

Iliac crest

Gluteus medius

Tensor fasciae latae

Gluteus maximus

Adductor magnus

Gracilis

Iliotibial band

Semitendinosus

Biceps femoris long head

Biceps femoris short head

Semimembranosus

Popliteal artery

Popliteal vein

Tibial nerve

Common fibular nerve

Sartorius

Plantaris

Gastrocnemius

Gastrocnemius

Soleus

Soleus

MEDIAL

LATERAL

DISTAL

POSTERIOR VIEW OF THE RIGHT THIGH (DEEP)

PROXIMAL

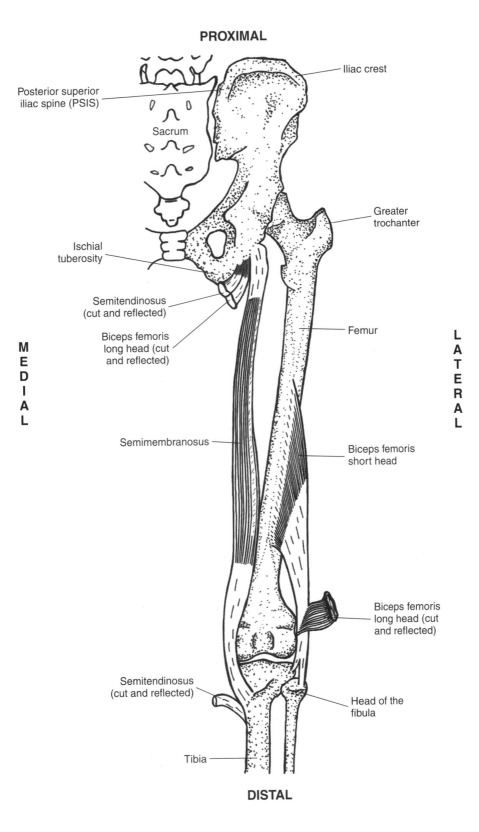

Iliac crest

Posterior superior
iliac spine (PSIS)

Sacrum

Greater
trochanter

Ischial
tuberosity

Semitendinosus
(cut and reflected)

Biceps femoris
long head (cut
and reflected)

Femur

**M
E
D
I
A
L**

**L
A
T
E
R
A
L**

Semimembranosus

Biceps femoris
short head

Biceps femoris
long head (cut
and reflected)

Semitendinosus
(cut and reflected)

Head of the
fibula

Tibia

DISTAL

Muscles of the Thigh

LATERAL VIEW OF THE RIGHT THIGH

PROXIMAL

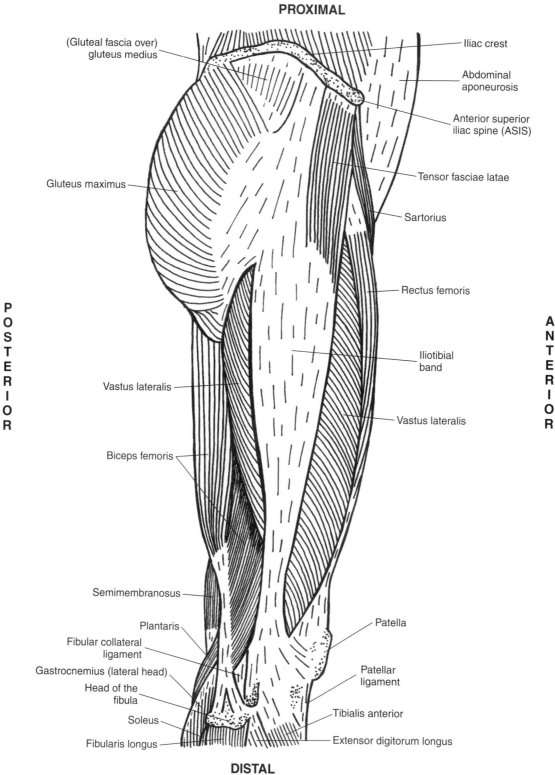

(Gluteal fascia over)
gluteus medius

Iliac crest

Abdominal
aponeurosis

Anterior superior
iliac spine (ASIS)

Gluteus maximus

Tensor fasciae latae

Sartorius

Rectus femoris

P O S T E R I O R

A N T E R I O R

Iliotibial
band

Vastus lateralis

Vastus lateralis

Biceps femoris

Semimembranosus

Plantaris

Patella

Fibular collateral
ligament

Gastrocnemius (lateral head)

Head of the
fibula

Patellar
ligament

Soleus

Tibialis anterior

Fibularis longus

Extensor digitorum longus

DISTAL

MEDIAL VIEW OF THE RIGHT THIGH

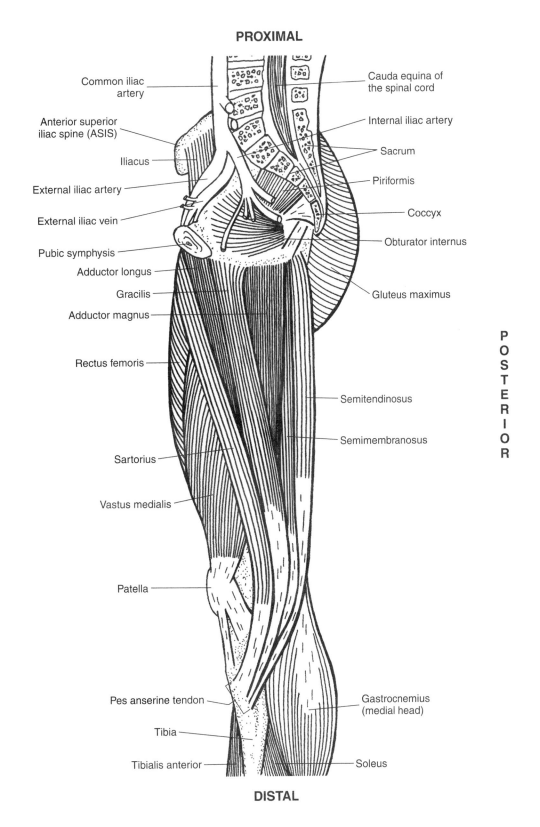

PROXIMAL

Common iliac artery

Anterior superior iliac spine (ASIS)

Iliacus

External iliac artery

External iliac vein

Pubic symphysis

Adductor longus

Gracilis

Adductor magnus

Rectus femoris

Sartorius

Vastus medialis

Patella

Pes anserine tendon

Tibia

Tibialis anterior

Cauda equina of the spinal cord

Internal iliac artery

Sacrum

Piriformis

Coccyx

Obturator internus

Gluteus maximus

Semitendinosus

Semimembranosus

Gastrocnemius (medial head)

Soleus

ANTERIOR

POSTERIOR

DISTAL

Muscles of the Thigh

TENSOR FASCIAE LATAE ("TFL")

ten-sor **fash**-ee-a **la**-tee

Actions
Flexion of the thigh at
   the hip joint
Abduction of the thigh at
   the hip joint
Medial rotation of the
   thigh at the hip joint
Anterior tilt of the pelvis
   at the hip joint
Depression (lateral tilt)
   of the pelvis at the hip
   joint
Ipsilateral rotation of the
   pelvis at the hip joint
Extension of the leg at
   the knee joint

Innervation
The superior gluteal
   nerve

Arterial Supply
The superior gluteal
   artery

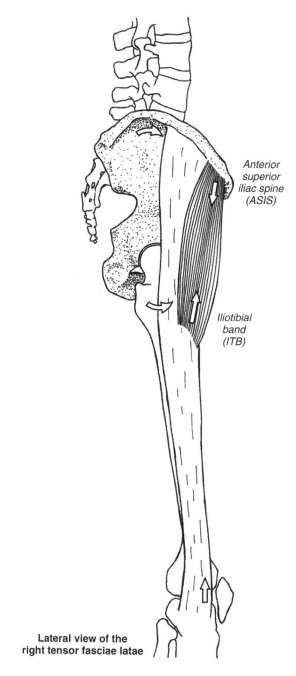

Anterior
superior
iliac spine
(ASIS)

Iliotibial
band
(ITB)

**Lateral view of the
right tensor fasciae latae**

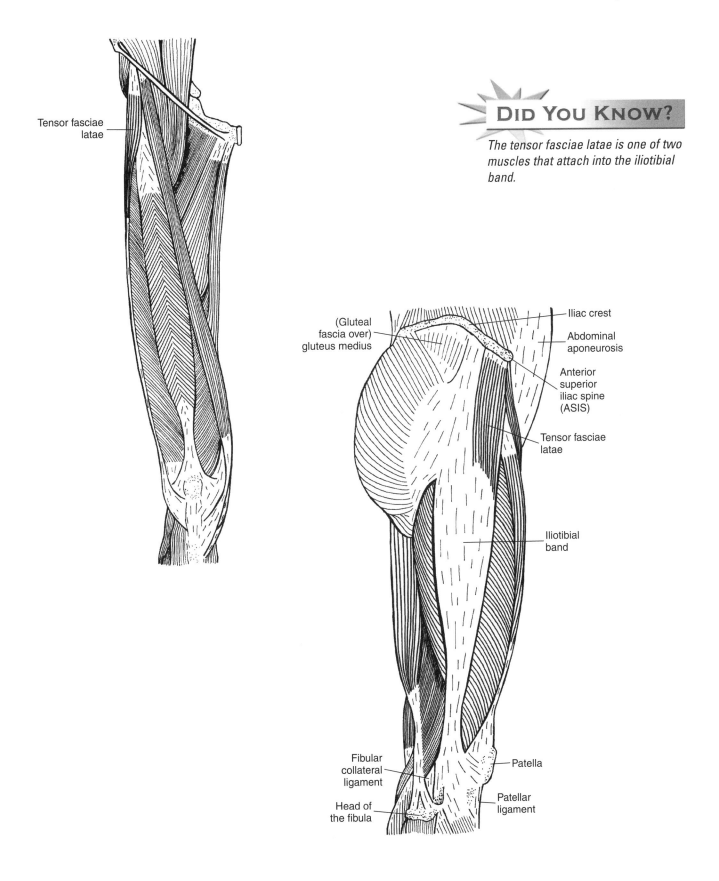

Tensor fasciae latae

DID YOU KNOW?

The tensor fasciae latae is one of two muscles that attach into the iliotibial band.

(Gluteal fascia over) gluteus medius

Iliac crest

Abdominal aponeurosis

Anterior superior iliac spine (ASIS)

Tensor fasciae latae

Iliotibial band

Fibular collateral ligament

Head of the fibula

Patella

Patellar ligament

Muscles of the Thigh

SARTORIUS

sar-**tor**-ee-us

Actions
Flexion of the thigh at the hip joint
Abduction of the thigh at the hip joint
Lateral rotation of the thigh at the hip joint
Flexion of the leg at the knee joint
Anterior tilt of the pelvis at the hip joint
Medial rotation of the leg at the knee joint
Depression (lateral tilt) of the pelvis at the hip joint
Contralateral rotation of the pelvis at the hip joint

Innervation
The femoral nerve

Arterial Supply
The femoral artery

Anterior superior iliac spine (ASIS)

Anterior view of the right sartorius

Pes anserine tendon

Muscles of the Thigh

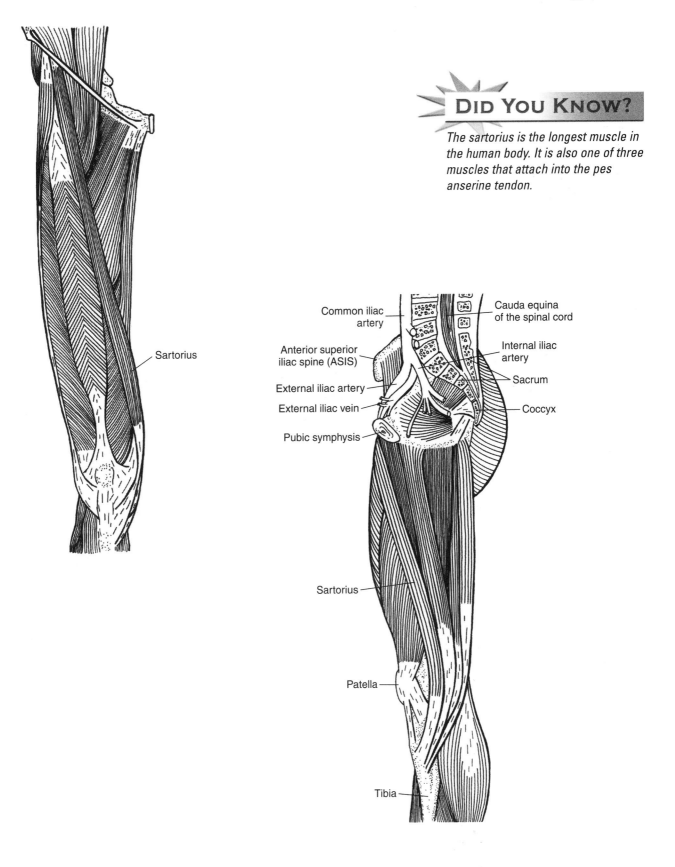

Sartorius

DID YOU KNOW?

The sartorius is the longest muscle in the human body. It is also one of three muscles that attach into the pes anserine tendon.

Common iliac artery

Cauda equina of the spinal cord

Anterior superior iliac spine (ASIS)

Internal iliac artery

External iliac artery

Sacrum

External iliac vein

Coccyx

Pubic symphysis

Sartorius

Patella

Tibia

Muscles of the Thigh

RECTUS FEMORIS

(OF THE QUADRICEPS FEMORIS GROUP)

rek-tus **fem**-o-ris

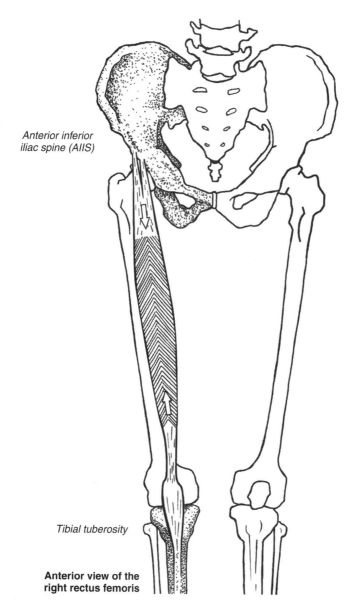

Anterior inferior
iliac spine (AIIS)

Tibial tuberosity

**Anterior view of the
right rectus femoris**

Actions
Extension of the leg at the
knee joint
Flexion of the thigh at the
hip joint
Anterior tilt of the pelvis
at the hip joint

Innervation
The femoral nerve

Arterial Supply
The femoral artery and the
deep femoral artery

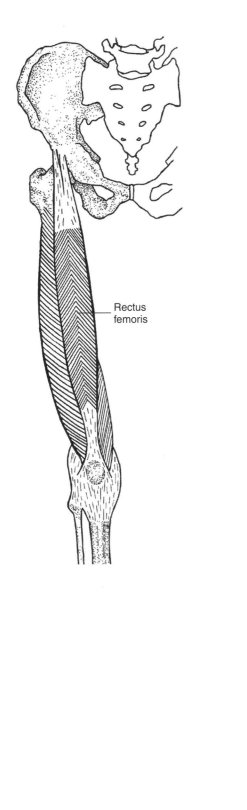

Rectus
femoris

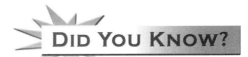

DID YOU KNOW?

The rectus femoris is the only quadriceps femoris muscle that can create movement of the thigh or pelvis at the hip joint, because it is the only one that crosses the hip joint.

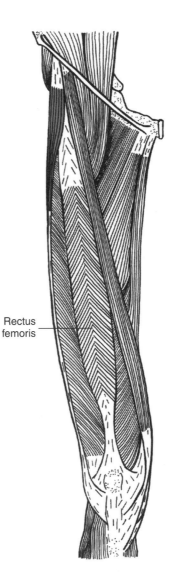

Rectus
femoris

Muscles of the Thigh

VASTUS LATERALIS

(OF THE QUADRICEPS FEMORIS GROUP)

vas-tus lat-er-**a**-lis

Action
Extension of the leg at the knee joint
Innervation
The femoral nerve
Arterial Supply
The femoral artery and the deep femoral artery

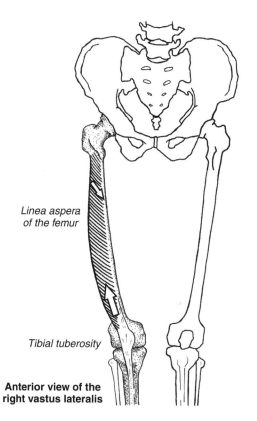

Linea aspera of the femur

Tibial tuberosity

Anterior view of the right vastus lateralis

VASTUS MEDIALIS

(OF THE QUADRICEPS FEMORIS GROUP)

vas-tus mee-dee-**a**-lis

Action
Extension of the leg at the knee joint
Innervation
The femoral nerve
Arterial Supply
The femoral artery

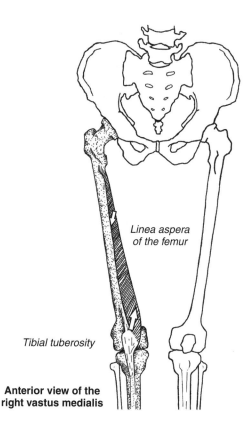

Linea aspera of the femur

Tibial tuberosity

Anterior view of the right vastus medialis

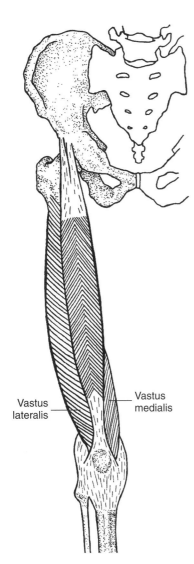

Vastus
lateralis

Vastus
medialis

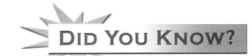

DID YOU KNOW?

The vastus lateralis is the largest of the four quadriceps femoris muscles. Pain attributed to the iliotibial band is often due to this large muscle that lies deep to it.

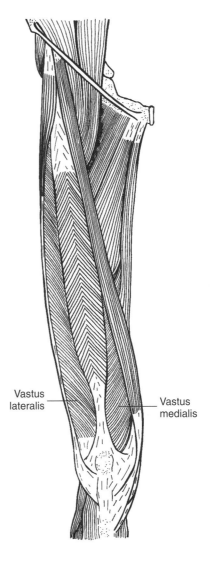

Vastus
lateralis

Vastus
medialis

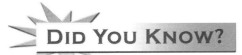

DID YOU KNOW?

The most distal aspect of the vastus medialis is bulky and may form a bulge in well-toned individuals.

Muscles of the Thigh

VASTUS INTERMEDIUS
(OF THE QUADRICEPS FEMORIS GROUP)

vas-tus in-ter-**mee**-dee-us

Action
Extension of the leg at
  the knee joint

Innervation
The femoral nerve

Arterial supply
The deep femoral artery

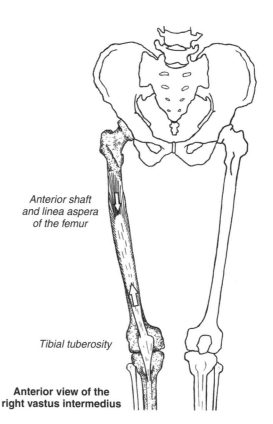

Anterior shaft
and linea aspera
of the femur

Tibial tuberosity

**Anterior view of the
right vastus intermedius**

ARTICULARIS GENUS

ar-**tik**-you-**la**-ris **je**-new

Action
Tenses and pulls the
  joint capsule of the
  knee joint proximally

Innervation
The femoral nerve

Arterial Supply
The deep femoral artery

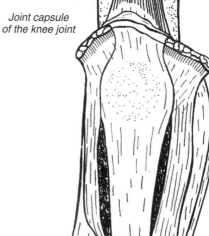

Anterior distal
femoral shaft

Joint capsule
of the knee joint

**Anterior view of the
right articularis genus**

Muscles of the Thigh

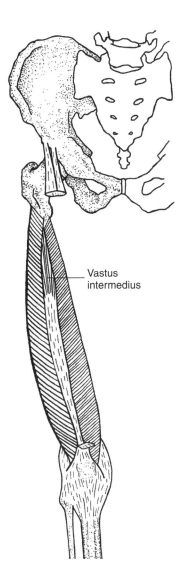

Vastus
intermedius

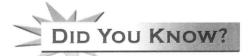

From most perspectives, the vastus intermedius is the deepest of the four quadriceps femoris muscles.

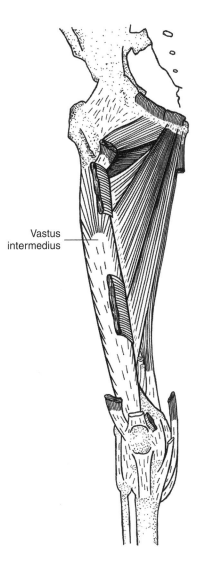

Vastus
intermedius

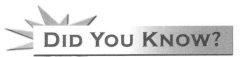

The articularis genus has no skeletal function to move bones. It acts to move the joint capsule of the knee so that it doesn't get pinched between the femur and tibia when the knee joint moves.

Muscles of the Thigh

PECTINEUS

(OF THE ADDUCTOR GROUP)

pek-**tin**-ee-us

Actions
Adduction of the thigh at
the hip joint
Flexion of the thigh at
the hip joint
Anterior tilt of the pelvis
at the hip joint
Elevation of the pelvis at
the hip joint

Innervation
The femoral nerve

Arterial Supply
The femoral artery and
the deep femoral
artery

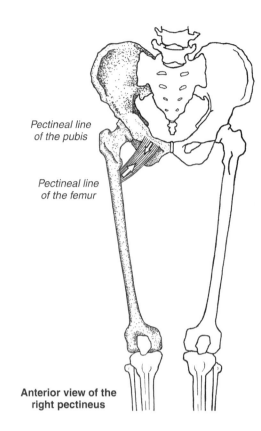

*Pectineal line
of the pubis*

*Pectineal line
of the femur*

**Anterior view of the
right pectineus**

GRACILIS

(OF THE ADDUCTOR GROUP)

gra-**sil**-is

Actions
Adduction of the thigh at
the hip joint
Flexion of the thigh at
the hip joint
Flexion of the leg at the
knee joint
Anterior tilt of the pelvis
at the hip joint
Medial rotation of the
leg at the knee joint
Elevation of the pelvis at
the hip joint

Innervation
The obturator nerve

Arterial Supply
The deep femoral artery

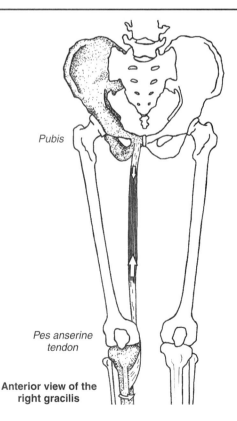

Pubis

*Pes anserine
tendon*

**Anterior view of the
right gracilis**

Muscles of the Thigh

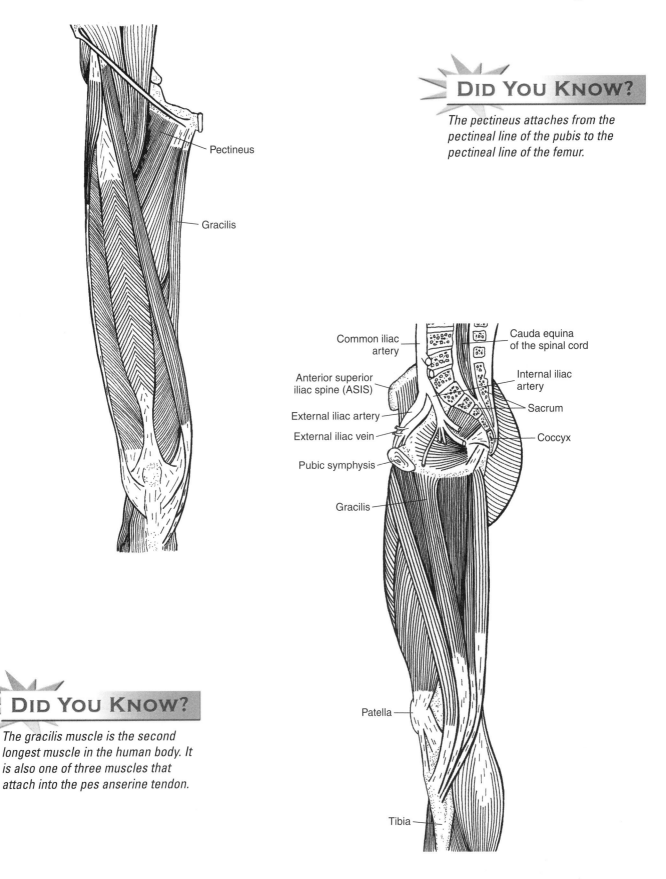

Pectineus

Gracilis

Common iliac artery

Cauda equina of the spinal cord

Anterior superior iliac spine (ASIS)

Internal iliac artery

External iliac artery

Sacrum

External iliac vein

Coccyx

Pubic symphysis

Gracilis

Patella

Tibia

Muscles of the Thigh

ADDUCTOR LONGUS

(OF THE ADDUCTOR GROUP)

ad-**duk**-tor **long**-us

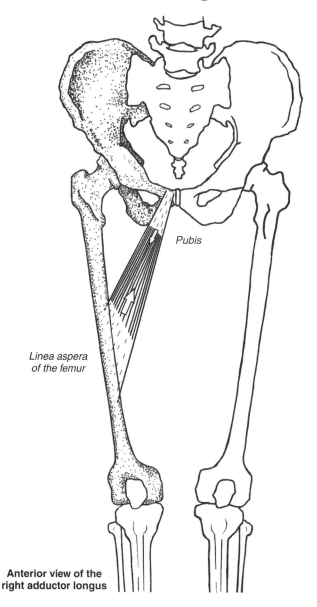

Pubis

Linea aspera
of the femur

**Anterior view of the
right adductor longus**

Actions	**Innervation**	**Arterial Supply**
Adduction of the thigh at the hip joint	The obturator nerve	The femoral artery and the deep femoral artery
Flexion of the thigh at the hip joint		
Anterior tilt of the pelvis at the hip joint		
Elevation of the pelvis at the hip joint		

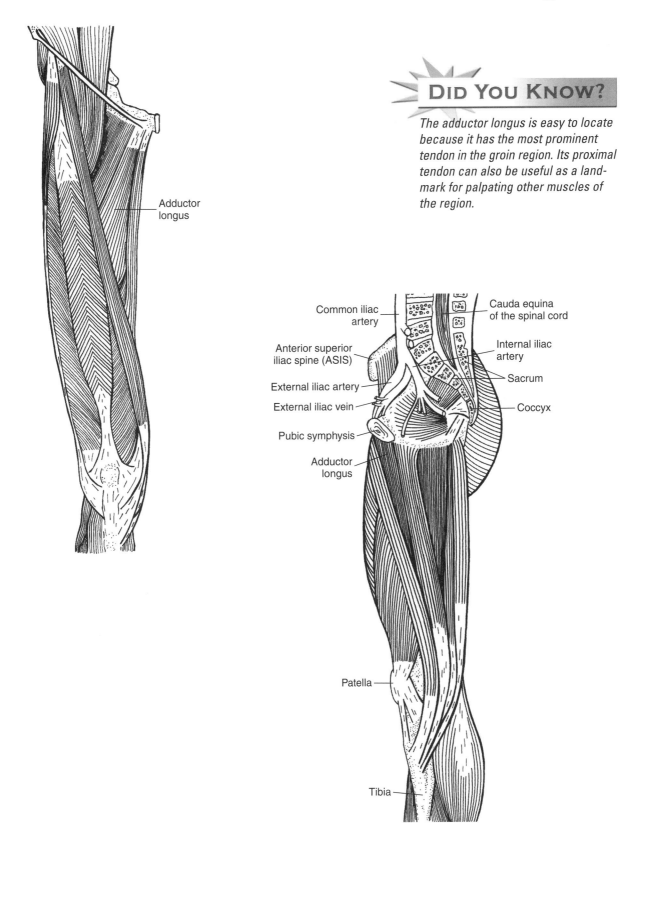

Adductor
longus

DID YOU KNOW?

The adductor longus is easy to locate because it has the most prominent tendon in the groin region. Its proximal tendon can also be useful as a landmark for palpating other muscles of the region.

Common iliac
artery

Cauda equina
of the spinal cord

Anterior superior
iliac spine (ASIS)

Internal iliac
artery

External iliac artery

Sacrum

External iliac vein

Coccyx

Pubic symphysis

Adductor
longus

Patella

Tibia

Muscles of the Thigh

ADDUCTOR BREVIS
(OF THE ADDUCTOR GROUP)

ad-**duk**-tor **bre**-vis

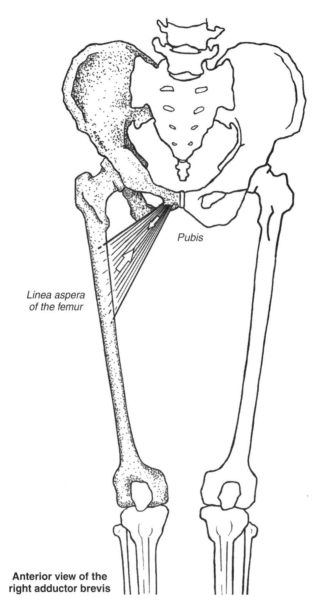

Pubis

Linea aspera
of the femur

**Anterior view of the
right adductor brevis**

Actions	Innervation	Arterial Supply
Adduction of the thigh at the hip joint Flexion of the thigh at the hip joint Anterior tilt of the pelvis at the hip joint Elevation of the pelvis at the hip joint	The obturator nerve	The femoral artery and the deep femoral artery

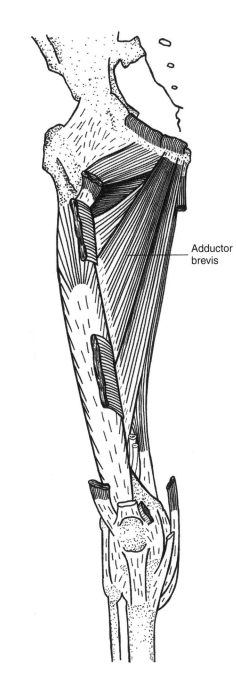

Adductor
brevis

Muscles of the Thigh

ADDUCTOR MAGNUS

(OF THE ADDUCTOR GROUP)

ad-**duk**-tor **mag**-nus

Actions
Adduction of the thigh at
  the hip joint
Extension of the thigh at
  the hip joint
Posterior tilt of the
  pelvis at the hip joint
Elevation of the pelvis
  at the hip joint

Innervation
The obturator nerve and
  the sciatic nerve

Arterial Supply
Anterior head: the
  femoral artery and the
  deep femoral artery
Posterior head: the deep
  femoral artery and the
  inferior gluteal artery

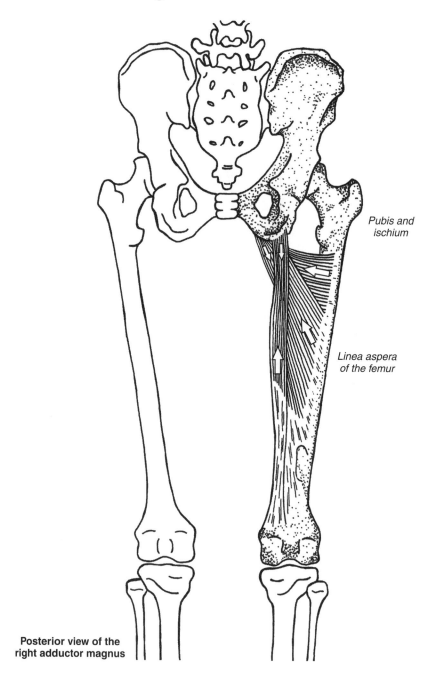

Pubis and
ischium

Linea aspera
of the femur

**Posterior view of the
right adductor magnus**

Muscles of the Thigh

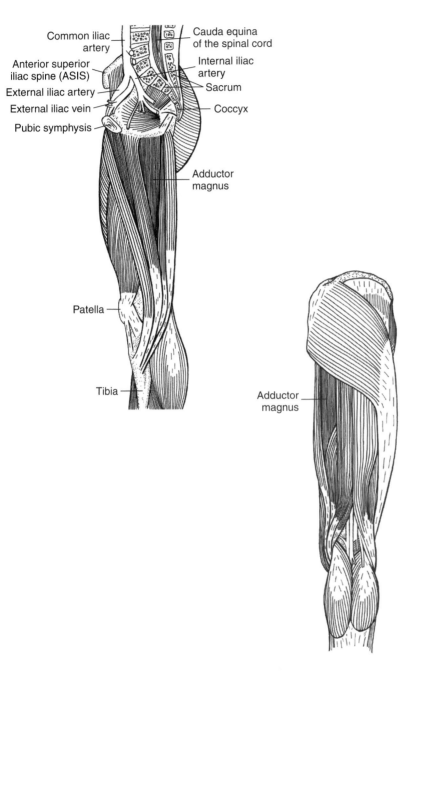

Common iliac artery

Cauda equina of the spinal cord

Anterior superior iliac spine (ASIS)

Internal iliac artery

External iliac artery

Sacrum

External iliac vein

Coccyx

Pubic symphysis

Adductor magnus

Patella

Tibia

Adductor magnus

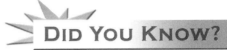

DID YOU KNOW?

Because the adductor magnus is so far posterior, attaches to the ischial tuberosity, and can extend the thigh at the hip joint, it is sometimes called the 4th hamstring.

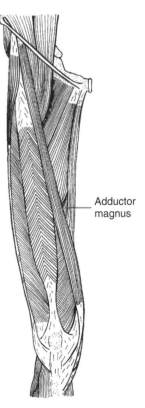

Adductor magnus

Muscles of the Thigh

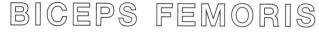

BICEPS FEMORIS

(OF THE HAMSTRING GROUP)

by-seps **fem**-o-ris

Actions
Flexion of the leg at the knee joint (entire muscle)

Extension of the thigh at the hip joint (long head)

Posterior tilt of the pelvis at the hip joint (long head)

Lateral rotation of the leg at the knee joint (entire muscle)

Adduction of the thigh at the hip joint (long head)

Lateral rotation of the thigh at the hip joint (long head)

Innervation
The sciatic nerve

Arterial Supply
Long head: the inferior gluteal artery and perforating branches of the deep femoral artery

Short head: perforating branches of the deep femoral artery

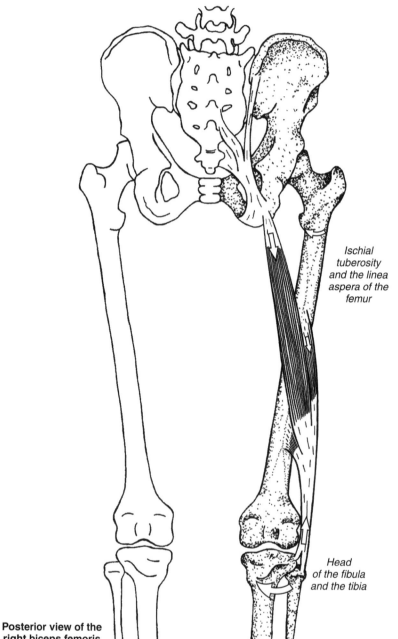

Ischial tuberosity and the linea aspera of the femur

Head of the fibula and the tibia

Posterior view of the right biceps femoris

Muscles of the Thigh

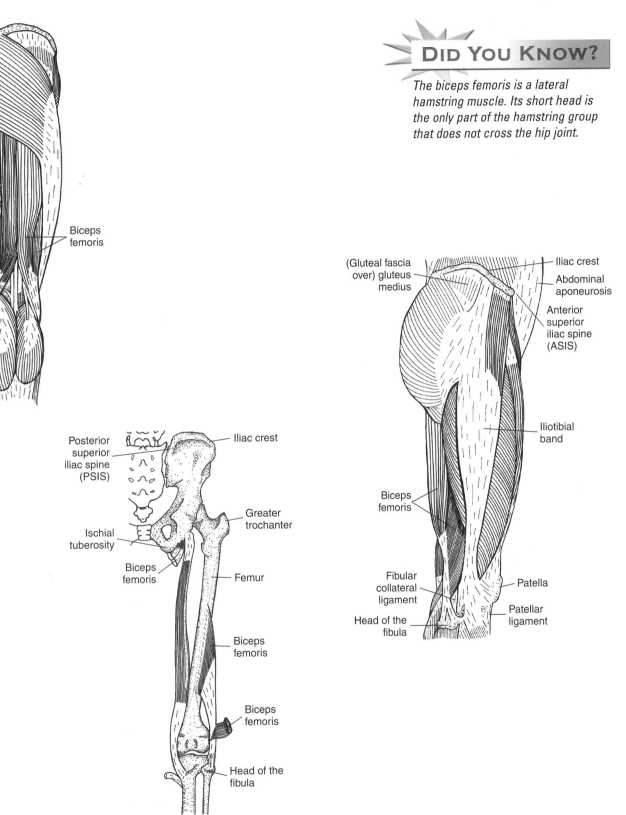

DID YOU KNOW?

The biceps femoris is a lateral hamstring muscle. Its short head is the only part of the hamstring group that does not cross the hip joint.

Biceps femoris

(Gluteal fascia over) gluteus medius

Iliac crest

Abdominal aponeurosis

Anterior superior iliac spine (ASIS)

Iliotibial band

Biceps femoris

Posterior superior iliac spine (PSIS)

Iliac crest

Greater trochanter

Ischial tuberosity

Biceps femoris

Femur

Biceps femoris

Biceps femoris

Head of the fibula

Fibular collateral ligament

Head of the fibula

Patella

Patellar ligament

Muscles of the Thigh

Actions
Flexion of the leg at the
  knee joint
Extension of the thigh at
  the hip joint
Posterior tilt of the
  pelvis at the hip joint
Medial rotation of the
  leg at the knee joint
Medial rotation of the
  thigh at the hip joint

Innervation
The sciatic nerve

Arterial Supply
The inferior gluteal
  artery and perforating
  branches of the deep
  femoral artery

SEMITENDINOSUS
(OF THE HAMSTRING GROUP)

sem-i-ten-di-no-sus

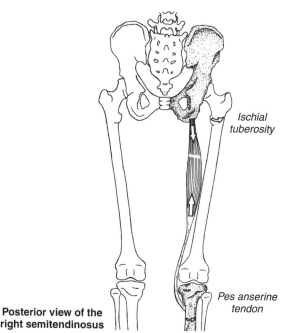

Ischial
tuberosity

Pes anserine
tendon

**Posterior view of the
right semitendinosus**

Actions
Flexion of the leg at the
  knee joint
Extension of the thigh at
  the hip joint
Posterior tilt of the
  pelvis at the hip joint
Medial rotation of the
  leg at the knee joint
Medial rotation of the
  thigh at the hip joint

Innervation
The sciatic nerve

Arterial Supply
The inferior gluteal
  artery and perforating
  branches of the deep
  femoral artery

SEMIMEMBRANOSUS
(OF THE HAMSTRING GROUP)

sem-i-mem-bra-no-sus

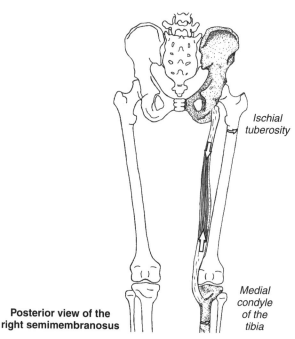

Ischial
tuberosity

Medial
condyle
of the
tibia

**Posterior view of the
right semimembranosus**

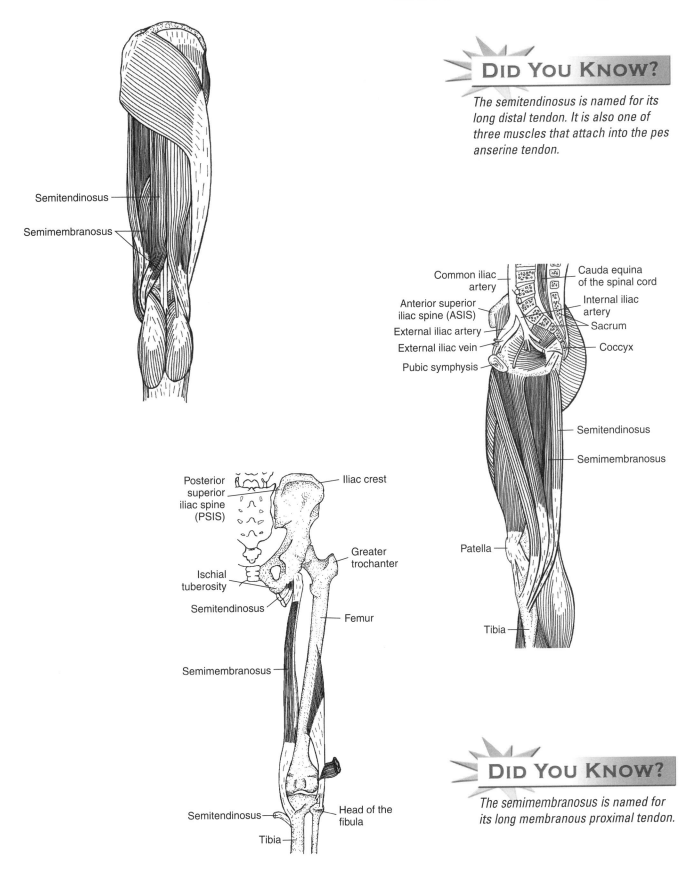

Semitendinosus

Semimembranosus

Common iliac artery

Anterior superior iliac spine (ASIS)

External iliac artery

External iliac vein

Pubic symphysis

Cauda equina of the spinal cord

Internal iliac artery

Sacrum

Coccyx

Semitendinosus

Semimembranosus

Patella

Tibia

Posterior superior iliac spine (PSIS)

Iliac crest

Greater trochanter

Ischial tuberosity

Semitendinosus

Femur

Semimembranosus

Semitendinosus

Head of the fibula

Tibia

Muscles of the Thigh

ANTERIOR VIEW OF THE RIGHT THIGH (SUPERFICIAL)

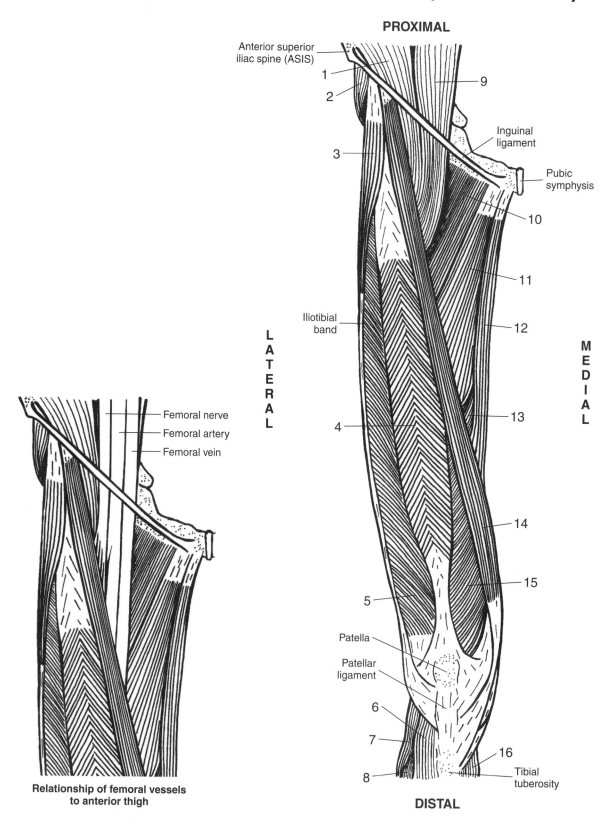

PROXIMAL

Anterior superior
iliac spine (ASIS)

1

2

3

9

Inguinal
ligament

Pubic
symphysis

10

11

12

Iliotibial
band

13

L
A
T
E
R
A
L

M
E
D
I
A
L

4

14

15

5

Patella

Patellar
ligament

6

7

8

16

Tibial
tuberosity

DISTAL

Femoral nerve

Femoral artery

Femoral vein

**Relationship of femoral vessels
to anterior thigh**

ANTERIOR VIEW OF THE RIGHT THIGH (DEEP)

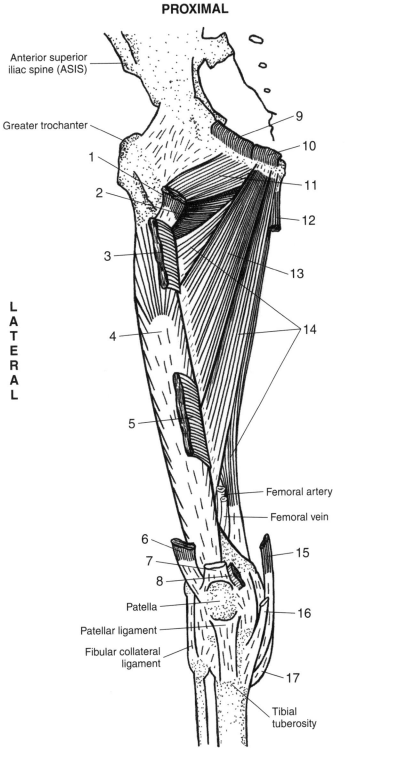

PROXIMAL

Anterior superior
iliac spine (ASIS)

Greater trochanter

1

2

3

4

5

6

7

8

Patella

Patellar ligament

Fibular collateral
ligament

9

10

11

12

13

14

Femoral artery

Femoral vein

15

16

17

Tibial
tuberosity

L
A
T
E
R
A
L

M
E
D
I
A
L

DISTAL

Muscles of the Thigh

POSTERIOR VIEW OF THE RIGHT THIGH (SUPERFICIAL)

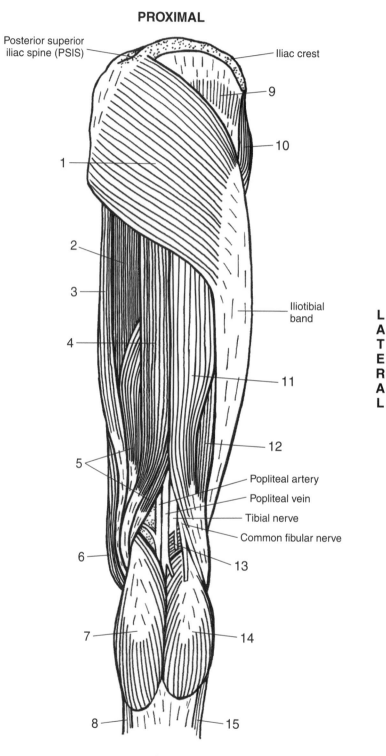

PROXIMAL

Posterior superior iliac spine (PSIS)

Iliac crest

9

10

1

2

3

4

Iliotibial band

11

12

Popliteal artery

Popliteal vein

Tibial nerve

Common fibular nerve

5

6

13

7

14

8

15

MEDIAL

LATERAL

DISTAL

POSTERIOR VIEW OF THE RIGHT THIGH (DEEP)

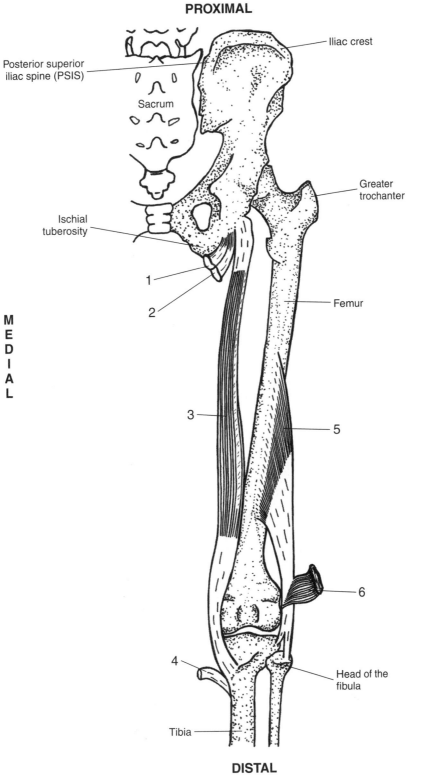

PROXIMAL

Iliac crest

Posterior superior
iliac spine (PSIS)

Sacrum

Greater
trochanter

Ischial
tuberosity

1

2

Femur

M E D I A L

L A T E R A L

3

5

6

4

Head of the
fibula

Tibia

DISTAL

Muscles of the Thigh

LATERAL VIEW OF THE RIGHT THIGH

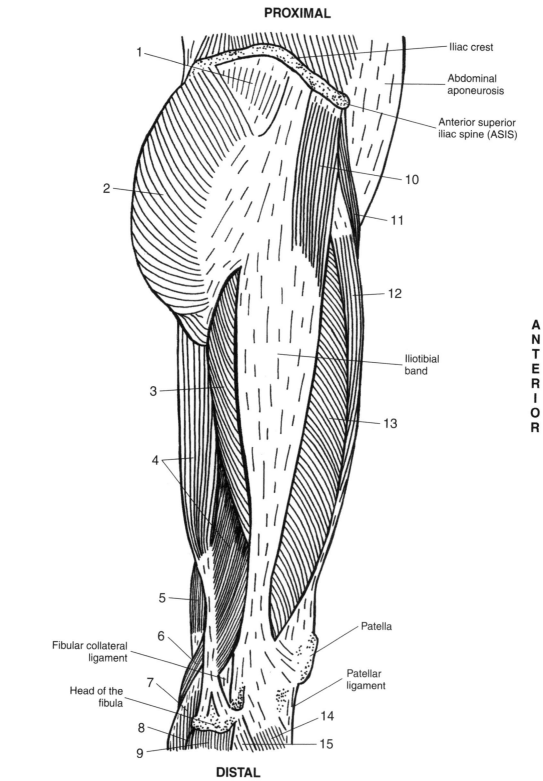

PROXIMAL

1

2

3

4

5

6

7

8

9

POSTERIOR

ANTERIOR

Iliac crest

Abdominal aponeurosis

Anterior superior iliac spine (ASIS)

10

11

12

Iliotibial band

13

Patella

Patellar ligament

14

15

Fibular collateral ligament

Head of the fibula

DISTAL

MEDIAL VIEW OF THE RIGHT THIGH

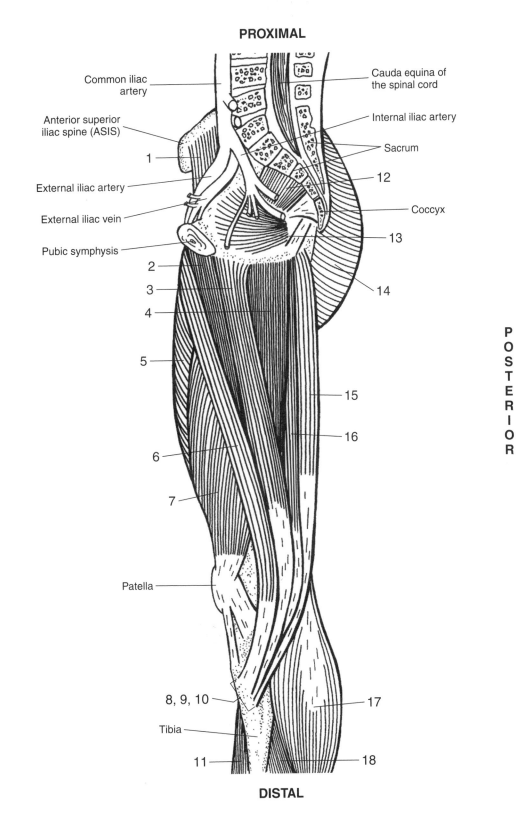

PROXIMAL

Common iliac artery

Cauda equina of the spinal cord

Anterior superior iliac spine (ASIS)

Internal iliac artery

1

Sacrum

External iliac artery

12

External iliac vein

Coccyx

Pubic symphysis

13

2

14

3

4

ANTERIOR

POSTERIOR

5

15

16

6

7

Patella

8, 9, 10

17

Tibia

11

18

DISTAL

Muscles of the Leg

ANTERIOR VIEW OF THE RIGHT LEG

PROXIMAL

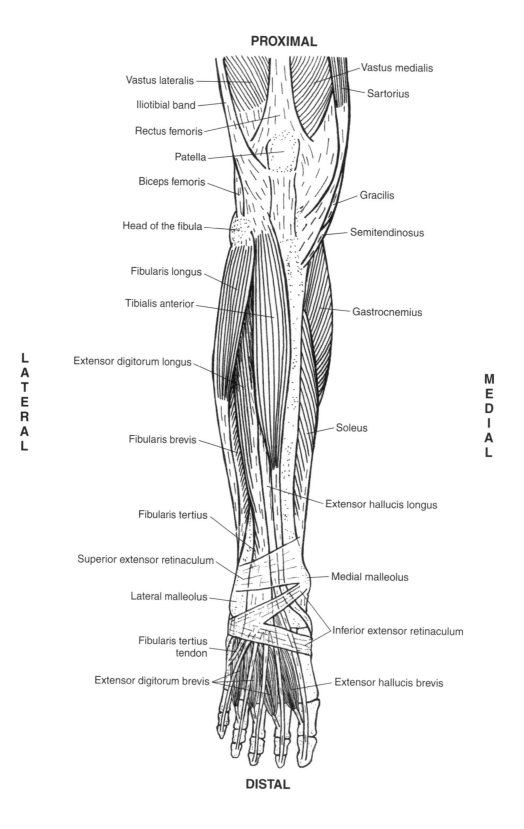

Vastus lateralis

Iliotibial band

Rectus femoris

Patella

Biceps femoris

Head of the fibula

Fibularis longus

Tibialis anterior

Extensor digitorum longus

Fibularis brevis

Fibularis tertius

Superior extensor retinaculum

Lateral malleolus

Fibularis tertius tendon

Extensor digitorum brevis

Vastus medialis

Sartorius

Gracilis

Semitendinosus

Gastrocnemius

Soleus

Extensor hallucis longus

Medial malleolus

Inferior extensor retinaculum

Extensor hallucis brevis

L A T E R A L

M E D I A L

DISTAL

POSTERIOR VIEW OF THE RIGHT LEG (SUPERFICIAL)

PROXIMAL

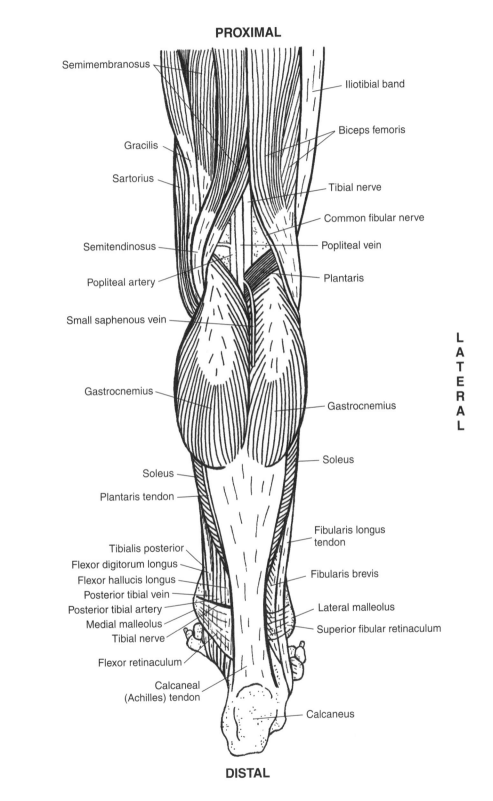

Semimembranosus

Gracilis

Sartorius

Semitendinosus

Popliteal artery

Small saphenous vein

MEDIAL

Gastrocnemius

Soleus

Plantaris tendon

Tibialis posterior
Flexor digitorum longus
Flexor hallucis longus
Posterior tibial vein
Posterior tibial artery
Medial malleolus
Tibial nerve

Flexor retinaculum

Calcaneal
(Achilles) tendon

Iliotibial band

Biceps femoris

Tibial nerve

Common fibular nerve

Popliteal vein

Plantaris

LATERAL

Gastrocnemius

Soleus

Fibularis longus
tendon

Fibularis brevis

Lateral malleolus

Superior fibular retinaculum

Calcaneus

DISTAL

Muscles of the Leg

POSTERIOR VIEW OF THE RIGHT LEG (INTERMEDIATE)

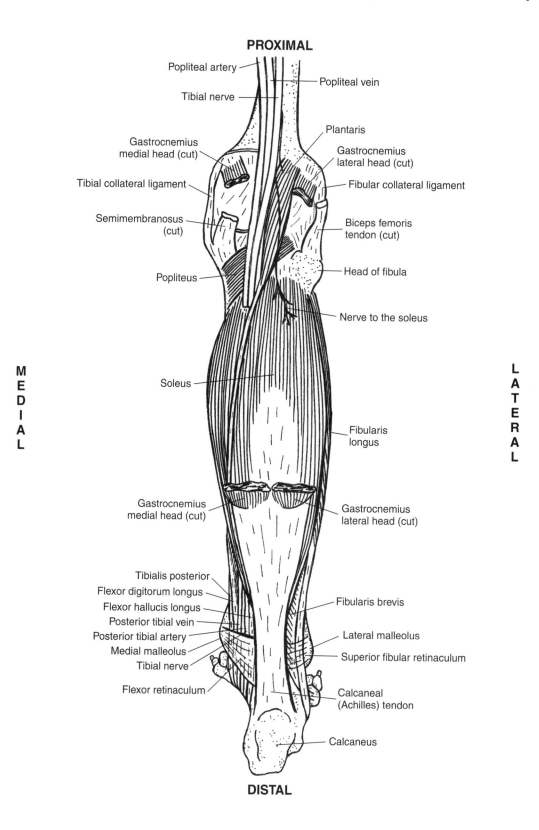

PROXIMAL

Popliteal artery

Tibial nerve

Popliteal vein

Plantaris

Gastrocnemius medial head (cut)

Gastrocnemius lateral head (cut)

Tibial collateral ligament

Fibular collateral ligament

Semimembranosus (cut)

Biceps femoris tendon (cut)

Popliteus

Head of fibula

Nerve to the soleus

MEDIAL

LATERAL

Soleus

Fibularis longus

Gastrocnemius medial head (cut)

Gastrocnemius lateral head (cut)

Tibialis posterior
Flexor digitorum longus
Flexor hallucis longus
Posterior tibial vein
Posterior tibial artery
Medial malleolus
Tibial nerve

Fibularis brevis

Lateral malleolus

Superior fibular retinaculum

Flexor retinaculum

Calcaneal (Achilles) tendon

Calcaneus

DISTAL

POSTERIOR VIEW OF THE RIGHT LEG (DEEP)

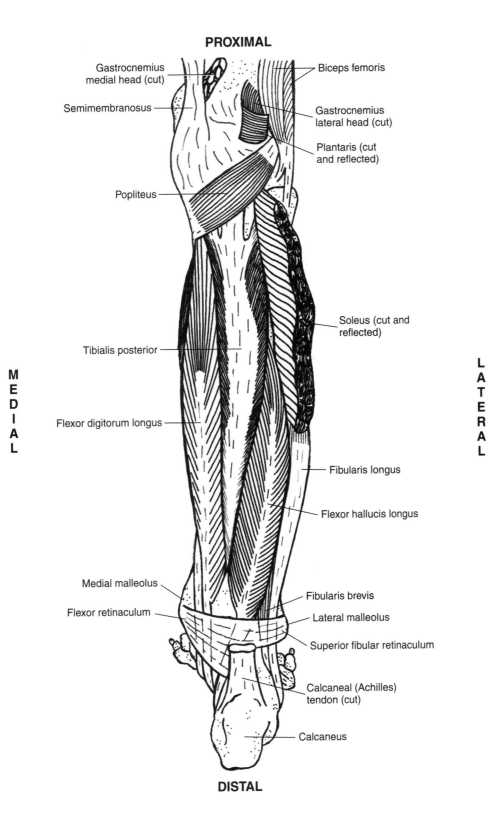

PROXIMAL

Gastrocnemius medial head (cut)

Semimembranosus

Popliteus

Tibialis posterior

Flexor digitorum longus

Biceps femoris

Gastrocnemius lateral head (cut)

Plantaris (cut and reflected)

Soleus (cut and reflected)

Fibularis longus

Flexor hallucis longus

Medial malleolus

Flexor retinaculum

Fibularis brevis

Lateral malleolus

Superior fibular retinaculum

Calcaneal (Achilles) tendon (cut)

Calcaneus

MEDIAL

LATERAL

DISTAL

Muscles of the Leg

LATERAL VIEW OF THE RIGHT LEG

PROXIMAL

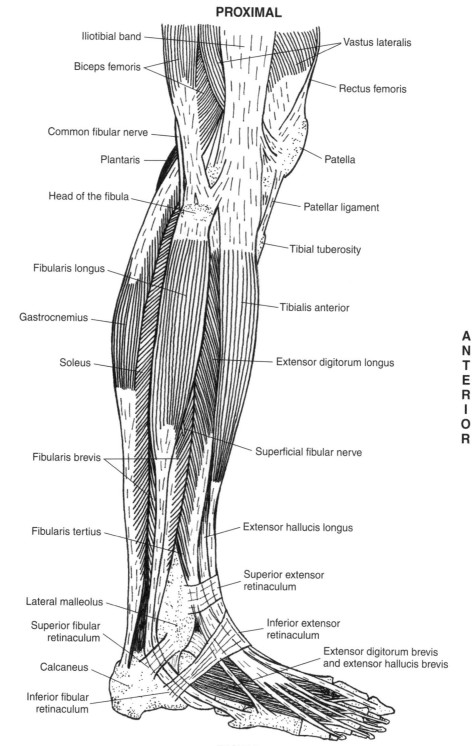

Iliotibial band

Biceps femoris

Common fibular nerve

Plantaris

Head of the fibula

Fibularis longus

Gastrocnemius

Soleus

Fibularis brevis

Fibularis tertius

Lateral malleolus

Superior fibular retinaculum

Calcaneus

Inferior fibular retinaculum

Vastus lateralis

Rectus femoris

Patella

Patellar ligament

Tibial tuberosity

Tibialis anterior

Extensor digitorum longus

Superficial fibular nerve

Extensor hallucis longus

Superior extensor retinaculum

Inferior extensor retinaculum

Extensor digitorum brevis and extensor hallucis brevis

POSTERIOR

ANTERIOR

DISTAL

MEDIAL VIEW OF THE RIGHT LEG

PROXIMAL

Gracilis

Rectus femoris

Sartorius

Vastus medialis

Patella

Patellar ligament

Tibial tuberosity

Pes anserine tendon

Tibialis anterior

Tibia

Superior extensor retinaculum

Inferior extensor retinaculum

Extensor hallucis longus

Extensor digitorum longus

Adductor magnus

Semitendinosus

Semimembranosus

Gastrocnemius

Soleus

Plantaris

Flexor digitorum longus

Medial malleolus

Tibialis posterior

Flexor hallucis longus

Calcaneal (Achilles) tendon

Flexor retinaculum

Calcaneus

ANTERIOR

POSTERIOR

DISTAL

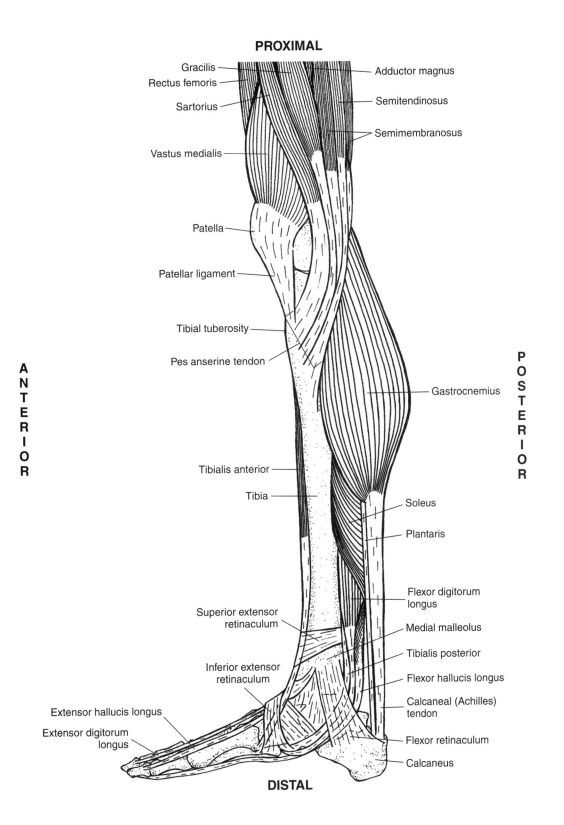

Muscles of the Leg

TIBIALIS ANTERIOR
(IN THE ANTERIOR COMPARTMENT)

tib-ee-**a**-lis an-**tee**-ri-or

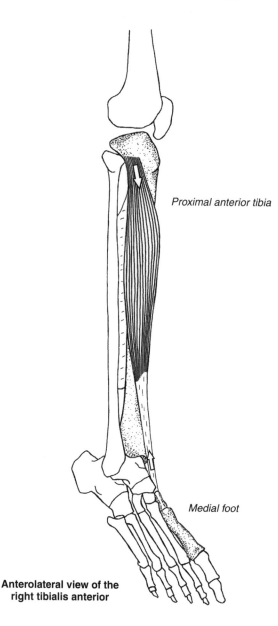

Proximal anterior tibia

Medial foot

**Anterolateral view of the
right tibialis anterior**

Actions	**Innervation**	**Arterial Supply**
Dorsiflexion of the foot at the ankle joint Inversion of the foot at the tarsal joints	The deep fibular nerve	The anterior tibial artery

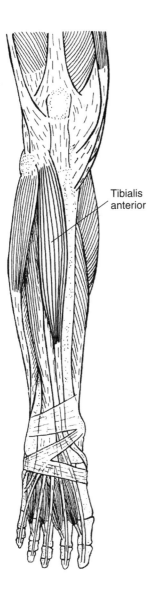

Tibialis
anterior

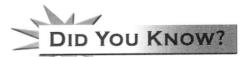

DID YOU KNOW?

The tibialis anterior is the most commonly affected muscle when a person has shin splints. The tibialis anterior is also one of the two 'stirrup muscles'.

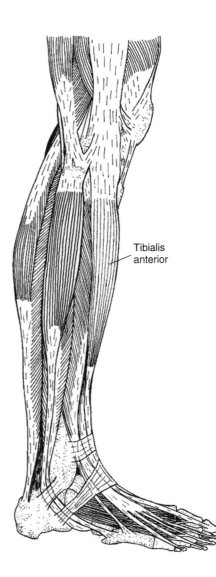

Tibialis
anterior

Muscles of the Leg

EXTENSOR HALLUCIS LONGUS

(IN THE ANTERIOR COMPARTMENT)

eks-**ten**-sor hal-**oo**-sis **long**-us

Actions
Extension of the big toe (toe #1) at the meta-tarsophalangeal joint and the interphalan-geal joint
Dorsiflexion of the foot at the ankle joint
Inversion of the foot at the tarsal joints

Innervation
The deep fibular nerve

Arterial Supply
The anterior tibial artery

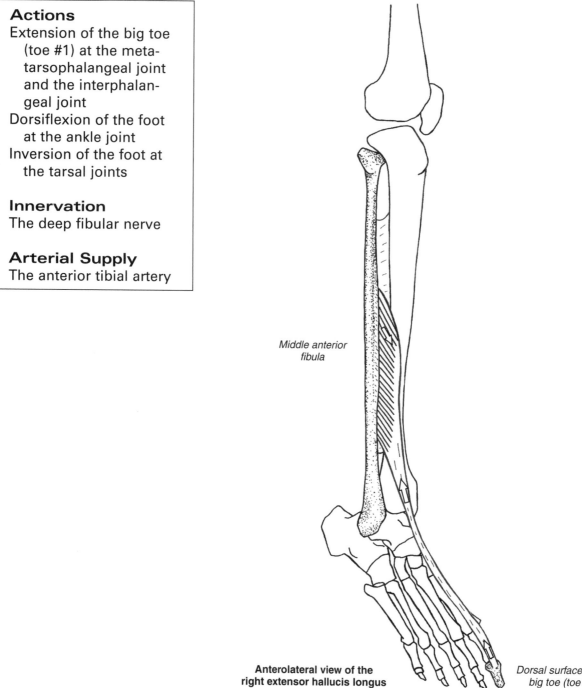

Middle anterior fibula

Anterolateral view of the right extensor hallucis longus

Dorsal surface of the big toe (toe #1)

Muscles of the Leg

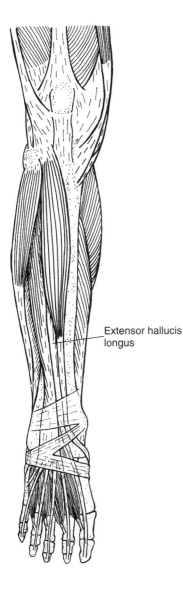

Extensor hallucis longus

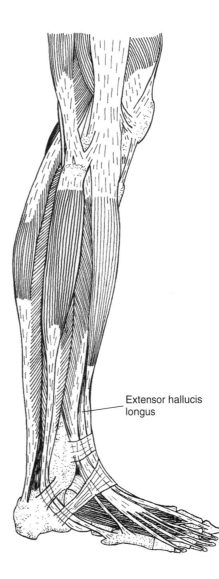

Extensor hallucis longus

Muscles of the Leg

EXTENSOR DIGITORUM LONGUS

(IN THE ANTERIOR COMPARTMENT)

eks-**ten**-sor dij-i-**toe**-rum **long**-us

Actions
Extension of toes #2-5 at
the metatarsophalan-
geal joint and the
proximal and distal
interphalangeal joints
Dorsiflexion of the foot
at the ankle joint
Eversion of the foot at
the tarsal joints

Innervation
The deep fibular nerve

Arterial Supply
The anterior tibial artery

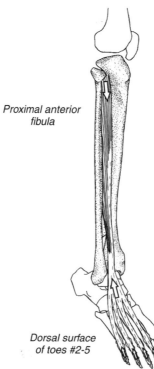

Proximal anterior
fibula

Dorsal surface
of toes #2-5

**Anterolateral view of the
right extensor digitorum longus**

FIBULARIS TERTIUS

(IN THE ANTERIOR COMPARTMENT)

fib-you **la**-ris **ter**-she-us

Actions
Dorsiflexion of the foot
at the ankle joint
Eversion of the foot at
the tarsal joints

Innervation
The deep fibular nerve

Arterial Supply
The anterior tibial artery

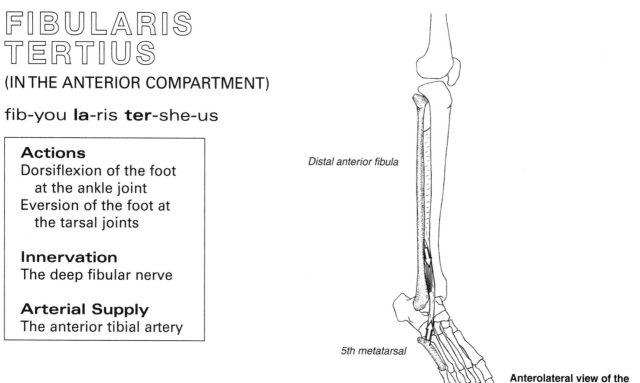

Distal anterior fibula

5th metatarsal

**Anterolateral view of the
right fibularis tertius**

Muscles of the Leg

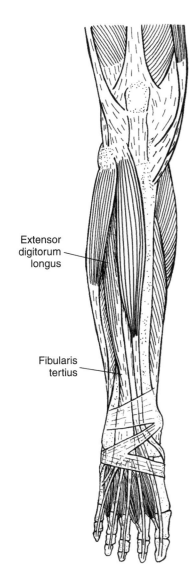

Extensor
digitorum
longus

Fibularis
tertius

The most distal and lateral part of the extensor digitorum longus does not attach onto 'digits', therefore it is given another name, the fibularis tertius. Therefore, the fibularis tertius is actually the most distal and lateral part of the extensor digitorum longus. It is given a separate name because it does not attach onto 'digits'.

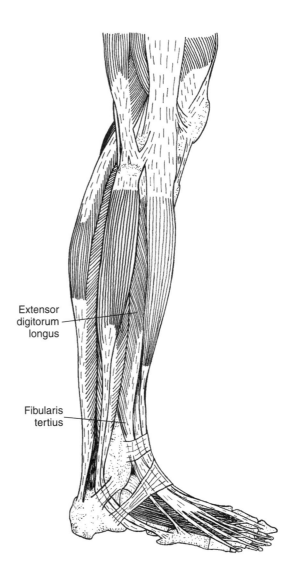

Extensor
digitorum
longus

Fibularis
tertius

Muscles of the Leg

FIBULARIS LONGUS

(IN THE LATERAL COMPARTMENT)

fib-you-**la**-ris **long**-us

Actions
Eversion of the foot at
the tarsal joints
Plantarflexion of the foot
at the ankle joint

Innervation
The superficial fibular
nerve

Arterial Supply
The fibular artery

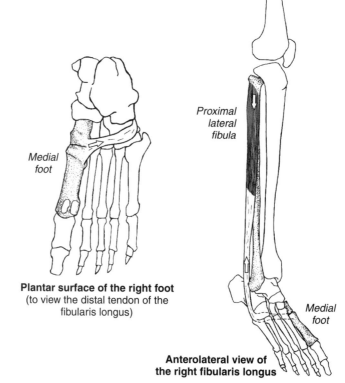

Medial foot

Proximal lateral fibula

Medial foot

Plantar surface of the right foot
(to view the distal tendon of the
fibularis longus)

**Anterolateral view of
the right fibularis longus**

FIBULARIS BREVIS

(IN THE LATERAL COMPARTMENT)

fib-you-**la**-ris **bre**-vis

Actions
Eversion of the foot at
the tarsal joints
Plantarflexion of the foot
at the ankle joint

Innervation
The superficial fibular
nerve

Arterial Supply
The fibular artery

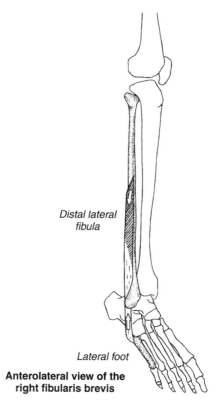

Distal lateral fibula

Lateral foot

**Anterolateral view of the
right fibularis brevis**

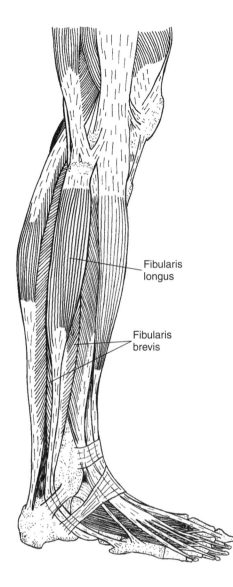

Fibularis
longus

Fibularis
brevis

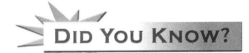

DID YOU KNOW?

The fibularis longus, along with the tibialis anterior, are often called the 'stirrup muscles' because their distal tendons form a stirrup around the foot.

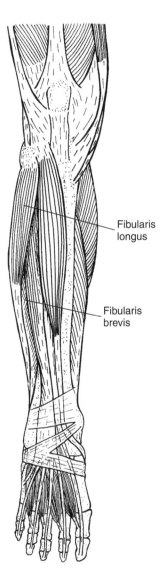

Fibularis
longus

Fibularis
brevis

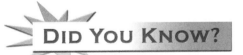

DID YOU KNOW?

The fibularis brevis is located deep to the fibularis longus and has the same actions as the fibularis longus.

Muscles of the Leg

GASTROCNEMIUS ("GASTROCS")

(OF THE TRICEPS SURAE AND IN THE SUPERFICIAL POSTERIOR COMPARTMENT)

gas-trok-**nee**-me-us

Actions
Plantarflexion of the foot at the ankle joint
Flexion of the leg at the knee joint
Inversion of the foot at the tarsal joints

Innervation
The tibial nerve

Arterial Supply
Sural branches of the popliteal artery

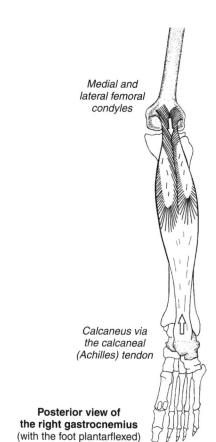

Medial and lateral femoral condyles

Calcaneus via the calcaneal (Achilles) tendon

Posterior view of the right gastrocnemius
(with the foot plantarflexed)

SOLEUS

(OF THE TRICEPS SURAE AND IN THE SUPERFICIAL POSTERIOR COMPARTMENT)

so-lee-us

Actions
Plantarflexion of the foot at the ankle joint
Inversion of the foot at the tarsal joints

Innervation
The tibial nerve

Arterial Supply
Sural branches of the popliteal artery

Posterior tibia and fibula

Calcaneus via the calcaneal (Achilles) tendon

Posterior view of the right soleus
(with the foot plantarflexed)

Muscles of the Leg

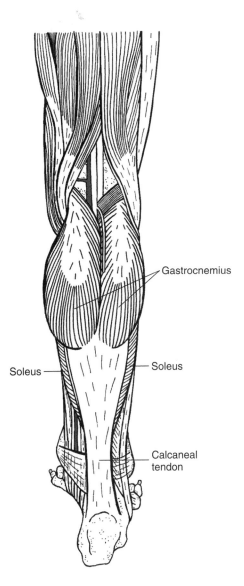

Gastrocnemius

Soleus

Soleus

Calcaneal tendon

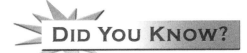

The gastrocnemius (and soleus) attaches into the calcaneus via the calcaneal tendon, which is more well known as the **Achilles** tendon.

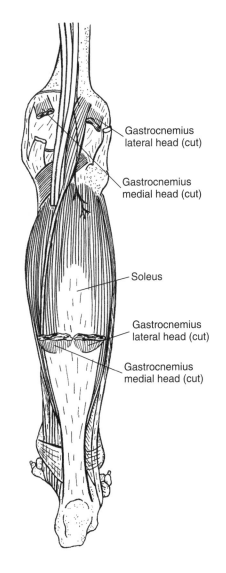

Gastrocnemius lateral head (cut)

Gastrocnemius medial head (cut)

Soleus

Gastrocnemius lateral head (cut)

Gastrocnemius medial head (cut)

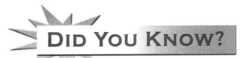

The soleus is actually quite large and massive, accounting for the contours of the gastrocnemius being so visible. "Behind every great gastrocnemius is a great soleus ☺."

Muscles of the Leg

PLANTARIS
(IN THE SUPERFICIAL POSTERIOR COMPARTMENT)

plan-**ta**-ris

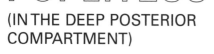

Actions
Plantarflexion of the foot
  at the ankle joint
Flexion of the leg at the
  knee joint

Innervation
The tibial nerve

Arterial Supply
Sural branches of the
  popliteal artery

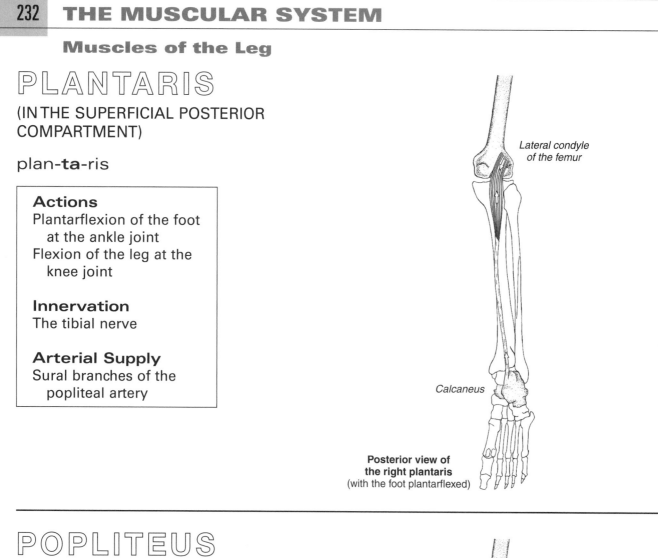

*Lateral condyle
of the femur*

Calcaneus

**Posterior view of
the right plantaris**
(with the foot plantarflexed)

POPLITEUS
(IN THE DEEP POSTERIOR COMPARTMENT)

pop-**lit**-ee-us

Actions
Medial rotation of the
  leg at the knee joint
Flexion of the leg at the
  knee joint
Lateral rotation of the
  thigh at the knee joint

Innervation
The tibial nerve

Arterial Supply
Branches of the popliteal
  artery

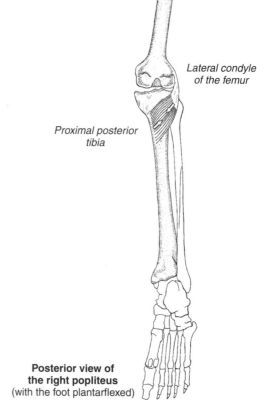

*Lateral condyle
of the femur*

*Proximal posterior
tibia*

**Posterior view of
the right popliteus**
(with the foot plantarflexed)

Muscles of the Leg

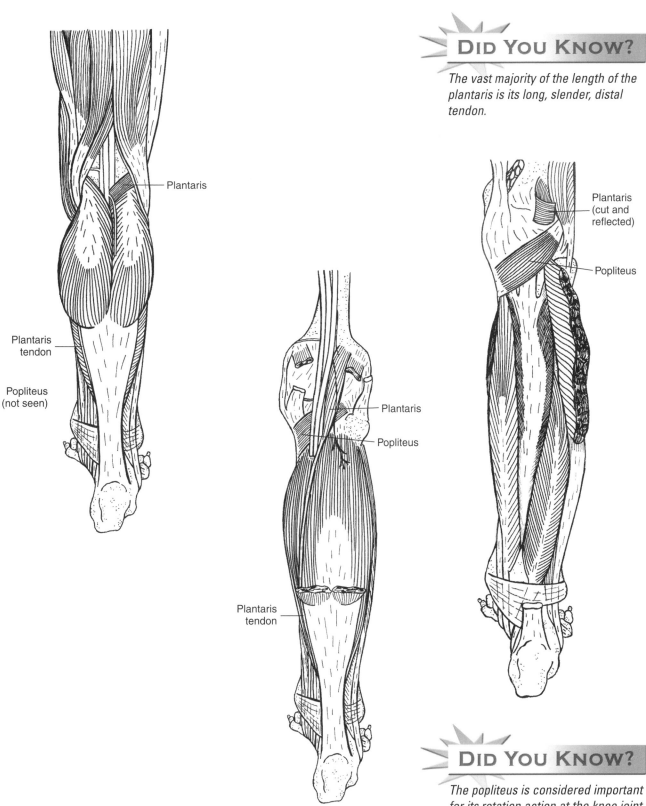

Plantaris

Plantaris
tendon

Popliteus
(not seen)

Plantaris

Popliteus

Plantaris
tendon

Plantaris
(cut and
reflected)

Popliteus

DID YOU KNOW?

The vast majority of the length of the plantaris is its long, slender, distal tendon.

DID YOU KNOW?

The popliteus is considered important for its rotation action at the knee joint, which is said to "unlock" the extended knee.

Muscles of the Leg

TIBIALIS POSTERIOR
(IN THE DEEP POSTERIOR COMPARTMENT)

tib-ee-**a**-lis pos-**tee**-ri-or

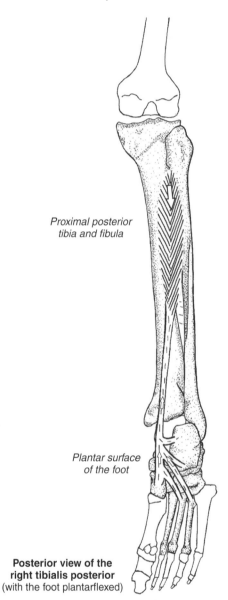

Proximal posterior tibia and fibula

Plantar surface of the foot

Posterior view of the right tibialis posterior
(with the foot plantarflexed)

Actions	**Innervation**	**Arterial Supply**
Plantarflexion of the foot at the ankle joint	The tibial nerve	The posterior tibial artery
Inversion of the foot at the tarsal joints		

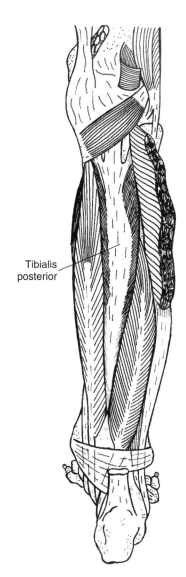

Tibialis
posterior

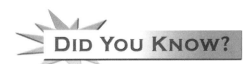

DID YOU KNOW?

*The tibialis posterior is 'Tom' of the
'Tom, Dick, and Harry muscles.'
'Tom, Dick, and Harry muscles' are
grouped together because their distal
tendons all cross posterior to the
medial malleolus of the tibia.*

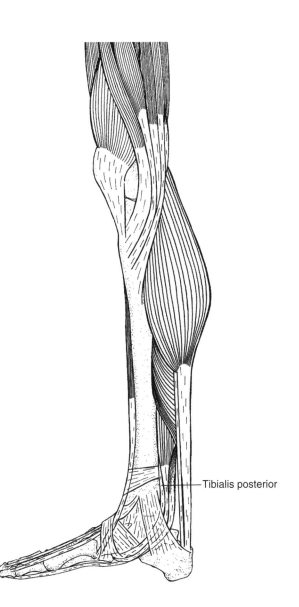

Tibialis posterior

Muscles of the Leg

FLEXOR DIGITORUM LONGUS

(IN THE DEEP POSTERIOR COMPARTMENT)

fleks-or dij-i-**toe**-rum **long**-us

Actions
Flexion of toes #2-5 at
the metatarsophalan-
geal joint and the
proximal and distal
interphalangeal joints
Plantarflexion of the foot
at the ankle joint
Inversion of the foot at
the tarsal joints

Innervation
The tibial nerve

Arterial Supply
The posterior tibial
artery

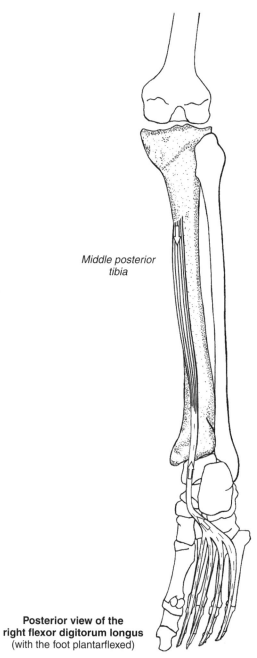

*Middle posterior
tibia*

**Posterior view of the
right flexor digitorum longus**
(with the foot plantarflexed)

Plantar surface of toes #2-5

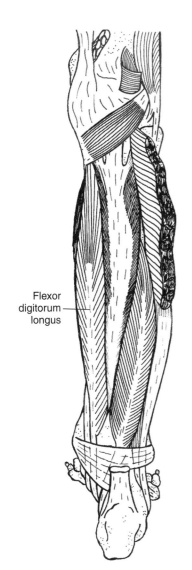

Flexor
digitorum
longus

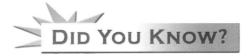

DID YOU KNOW?

The flexor digitorum longus is 'Dick' of the 'Tom, Dick, and Harry muscles.' 'Tom, Dick, and Harry muscles' are grouped together because their distal tendons all cross posterior to the medial malleolus of the tibia.

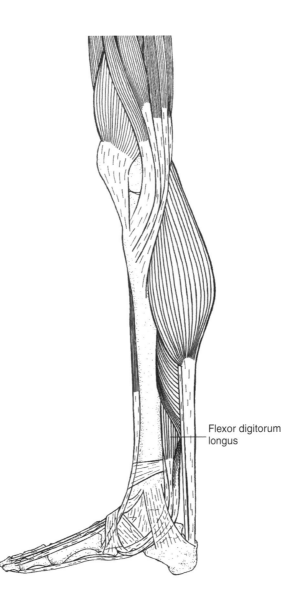

Flexor digitorum
longus

Muscles of the Leg

FLEXOR HALLUCIS LONGUS
(IN THE DEEP POSTERIOR COMPARTMENT)

fleks-or hal-**oo**-sis **long**-us

Actions
Flexion of the big toe
(toe #1) at the meta-
tarsophalangeal joint
and the interphalan-
geal joint
Plantarflexion of the foot
at the ankle joint
Inversion of the foot at
the tarsal joints

Innervation
The tibial nerve

Arterial Supply
The posterior tibial
artery

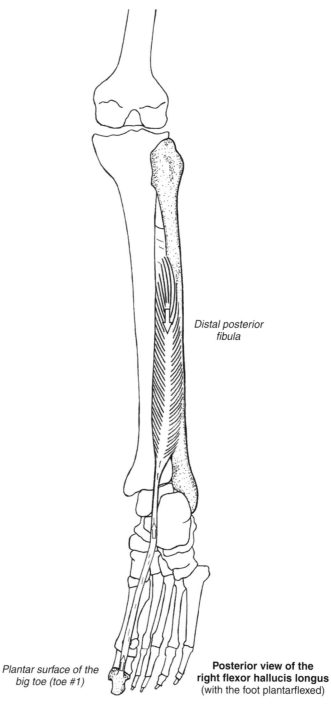

*Distal posterior
fibula*

*Plantar surface of the
big toe (toe #1)*

**Posterior view of the
right flexor hallucis longus**
(with the foot plantarflexed)

Muscles of the Leg

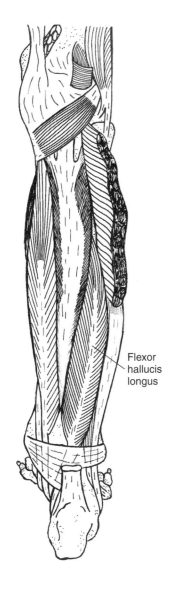

Flexor
hallucis
longus

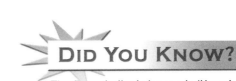

DID YOU KNOW?

The flexor hallucis longus is 'Harry' of the 'Tom, Dick, and Harry muscles.' 'Tom, Dick, and Harry muscles' are grouped together because their distal tendons all cross posterior to the medial malleolus of the tibia.

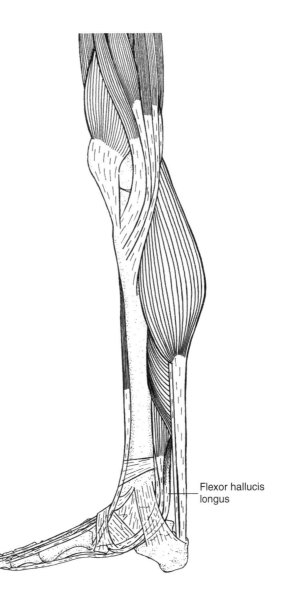

Flexor hallucis
longus

Muscles of the Leg

ANTERIOR VIEW OF THE RIGHT LEG

PROXIMAL

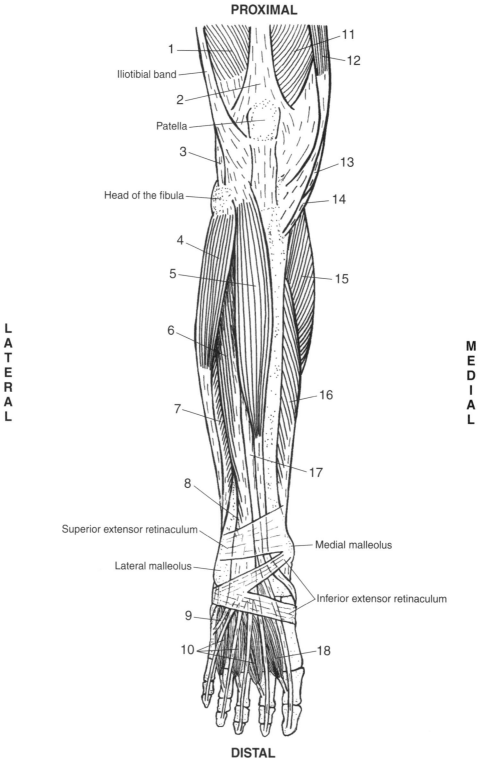

1

Iliotibial band

2

Patella

3

Head of the fibula

4

5

6

7

8

Superior extensor retinaculum

Lateral malleolus

9

10

11

12

13

14

15

16

17

Medial malleolus

Inferior extensor retinaculum

18

L
A
T
E
R
A
L

M
E
D
I
A
L

DISTAL

POSTERIOR VIEW OF THE RIGHT LEG (SUPERFICIAL)

PROXIMAL

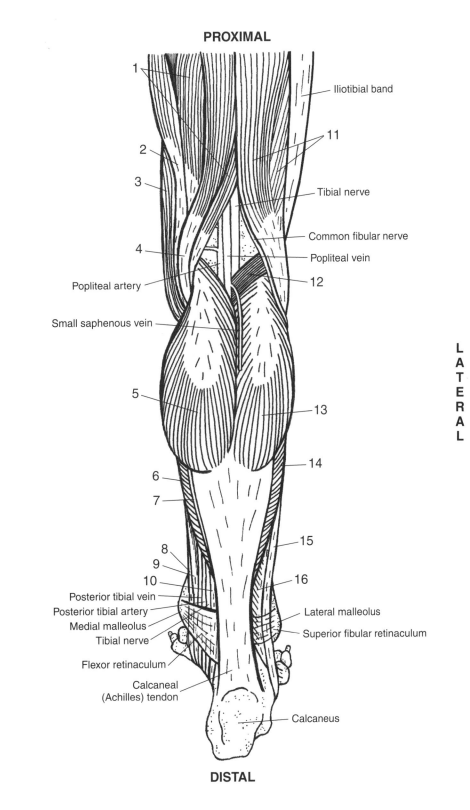

Iliotibial band

11

Tibial nerve

Common fibular nerve

Popliteal vein

12

Popliteal artery

Small saphenous vein

MEDIAL

LATERAL

13

14

6
7

15

8
9
10
Posterior tibial vein
Posterior tibial artery
Medial malleolus
Tibial nerve

16

Lateral malleolus

Superior fibular retinaculum

Flexor retinaculum

Calcaneal
(Achilles) tendon

Calcaneus

DISTAL

Muscles of the Leg

POSTERIOR VIEW OF THE RIGHT LEG (INTERMEDIATE)

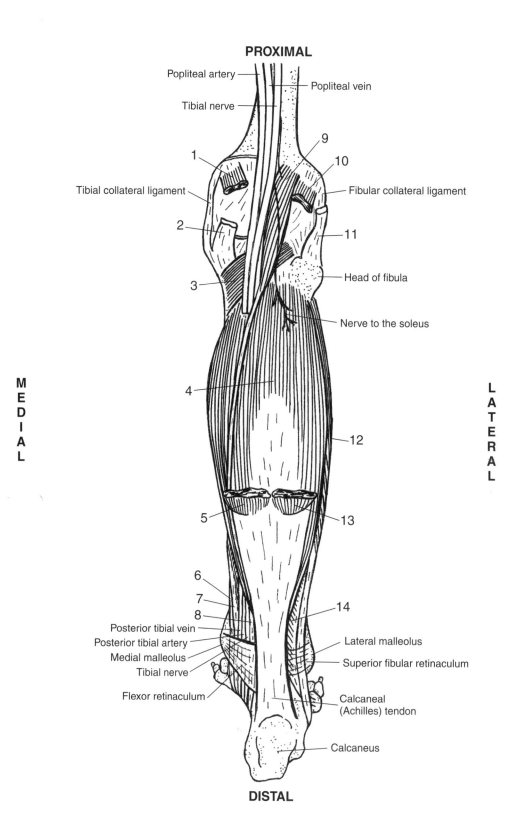

PROXIMAL

Popliteal artery

Popliteal vein

Tibial nerve

9

1

10

Tibial collateral ligament

Fibular collateral ligament

2

11

3

Head of fibula

Nerve to the soleus

MEDIAL

LATERAL

4

12

5

13

6

7

8

14

Posterior tibial vein

Posterior tibial artery

Lateral malleolus

Medial malleolus

Superior fibular retinaculum

Tibial nerve

Flexor retinaculum

Calcaneal
(Achilles) tendon

Calcaneus

DISTAL

POSTERIOR VIEW OF THE RIGHT LEG (DEEP)

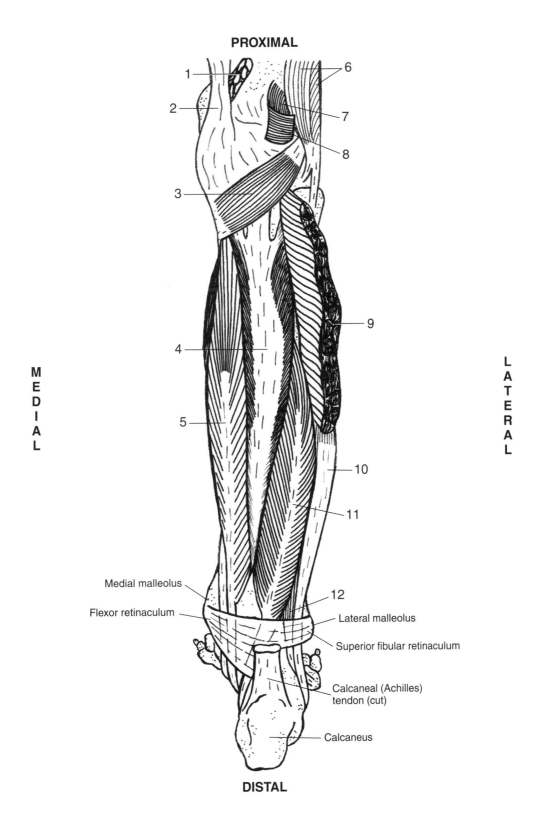

PROXIMAL

1

2

3

4

5

6

7

8

9

10

11

12

MEDIAL

LATERAL

Medial malleolus

Flexor retinaculum

Lateral malleolus

Superior fibular retinaculum

Calcaneal (Achilles) tendon (cut)

Calcaneus

DISTAL

LATERAL VIEW OF THE RIGHT LEG

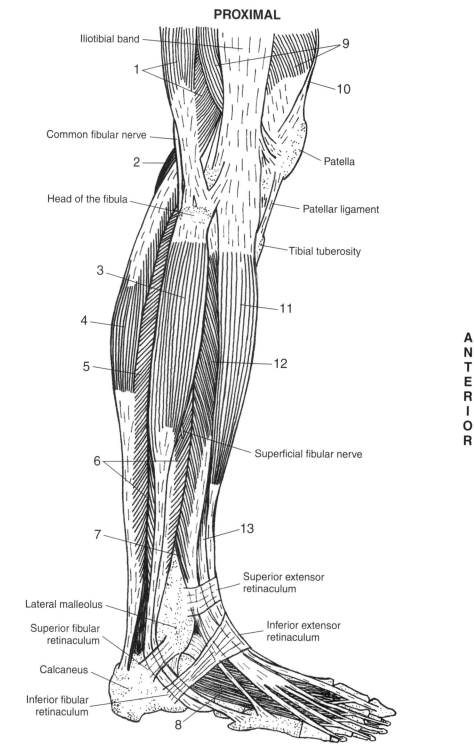

PROXIMAL

Iliotibial band

1

Common fibular nerve

2

Head of the fibula

3

4

5

6

7

Lateral malleolus

Superior fibular
retinaculum

Calcaneus

Inferior fibular
retinaculum

8

9

10

Patella

Patellar ligament

Tibial tuberosity

11

12

Superficial fibular nerve

13

Superior extensor
retinaculum

Inferior extensor
retinaculum

POSTERIOR

ANTERIOR

DISTAL

MEDIAL VIEW OF THE RIGHT LEG

PROXIMAL

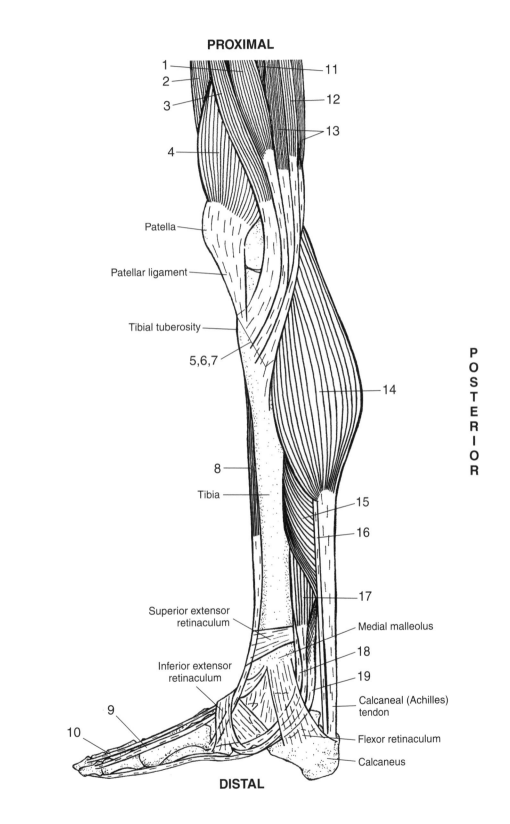

1
2
3
4

11
12
13

Patella

Patellar ligament

Tibial tuberosity

5,6,7

A N T E R I O R

P O S T E R I O R

14

8

Tibia

15

16

17

Superior extensor
retinaculum

Medial malleolus

18

Inferior extensor
retinaculum

19

9

Calcaneal (Achilles)
tendon

10

Flexor retinaculum

Calcaneus

DISTAL

Intrinsic Muscles of the Foot

DORSAL VIEW OF THE RIGHT FOOT

PROXIMAL

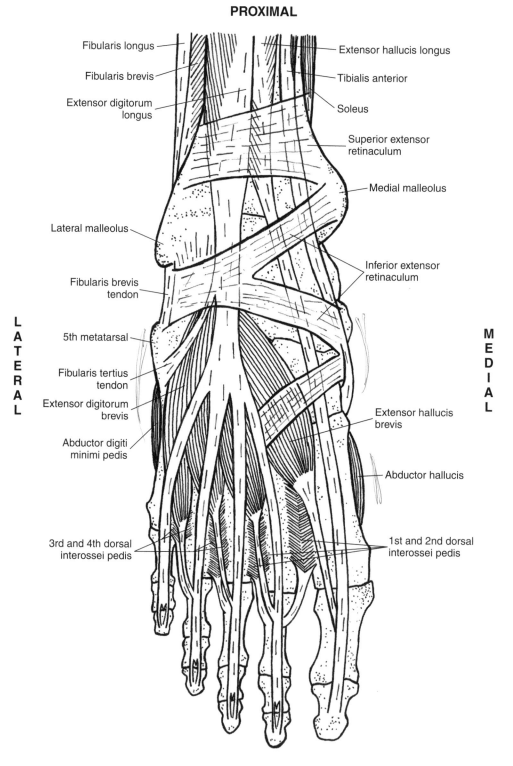

Fibularis longus

Fibularis brevis

Extensor digitorum longus

Lateral malleolus

Fibularis brevis tendon

5th metatarsal

Fibularis tertius tendon

Extensor digitorum brevis

Abductor digiti minimi pedis

3rd and 4th dorsal interossei pedis

Extensor hallucis longus

Tibialis anterior

Soleus

Superior extensor retinaculum

Medial malleolus

Inferior extensor retinaculum

Extensor hallucis brevis

Abductor hallucis

1st and 2nd dorsal interossei pedis

LATERAL

MEDIAL

DISTAL

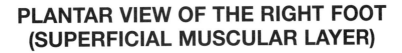

PLANTAR VIEW OF THE RIGHT FOOT
(SUPERFICIAL MUSCULAR LAYER)

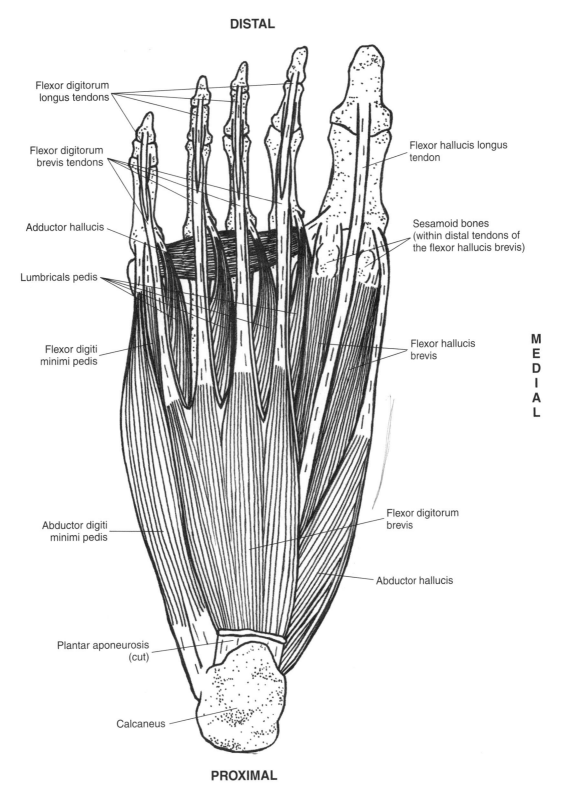

DISTAL

Flexor digitorum longus tendons

Flexor digitorum brevis tendons

Adductor hallucis

Lumbricals pedis

Flexor digiti minimi pedis

Abductor digiti minimi pedis

Plantar aponeurosis (cut)

Calcaneus

Flexor hallucis longus tendon

Sesamoid bones (within distal tendons of the flexor hallucis brevis)

Flexor hallucis brevis

Flexor digitorum brevis

Abductor hallucis

LATERAL

MEDIAL

PROXIMAL

Intrinsic Muscles of the Foot

PLANTAR VIEW OF THE RIGHT FOOT
(INTERMEDIATE MUSCULAR LAYER)

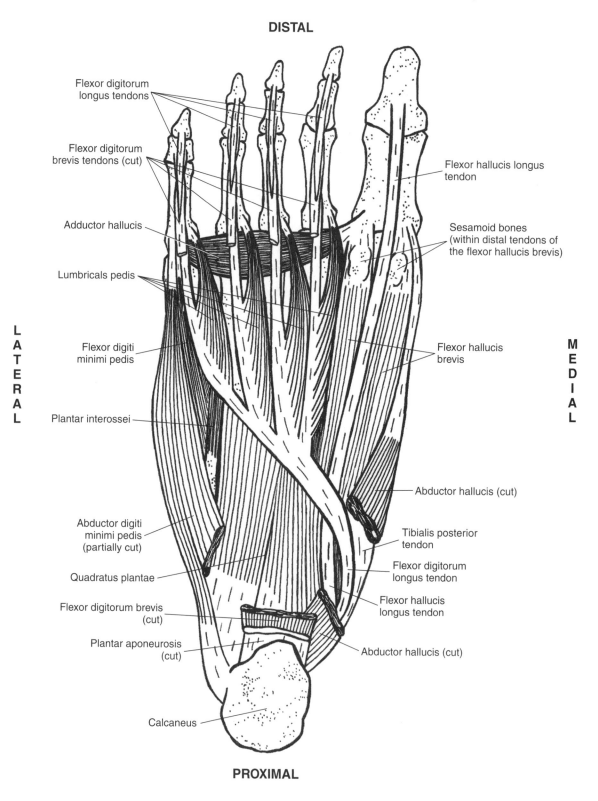

DISTAL

Flexor digitorum
longus tendons

Flexor digitorum
brevis tendons (cut)

Adductor hallucis

Lumbricals pedis

Flexor digiti
minimi pedis

Plantar interossei

Abductor digiti
minimi pedis
(partially cut)

Quadratus plantae

Flexor digitorum brevis
(cut)

Plantar aponeurosis
(cut)

Calcaneus

Flexor hallucis longus
tendon

Sesamoid bones
(within distal tendons of
the flexor hallucis brevis)

Flexor hallucis
brevis

Abductor hallucis (cut)

Tibialis posterior
tendon

Flexor digitorum
longus tendon

Flexor hallucis
longus tendon

Abductor hallucis (cut)

LATERAL

MEDIAL

PROXIMAL

PLANTAR VIEW OF THE RIGHT FOOT
(DEEP MUSCULAR LAYER)

DISTAL

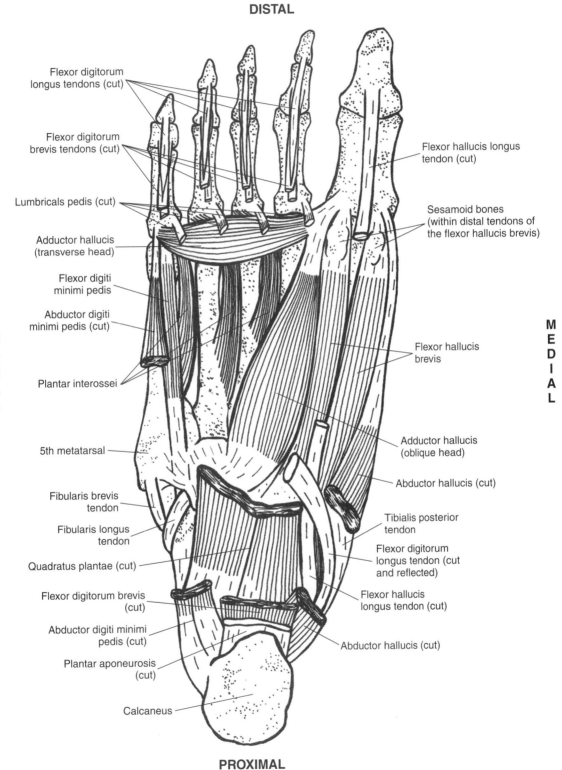

Flexor digitorum
longus tendons (cut)

Flexor digitorum
brevis tendons (cut)

Lumbricals pedis (cut)

Adductor hallucis
(transverse head)

Flexor digiti
minimi pedis

Abductor digiti
minimi pedis (cut)

Plantar interossei

5th metatarsal

Fibularis brevis
tendon

Fibularis longus
tendon

Quadratus plantae (cut)

Flexor digitorum brevis
(cut)

Abductor digiti minimi
pedis (cut)

Plantar aponeurosis
(cut)

Calcaneus

Flexor hallucis longus
tendon (cut)

Sesamoid bones
(within distal tendons of
the flexor hallucis brevis)

Flexor hallucis
brevis

Adductor hallucis
(oblique head)

Abductor hallucis (cut)

Tibialis posterior
tendon

Flexor digitorum
longus tendon (cut
and reflected)

Flexor hallucis
longus tendon (cut)

Abductor hallucis (cut)

LATERAL

MEDIAL

PROXIMAL

Intrinsic Muscles of the Foot

EXTENSOR DIGITORUM BREVIS

(DORSAL SURFACE)

eks-**ten**-sor
dij-i-**toe**-rum **bre**-vis

Action
Extension of toes #2-4 at the metatarso-phalangeal and proxi-mal and distal inter-phalangeal joints

Innervation
The deep fibular nerve

Arterial Supply
The dorsalis pedis artery

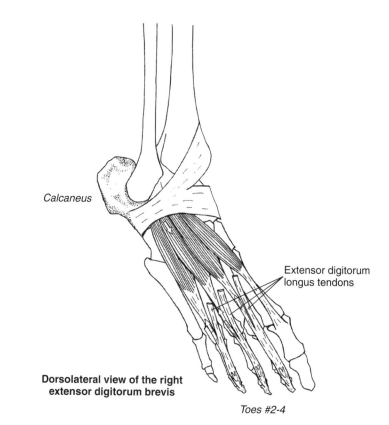

Calcaneus

Extensor digitorum longus tendons

Dorsolateral view of the right extensor digitorum brevis

Toes #2-4

EXTENSOR HALLUCIS BREVIS

(DORSAL SURFACE)

eks-**ten**-sor hal-**oo**-sis
bre-vis

Action
Extension of the big toe (toe #1) at the meta-tarsophalangeal joint

Innervation
The deep fibular nerve

Arterial Supply
The dorsalis pedis artery

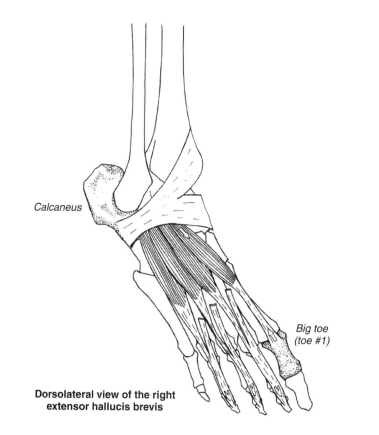

Calcaneus

Big toe (toe #1)

Dorsolateral view of the right extensor hallucis brevis

Intrinsic Muscles of the Foot

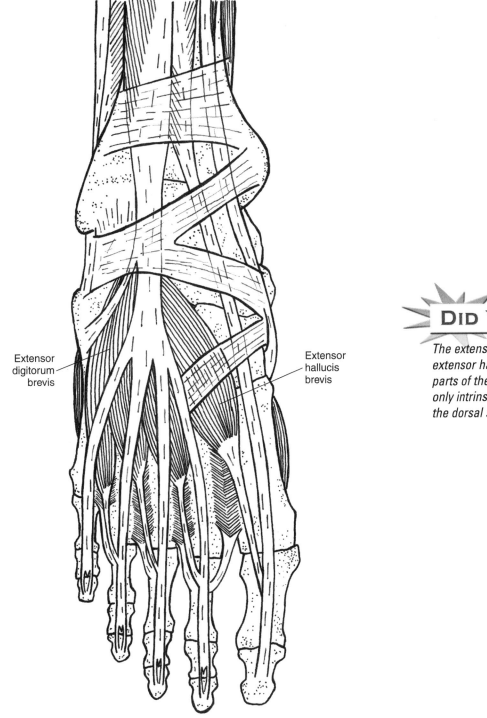

Extensor digitorum brevis

Extensor hallucis brevis

DID YOU KNOW?

The extensor digitorum brevis and extensor hallucis brevis are actually parts of the same muscle and are the only intrinsic foot muscles located on the dorsal side.

Intrinsic Muscles of the Foot

ABDUCTOR HALLUCIS

(PLANTAR SURFACE — LAYER I)

ab-**duk**-tor hal-**oo**-sis

Actions
Abduction of the big toe (toe #1) at the metatarsophalangeal joint
Flexion of the big toe (toe #1) at the metatarsophalangeal joint

Innervation
The medial plantar nerve

Arterial Supply
The medial plantar artery

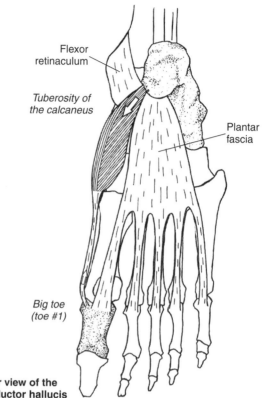

Flexor retinaculum

Tuberosity of the calcaneus

Plantar fascia

Big toe (toe #1)

Plantar view of the right abductor hallucis

ABDUCTOR DIGITI MINIMI PEDIS

(PLANTAR SURFACE — LAYER I)

ab-**duk**-tor **dij**-i-tee **min**-i-mee **peed**-us

Actions
Abduction of the little toe (toe #5) at the metatarsophalangeal joint
Flexion of the little toe (toe #5) at the metatarsophalangeal joint

Innervation
The lateral plantar nerve

Arterial Supply
The lateral plantar artery

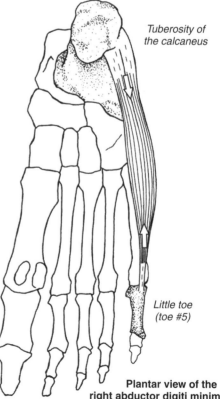

Tuberosity of the calcaneus

Little toe (toe #5)

Plantar view of the right abductor digiti minimi pedis

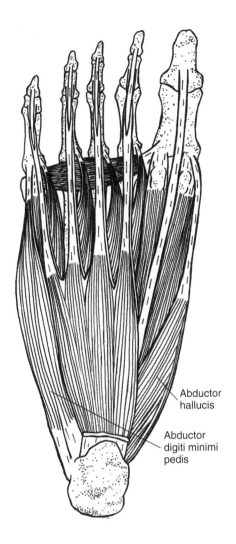

Abductor
hallucis

Abductor
digiti minimi
pedis

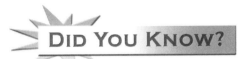

The abductor hallucis is easily
palpable on the medial side of the
plantar surface of the foot.

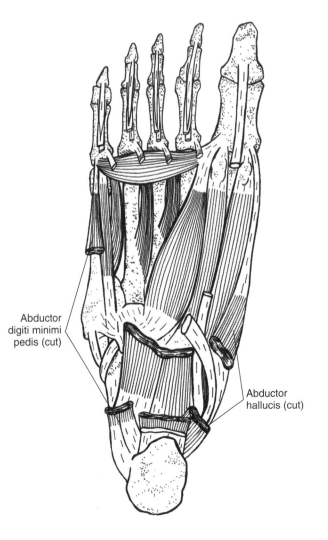

Abductor
digiti minimi
pedis (cut)

Abductor
hallucis (cut)

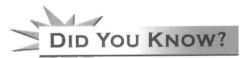

The abductor digiti minimi pedis is
often known simply as the abductor
digiti minimi. But there is an abductor
digiti minimi (manus) of the hand as
well and confusion can result.

Intrinsic Muscles of the Foot

FLEXOR DIGITORUM BREVIS

(PLANTAR SURFACE—LAYER I)

fleks-or dij-i-toe-rum bre-vis

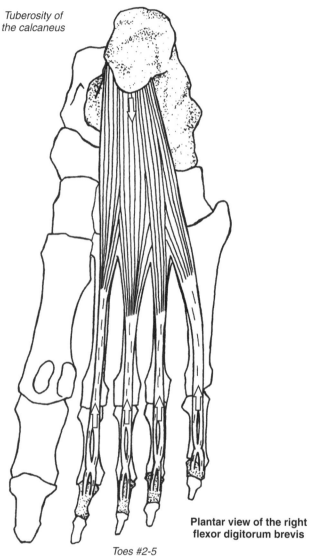

Tuberosity of
the calcaneus

Plantar view of the right
flexor digitorum brevis

Toes #2-5

Action	Innervation	Arterial Supply
Flexion of toes #2-5 at the metatarsophalangeal and the proximal interphalangeal joints	The medial plantar nerve	The medial and lateral plantar arteries

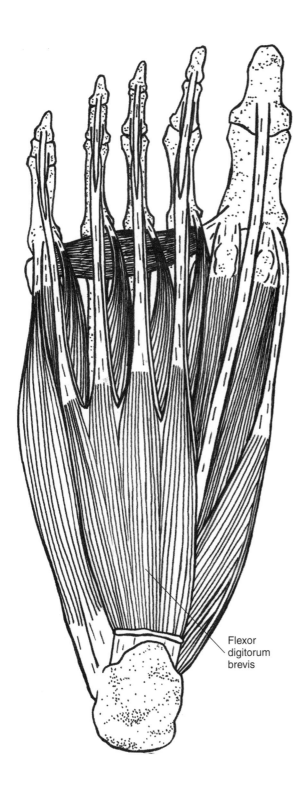

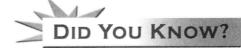

DID YOU KNOW?

The distal tendons of the flexor digitorum brevis split to allow passage of the distal tendons of the flexor digitorum longus to the distal phalanges of toes #2-5.

Flexor
digitorum
brevis

Intrinsic Muscles of the Foot

QUADRATUS PLANTAE
(PLANTAR SURFACE—LAYER II)

kwod-**ray**-tus **plan**-tee

Action
Flexion of toes #2-5 at the metatarsophalangeal and the proximal and distal interphalangeal joints

Innervation
The lateral plantar nerve

Arterial Supply
The medial and lateral plantar arteries

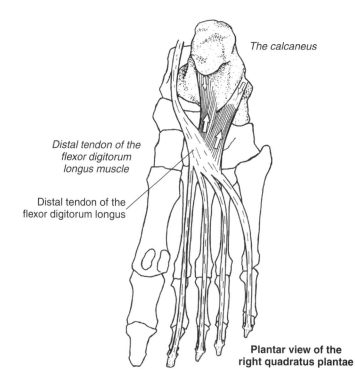

The calcaneus

Distal tendon of the flexor digitorum longus muscle

Distal tendon of the flexor digitorum longus

Plantar view of the right quadratus plantae

LUMBRICALS PEDIS
(PLANTAR SURFACE—LAYER II)

(There are four lumbrical pedis muscles, named #1, #2, #3, and #4.)

lum-bri-kuls **peed**-us

Actions
Extension of toes #2-5 at the proximal and distal interphalangeal joints
Flexion of toes #2-5 at the metatarsophalangeal joint

Innervation
The medial and lateral plantar nerves

Arterial Supply
The medial and lateral plantar arteries

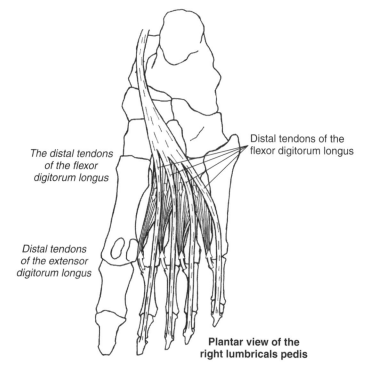

Distal tendons of the flexor digitorum longus

The distal tendons of the flexor digitorum longus

Distal tendons of the extensor digitorum longus

Plantar view of the right lumbricals pedis

Intrinsic Muscles of the Foot

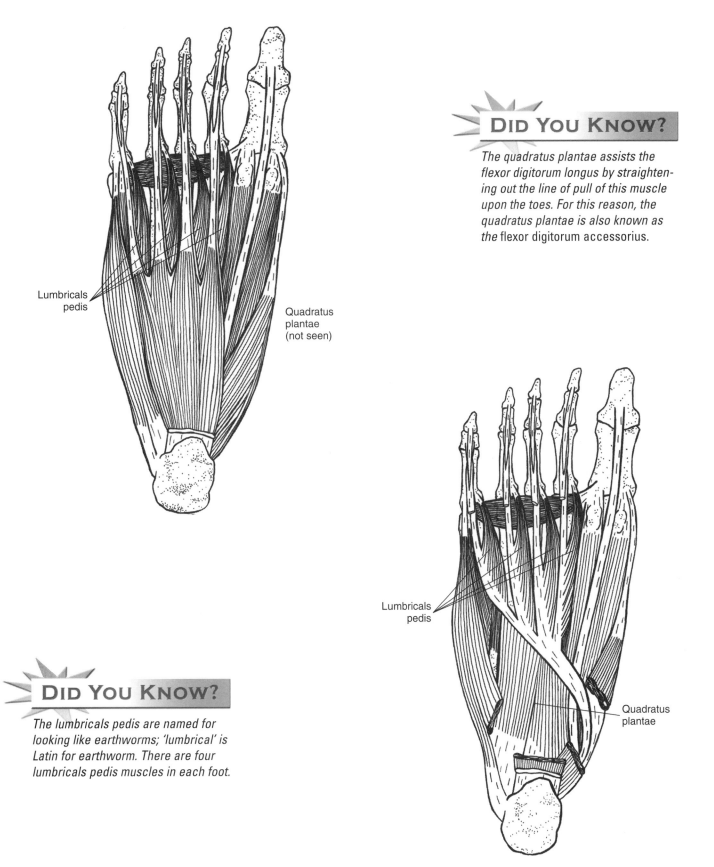

Lumbricals
pedis

Quadratus
plantae
(not seen)

Lumbricals
pedis

Quadratus
plantae

DID YOU KNOW?

The quadratus plantae assists the
flexor digitorum longus by straighten-
ing out the line of pull of this muscle
upon the toes. For this reason, the
quadratus plantae is also known as
the flexor digitorum accessorius.

DID YOU KNOW?

The lumbricals pedis are named for
looking like earthworms; 'lumbrical' is
Latin for earthworm. There are four
lumbricals pedis muscles in each foot.

Intrinsic Muscles of the Foot

FLEXOR HALLUCIS BREVIS

(PLANTAR SURFACE—LAYER III)

fleks-or hal-**oo**-sis **bre**-vis

Action
Flexion of the big toe (toe #1) at the metatarsophalangeal joint

Innervation
The medial plantar nerve

Arterial Supply
The medial plantar artery

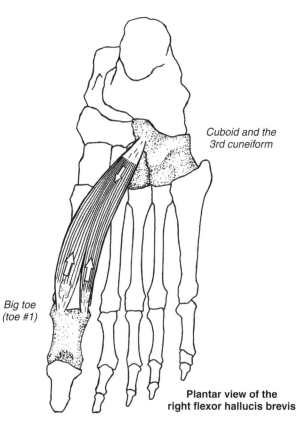

Cuboid and the 3rd cuneiform

Big toe (toe #1)

Plantar view of the right flexor hallucis brevis

FLEXOR DIGITI MINIMI PEDIS

(PLANTAR SURFACE—LAYER III)

fleks-or **dij**-i-tee **min**-i-mee **peed**-us

Action
Flexion of the little toe (toe #5) at the metatarsophalangeal joint

Innervation
The lateral plantar nerve

Arterial Supply
The lateral plantar artery

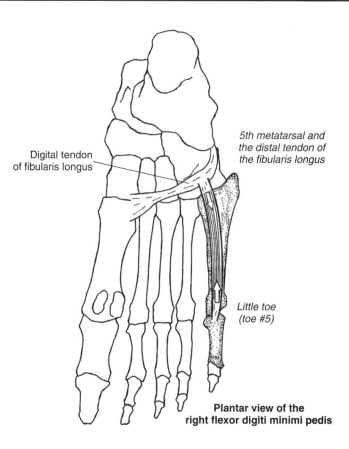

Digital tendon of fibularis longus

5th metatarsal and the distal tendon of the fibularis longus

Little toe (toe #5)

Plantar view of the right flexor digiti minimi pedis

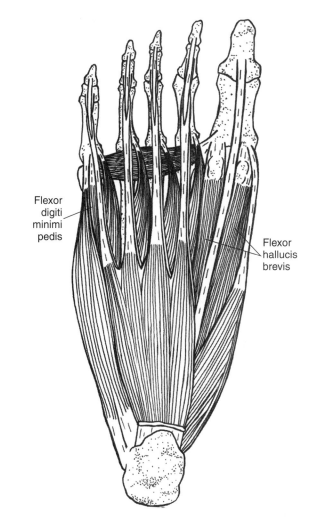

Flexor
digiti
minimi
pedis

Flexor
hallucis
brevis

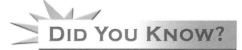

Distally, there is a sesamoid bone in the medial and lateral tendons of the flexor hallucis brevis.

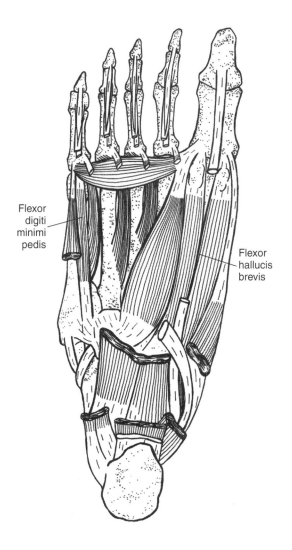

Flexor
digiti
minimi
pedis

Flexor
hallucis
brevis

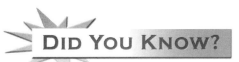

The flexor digiti minimi pedis is often known as simply the flexor digiti minimi or the flexor digiti minimi brevis. However, there is a flexor digiti minimi (manus) of the hand, and confusion can result.

Intrinsic Muscles of the Foot

ADDUCTOR HALLUCIS

(PLANTAR SURFACE—LAYER III)

ad-**duk**-tor hal-**oo**-sis

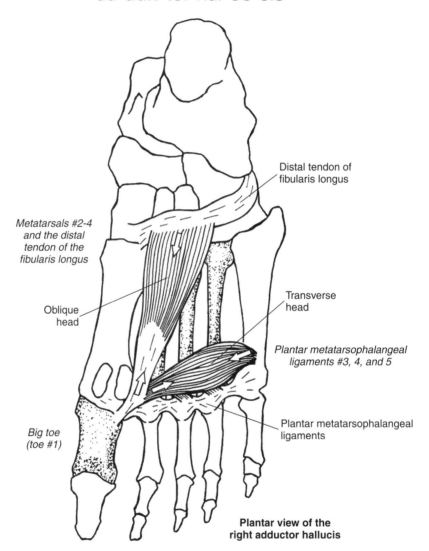

Distal tendon of
fibularis longus

*Metatarsals #2-4
and the distal
tendon of the
fibularis longus*

Oblique
head

Transverse
head

*Plantar metatarsophalangeal
ligaments #3, 4, and 5*

Plantar metatarsophalangeal
ligaments

*Big toe
(toe #1)*

**Plantar view of the
right adductor hallucis**

Actions	Innervation	Arterial Supply
Adduction of the big toe (toe #1) at the metatarsophalangeal joint Flexion of the big toe (toe #1) at the metatarsophalangeal joint	The lateral plantar nerve	Branches of the plantar arch

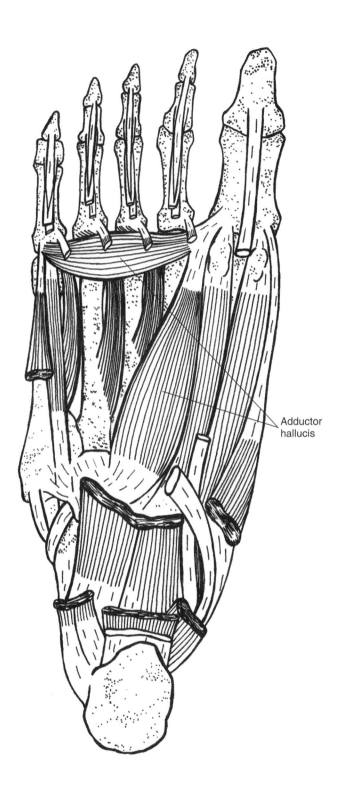

Adductor
hallucis

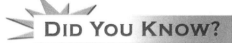

DID YOU KNOW?

The adductor hallucis occasionally has attachments onto the 1st metatarsal that can create opposition of the big toe toward the other toes. When this occurs, this muscle is called the opponens hallucis. *This arrangement is common in apes, whose feet are more 'handy' than ours ☺.*

Intrinsic Muscles of the Foot

PLANTAR INTEROSSEI

(PLANTAR SURFACE—LAYER IV)

(There are three plantar interossei muscles, named #1, #2, and #3.)

plan-tar in-ter-**oss**-ee-eye

Actions
Adduction of toes #3-5 at the metatarsophalangeal joint
Flexion of toes #3-5 at the metatarsophalangeal joint
Extension of toes #3-5 at the proximal and distal interphalangeal joints

Innervation
The lateral plantar nerve

Arterial Supply
Branches of the plantar arch

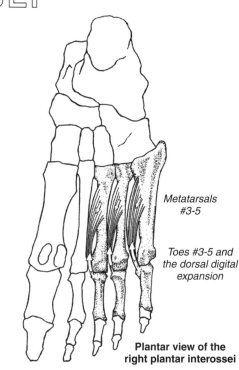

Metatarsals #3-5

Toes #3-5 and the dorsal digital expansion

Plantar view of the right plantar interossei

DORSAL INTEROSSEI PEDIS

(PLANTAR SURFACE—LAYER IV)

(There are four dorsal interossei pedis muscles, named #1, #2, #3, and #4.)

plan-tar in-ter-**oss**-ee-eye **peed**-us

Actions
Abduction of toes #2-4 at the metatarsophalangeal joint
Flexion of toes #2-4 at the metatarsophalangeal joint at the metatarsophalan-geal joint
Extension of toes #2-4 at the proximal and distal interphalangeal joints

Innervation
The lateral plantar nerve

Arterial Supply
Branches of the plantar arch

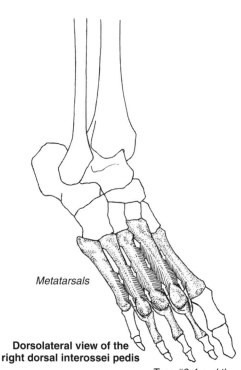

Metatarsals

Dorsolateral view of the right dorsal interossei pedis

Toes #2-4 and the dorsal digital expansion

Intrinsic Muscles of the Foot

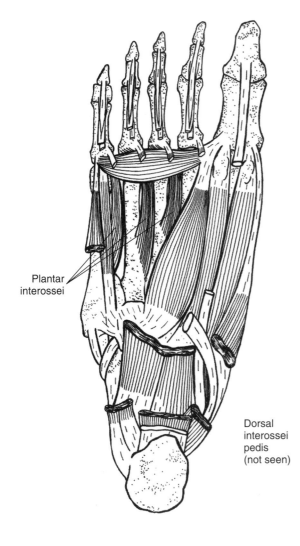

Plantar
interossei

Dorsal
interossei
pedis
(not seen)

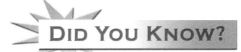

DID YOU KNOW?

*The main action of the dorsal interossei pedis is abduction of the toes at the metatarsophalangeal joints. The main action of the plantar interossei is adduction of the toes at the metatarsophalangeal joints. The mnemonic to remember these actions is **DAB PAD; D**orsals **AB**duct, **P**lantars **AD**duct.*

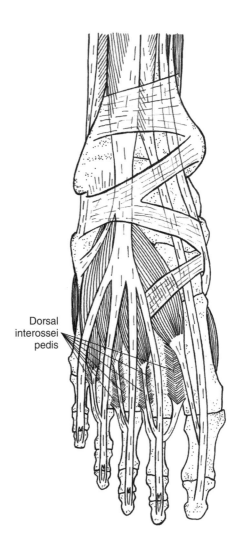

Dorsal
interossei
pedis

Intrinsic Muscles of the Foot

DORSAL VIEW OF THE RIGHT FOOT

PROXIMAL

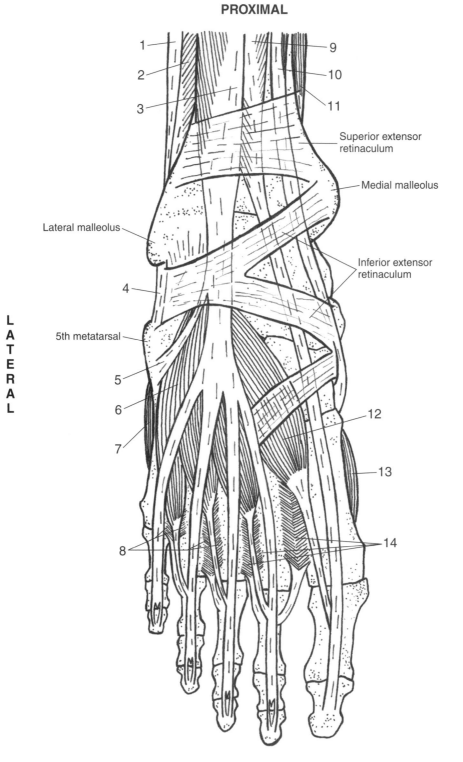

1

2

3

9

10

11

Superior extensor retinaculum

Medial malleolus

Lateral malleolus

Inferior extensor retinaculum

4

L A T E R A L

M E D I A L

5th metatarsal

5

6

7

12

13

8

14

DISTAL

PLANTAR VIEW OF THE RIGHT FOOT (SUPERFICIAL MUSCULAR LAYER)

DISTAL

LATERAL

MEDIAL

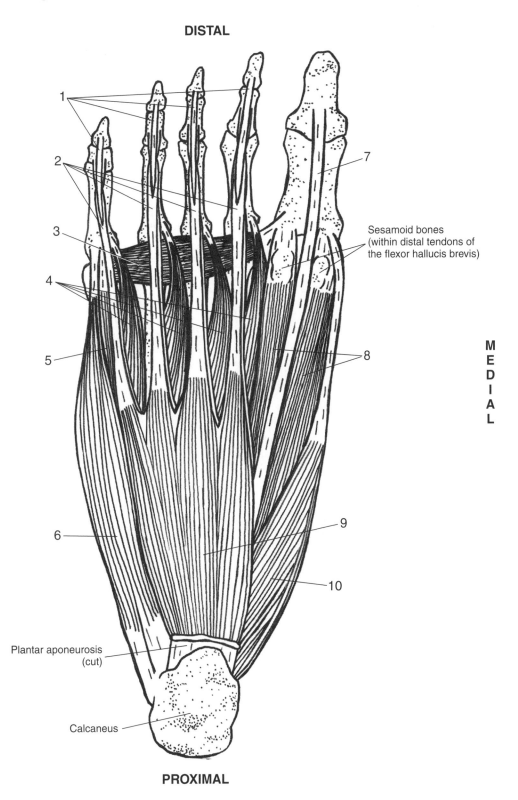

1

2

3

4

5

6

7

Sesamoid bones
(within distal tendons of
the flexor hallucis brevis)

8

9

10

Plantar aponeurosis
(cut)

Calcaneus

PROXIMAL

Intrinsic Muscles of the Foot

PLANTAR VIEW OF THE RIGHT FOOT
(INTERMEDIATE MUSCULAR LAYER)

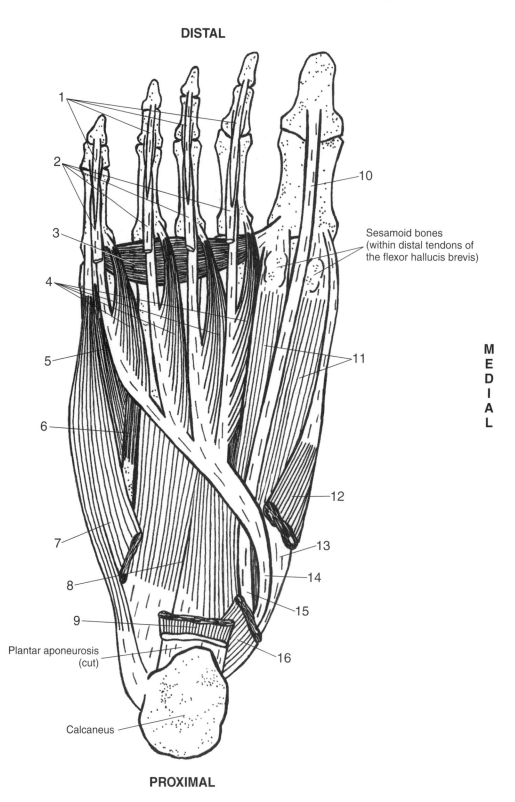

DISTAL

LATERAL

MEDIAL

Sesamoid bones
(within distal tendons of
the flexor hallucis brevis)

Plantar aponeurosis
(cut)

Calcaneus

PROXIMAL

PLANTAR VIEW OF THE RIGHT FOOT
(DEEP MUSCULAR LAYER)

DISTAL

LATERAL

MEDIAL

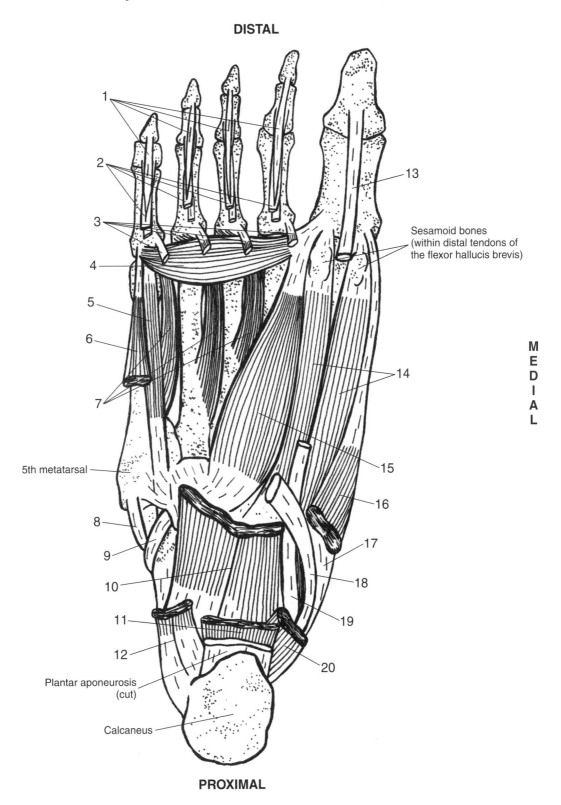

1

2

3

4

5

6

7

13

Sesamoid bones
(within distal tendons of
the flexor hallucis brevis)

14

15

16

17

18

19

20

5th metatarsal

8

9

10

11

12

Plantar aponeurosis
(cut)

Calcaneus

PROXIMAL

ANTERIOR VIEW OF THE RIGHT SHOULDER

SUPERIOR

LATERAL

MEDIAL

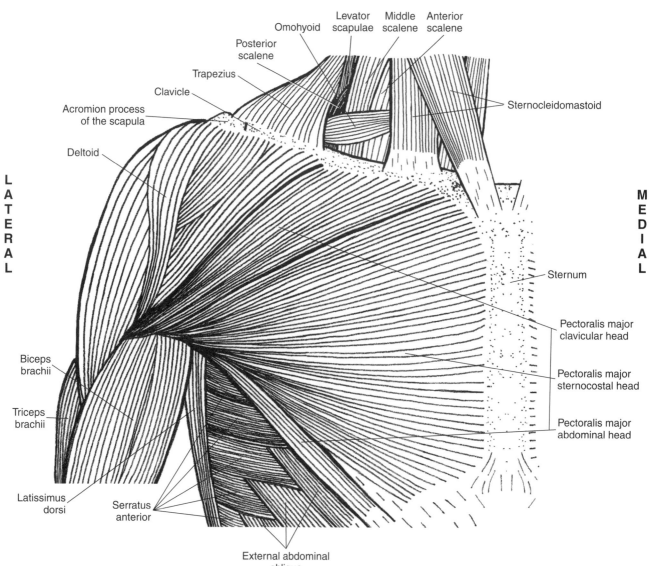

Omohyoid

Levator
scapulae

Middle
scalene

Anterior
scalene

Posterior
scalene

Trapezius

Clavicle

Acromion process
of the scapula

Deltoid

Sternocleidomastoid

Sternum

Pectoralis major
clavicular head

Biceps
brachii

Triceps
brachii

Pectoralis major
sternocostal head

Pectoralis major
abdominal head

Latissimus
dorsi

Serratus
anterior

External abdominal
oblique

INFERIOR

POSTERIOR VIEW OF THE SHOULDERS
(SUPERFICIAL AND INTERMEDIATE)

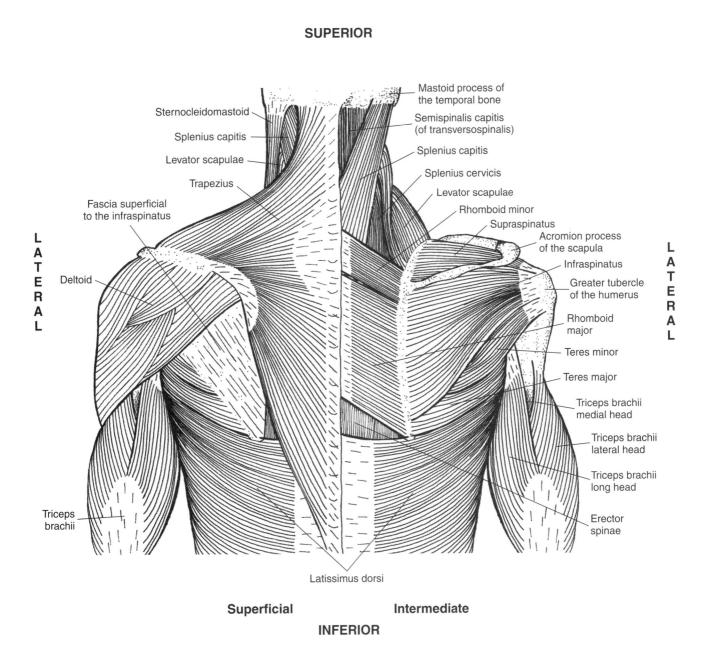

SUPERIOR

Sternocleidomastoid

Splenius capitis

Levator scapulae

Trapezius

Fascia superficial
to the infraspinatus

Deltoid

LATERAL

Triceps
brachii

Mastoid process of
the temporal bone

Semispinalis capitis
(of transversospinalis)

Splenius capitis

Splenius cervicis

Levator scapulae

Rhomboid minor

Supraspinatus

Acromion process
of the scapula

Infraspinatus

Greater tubercle
of the humerus

Rhomboid
major

Teres minor

Teres major

Triceps brachii
medial head

Triceps brachii
lateral head

Triceps brachii
long head

Erector
spinae

LATERAL

Latissimus dorsi

Superficial   Intermediate

INFERIOR

Muscles of the Scapula/Arm

ANTERIOR VIEW OF THE RIGHT ARM (SUPERFICIAL)

PROXIMAL

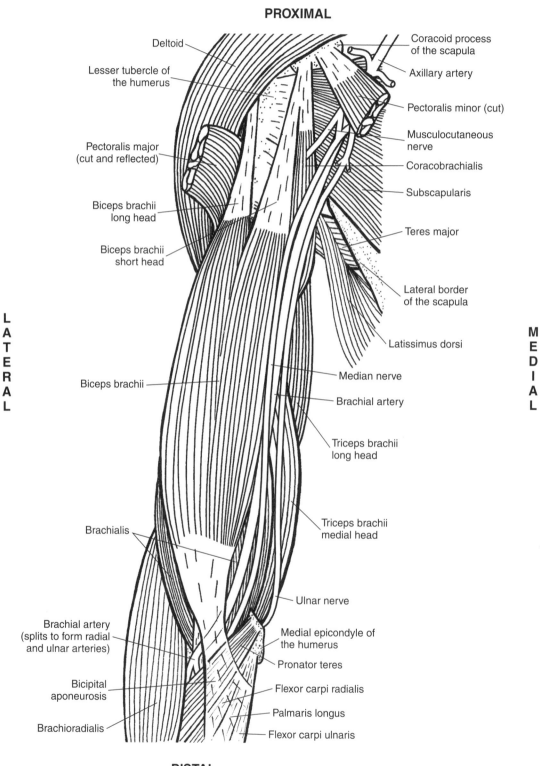

Deltoid

Lesser tubercle of the humerus

Pectoralis major (cut and reflected)

Biceps brachii long head

Biceps brachii short head

Coracoid process of the scapula

Axillary artery

Pectoralis minor (cut)

Musculocutaneous nerve

Coracobrachialis

Subscapularis

Teres major

Lateral border of the scapula

Latissimus dorsi

LATERAL

MEDIAL

Biceps brachii

Median nerve

Brachial artery

Triceps brachii long head

Brachialis

Triceps brachii medial head

Ulnar nerve

Brachial artery (splits to form radial and ulnar arteries)

Medial epicondyle of the humerus

Pronator teres

Bicipital aponeurosis

Flexor carpi radialis

Palmaris longus

Brachioradialis

Flexor carpi ulnaris

DISTAL

ANTERIOR VIEW OF THE RIGHT ARM (DEEP)

PROXIMAL

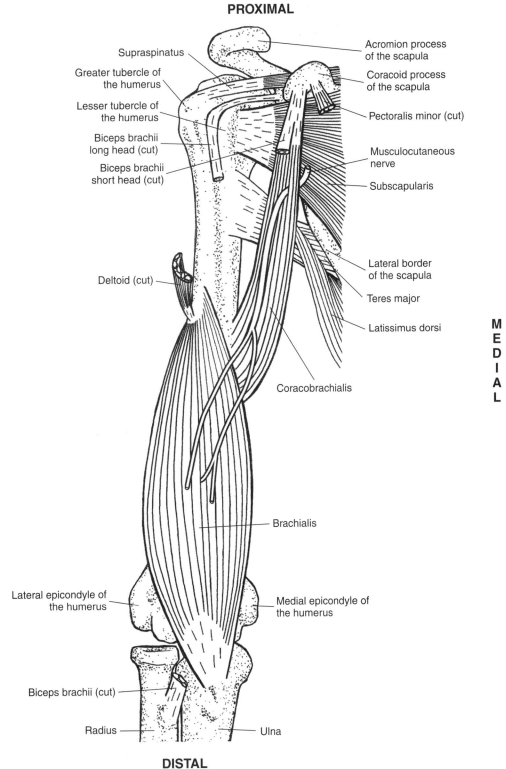

Supraspinatus

Greater tubercle of the humerus

Lesser tubercle of the humerus

Biceps brachii long head (cut)

Biceps brachii short head (cut)

Deltoid (cut)

Acromion process of the scapula

Coracoid process of the scapula

Pectoralis minor (cut)

Musculocutaneous nerve

Subscapularis

Lateral border of the scapula

Teres major

Latissimus dorsi

LATERAL

MEDIAL

Coracobrachialis

Brachialis

Lateral epicondyle of the humerus

Medial epicondyle of the humerus

Biceps brachii (cut)

Radius

Ulna

DISTAL

MEDIAL VIEW OF THE RIGHT ARM

PROXIMAL

Subdeltoid bursa

Biceps brachii
long head (cut)

Subscapularis
(cut)

Pectoralis major
(cut)

Biceps brachii
short head (cut)

Coracobrachialis
(cut)

Supraspinatus (cut)

Head of the humerus

Bursa

Infraspinatus (cut)

Shoulder joint capsule

Teres minor (cut)

Deltoid (cut)

Teres major (cut)

Latissimus dorsi (cut)

Deep brachial artery

Brachial artery

Ulnar nerve

Humerus

ANTERIOR

POSTERIOR

Median nerve

Biceps brachii

Triceps brachii
long head

Triceps brachii
medial head

Brachialis

Superior ulnar
collateral artery

Bicipital aponeurosis
of the biceps brachii

Pronator teres

Brachioradialis

Palmaris longus

Flexor carpi radialis

Flexor carpi ulnaris

DISTAL

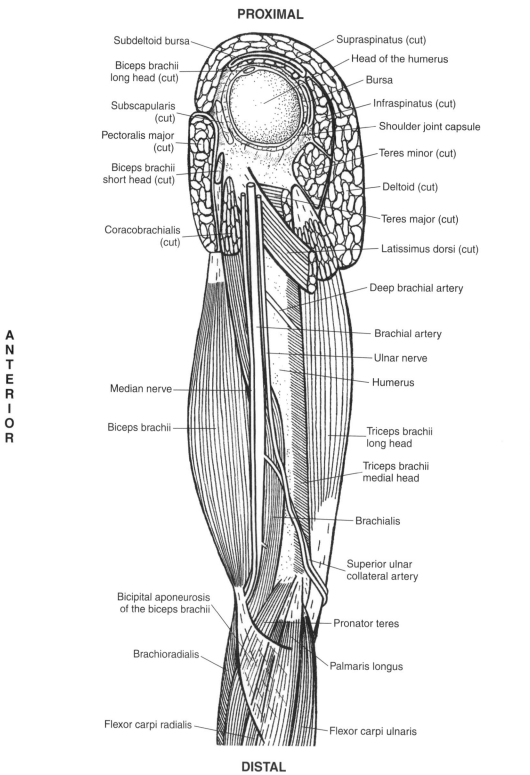

LATERAL VIEW OF THE RIGHT ARM

PROXIMAL

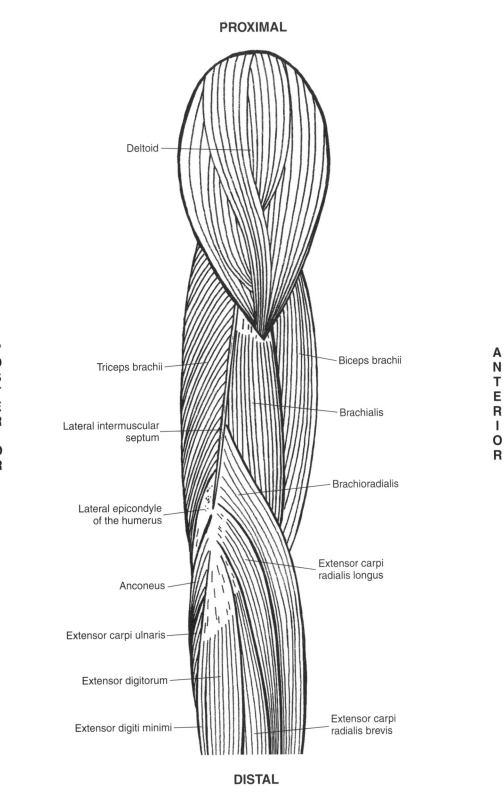

Deltoid

Triceps brachii

Biceps brachii

Brachialis

Lateral intermuscular septum

Brachioradialis

Lateral epicondyle of the humerus

Extensor carpi radialis longus

Anconeus

Extensor carpi ulnaris

Extensor digitorum

Extensor digiti minimi

Extensor carpi radialis brevis

POSTERIOR

ANTERIOR

DISTAL

Muscles of the Scapula/Arm

POSTERIOR VIEW OF THE RIGHT ARM

PROXIMAL

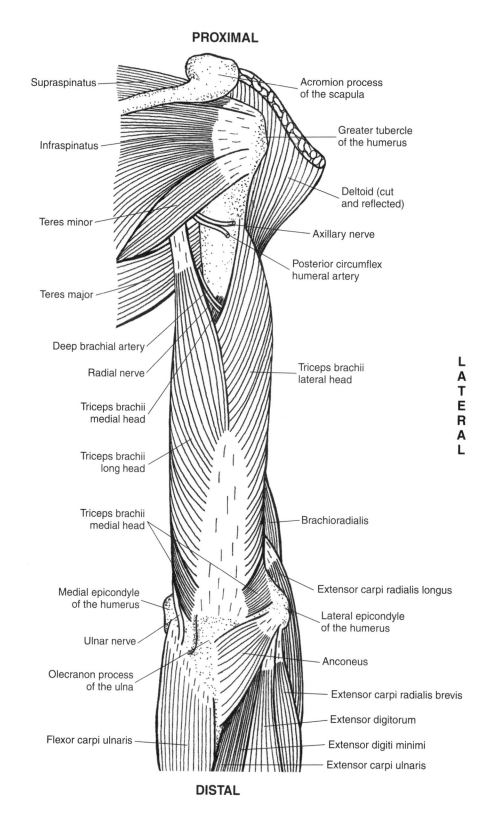

Supraspinatus

Infraspinatus

Teres minor

Teres major

Deep brachial artery

Radial nerve

Triceps brachii medial head

Triceps brachii long head

Triceps brachii medial head

Medial epicondyle of the humerus

Ulnar nerve

Olecranon process of the ulna

Flexor carpi ulnaris

Acromion process of the scapula

Greater tubercle of the humerus

Deltoid (cut and reflected)

Axillary nerve

Posterior circumflex humeral artery

Triceps brachii lateral head

Brachioradialis

Extensor carpi radialis longus

Lateral epicondyle of the humerus

Anconeus

Extensor carpi radialis brevis

Extensor digitorum

Extensor digiti minimi

Extensor carpi ulnaris

M E D I A L

L A T E R A L

DISTAL

ANTERIOR VIEW OF THE RIGHT GLENOHUMERAL JOINT

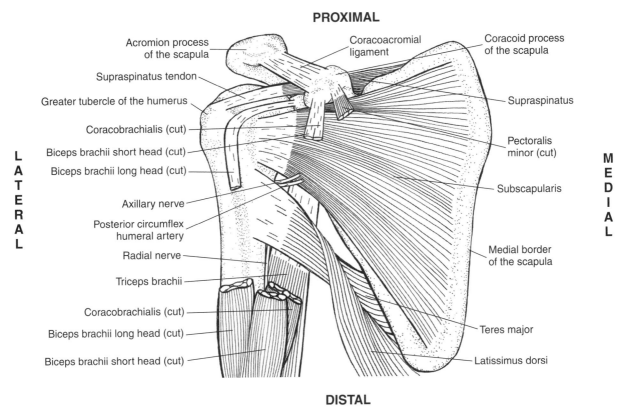

PROXIMAL

Acromion process of the scapula

Coracoacromial ligament

Coracoid process of the scapula

Supraspinatus tendon

Greater tubercle of the humerus

Supraspinatus

Coracobrachialis (cut)

Biceps brachii short head (cut)

Pectoralis minor (cut)

Biceps brachii long head (cut)

Subscapularis

Axillary nerve

Posterior circumflex humeral artery

Radial nerve

Medial border of the scapula

Triceps brachii

Coracobrachialis (cut)

Biceps brachii long head (cut)

Teres major

Biceps brachii short head (cut)

Latissimus dorsi

LATERAL

MEDIAL

DISTAL

POSTERIOR VIEW OF THE RIGHT GLENOHUMERAL JOINT

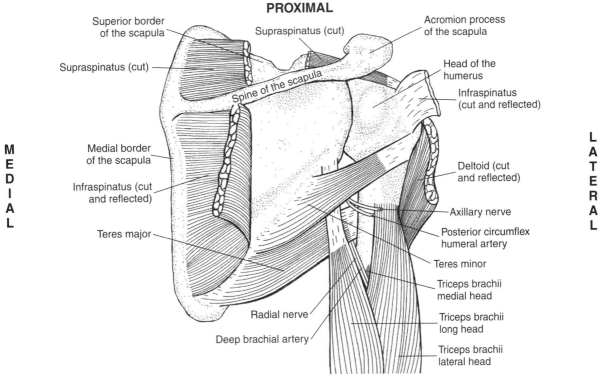

PROXIMAL

Superior border of the scapula

Supraspinatus (cut)

Acromion process of the scapula

Supraspinatus (cut)

Spine of the scapula

Head of the humerus

Infraspinatus (cut and reflected)

Medial border of the scapula

Deltoid (cut and reflected)

Infraspinatus (cut and reflected)

Axillary nerve

Teres major

Posterior circumflex humeral artery

Teres minor

Triceps brachii medial head

Radial nerve

Triceps brachii long head

Deep brachial artery

Triceps brachii lateral head

MEDIAL

LATERAL

DISTAL

Muscles of the Scapula/Arm

SUPRASPINATUS

(OF THE ROTATOR
CUFF GROUP)

soo-pra-spy-**nay**-tus

Action
Abduction of the arm at the shoulder joint
Innervation
The suprascapular nerve
Arterial Supply
The suprascapular artery

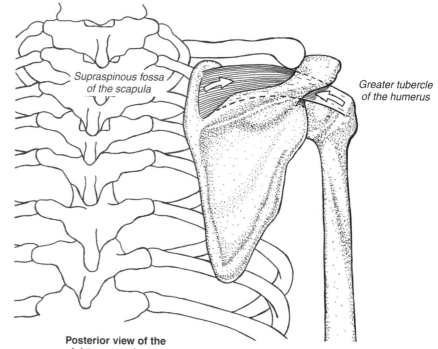

Supraspinous fossa of the scapula

Greater tubercle of the humerus

Posterior view of the right supraspinatus

INFRASPINATUS

(OF THE ROTATOR
CUFF GROUP)

in-fra-spy-**nay**-tus

Action
Lateral rotation of the arm at the shoulder joint
Innervation
The suprascapular nerve
Arterial Supply
The suprascapular artery

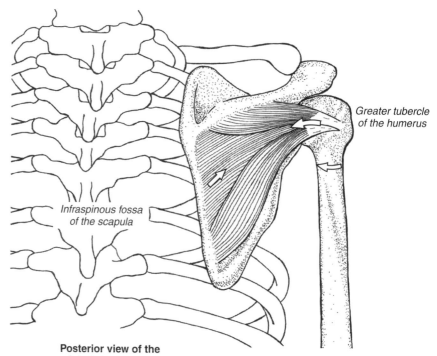

Infraspinous fossa of the scapula

Greater tubercle of the humerus

Posterior view of the right infraspinatus

Muscles of the Scapula/Arm

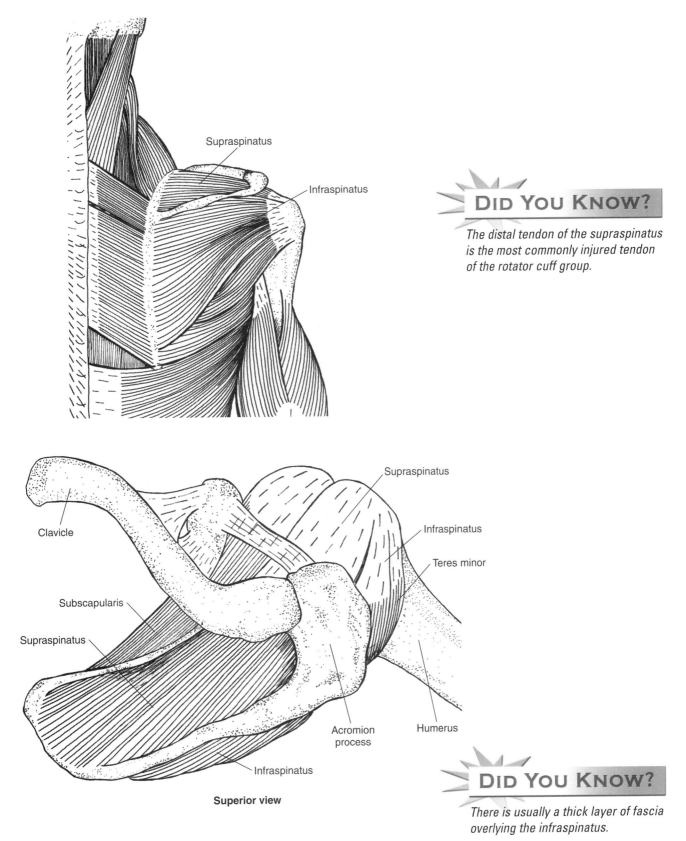

Supraspinatus

Infraspinatus

DID YOU KNOW?

The distal tendon of the supraspinatus is the most commonly injured tendon of the rotator cuff group.

Supraspinatus

Infraspinatus

Teres minor

Clavicle

Subscapularis

Supraspinatus

Acromion process

Humerus

Infraspinatus

Superior view

DID YOU KNOW?

There is usually a thick layer of fascia overlying the infraspinatus.

Muscles of the Scapula/Arm

TERES MINOR

(OF THE ROTATOR
CUFF GROUP)

te-reez **my**-nor

Action
Lateral rotation of the
  arm at the shoulder
  joint
Adduction of the arm at
  the shoulder joint

Innervation
The axillary nerve

Arterial Supply
The circumflex scapular
  artery

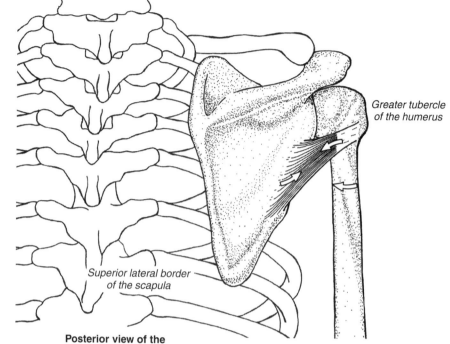

*Greater tubercle
of the humerus*

*Superior lateral border
of the scapula*

**Posterior view of the
right teres minor**

SUBSCAPULARIS

(OF THE ROTATOR
CUFF GROUP)

sub-skap-u-**la**-ris

Action
Medial rotation of the
  arm at the shoulder
  joint

Innervation
The upper and lower
  subscapular nerves

Arterial Supply
The circumflex scapular
artery and the dorsal
scapular and supra-
scapular arteries

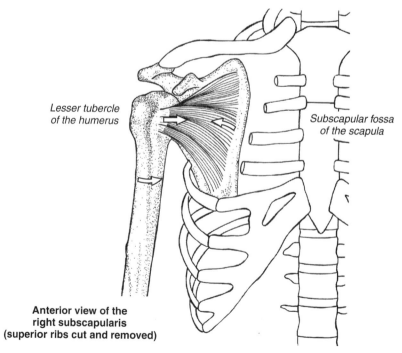

*Lesser tubercle
of the humerus*

*Subscapular fossa
of the scapula*

**Anterior view of the
right subscapularis
(superior ribs cut and removed)**

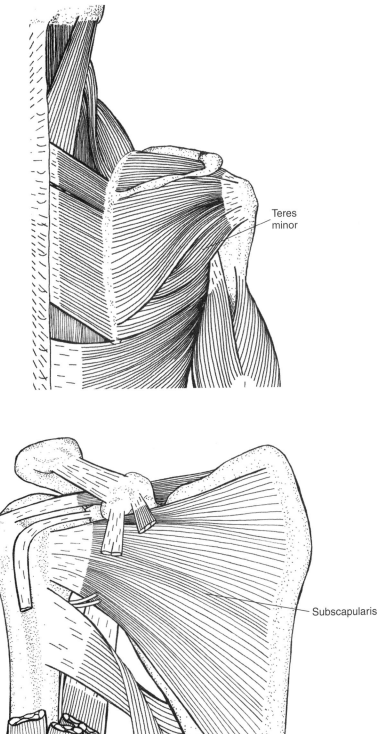

Teres minor

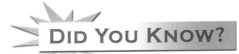

The teres minor often blends with the infraspinatus.

Subscapularis

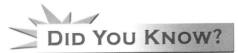

The subscapularis is the only muscle of the rotator cuff group that attaches onto the lesser tubercle of the humerus.

Muscles of the Scapula/Arm

TERES MAJOR

te-reez **may**-jor

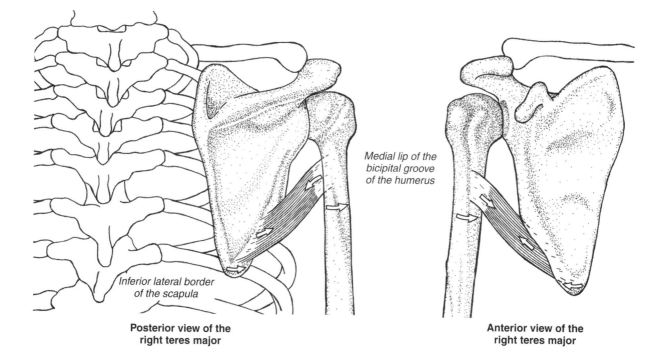

Medial lip of the bicipital groove of the humerus

Inferior lateral border of the scapula

Posterior view of the right teres major

Anterior view of the right teres major

Actions	Innervation	Arterial Supply
Medial rotation of the arm at the shoulder joint	The lower subscapular nerve	The circumflex scapular artery
Adduction of the arm at the shoulder joint		
Extension of the arm at the shoulder joint		
Upward rotation of the scapula at the scapulocostal joint		

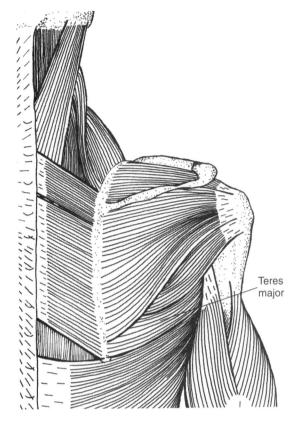

Teres
major

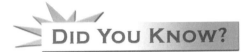

DID YOU KNOW?

The teres major can do all three actions of the arm at the shoulder joint (extension, adduction, and medial rotation) that the latissimus dorsi can. Therefore, these muscles often work together.

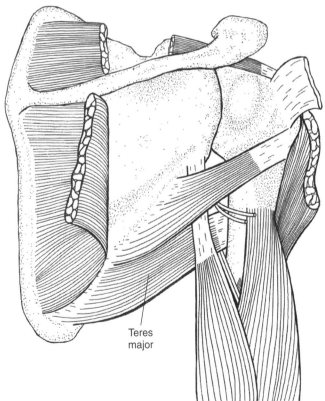

Teres
major

Muscles of the Scapula/Arm

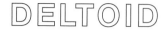

DELTOID

del-toid

Actions
Abduction of the arm at
the shoulder joint
(entire muscle)
Flexion of the arm at the
shoulder joint
(anterior deltoid)
Extension of the arm at
the shoulder joint
(posterior deltoid)
Medial rotation of the
arm at the shoulder
joint (anterior deltoid)
Lateral rotation of the
arm at the shoulder
joint (posterior deltoid)
Downward rotation of
the scapula at the
scapulocostal joint
(entire muscle)
Ipsilateral rotation of the
trunk at the shoulder
joint (anterior deltoid)
Contralateral rotation
of the trunk at the
shoulder joint
(posterior deltoid)

Innervation
The axillary nerve

Arterial Supply
The anterior and
posterior circumflex
humeral arteries

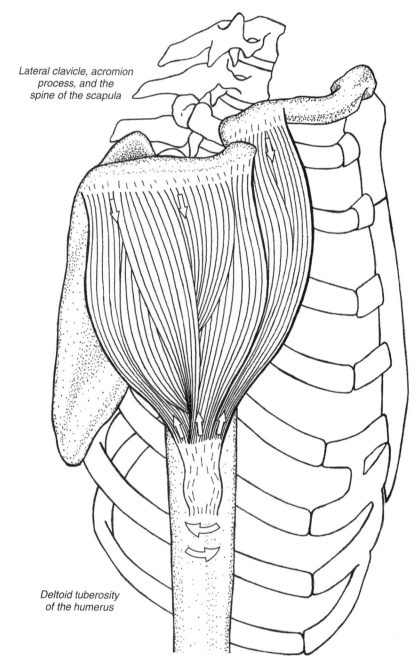

*Lateral clavicle, acromion
process, and the
spine of the scapula*

*Deltoid tuberosity
of the humerus*

Lateral view of the right deltoid

Muscles of the Scapula/Arm

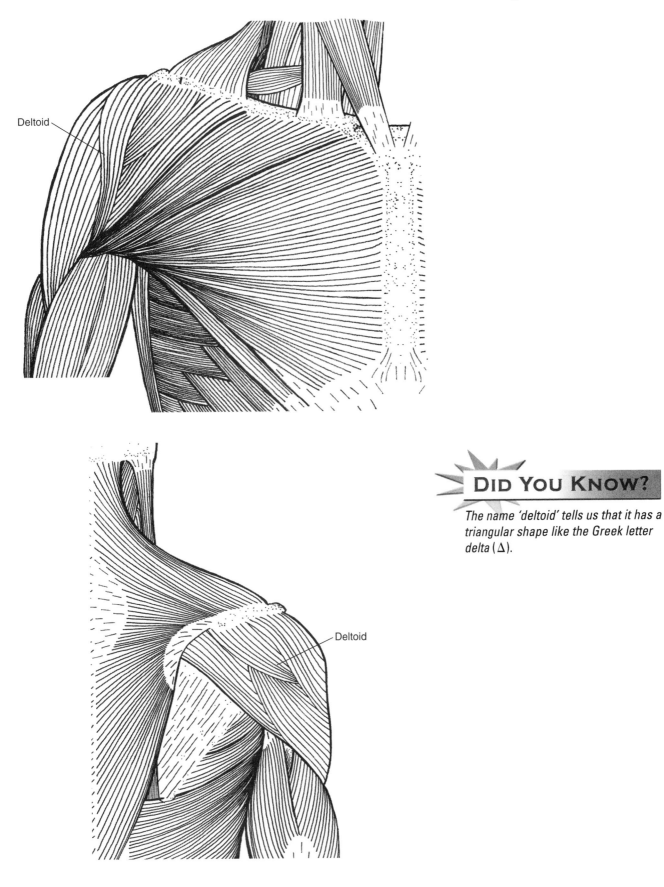

Deltoid

Deltoid

DID YOU KNOW?

The name 'deltoid' tells us that it has a triangular shape like the Greek letter delta (Δ).

Muscles of the Scapula/Arm

CORACOBRACHIALIS

kor-a-ko-**bray**-key-**al**-is

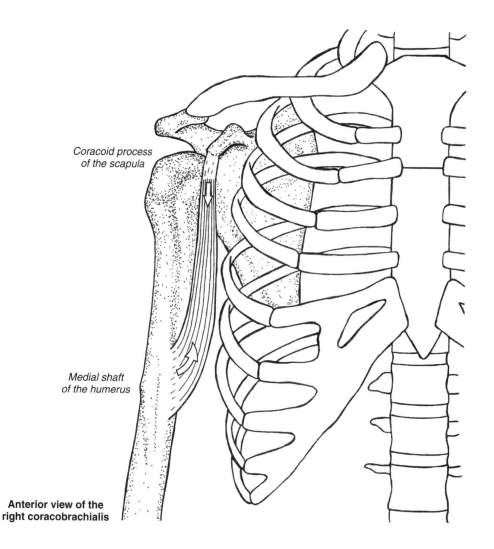

*Coracoid process
of the scapula*

*Medial shaft
of the humerus*

**Anterior view of the
right coracobrachialis**

Actions	**Innervation**	**Arterial Supply**
Flexion of the arm at the shoulder joint Adduction of the arm at the shoulder joint	The musculocutaneous nerve	The muscular branches of the brachial artery

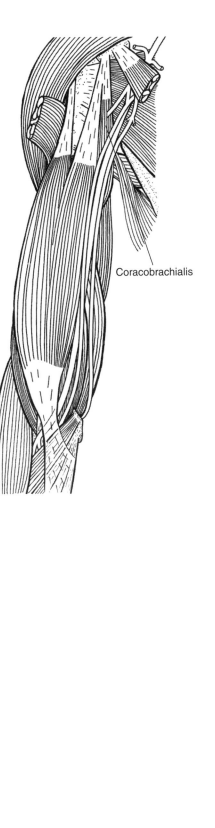

Coracobrachialis

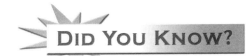

DID YOU KNOW?

The name coracobrachialis *tells us that this muscle attaches from the coracoid process of the scapula to the brachium (arm). That in turn, tells us that it crosses the shoulder joint so its actions must be at the shoulder joint.*

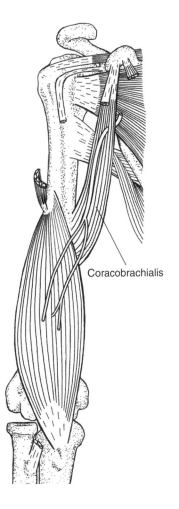

Coracobrachialis

Muscles of the Scapula/Arm

BICEPS BRACHII

by-seps **bray**-key-eye

Actions
Flexion of the forearm at the elbow joint (entire muscle)
Supination of the forearm at the radioulnar joints (entire muscle)
Flexion of the arm at the shoulder joint (entire muscle)
Abduction of the arm at the shoulder joint (long head)
Adduction of the arm at the shoulder joint (short head)

Innervation
The musculocutaneous nerve

Arterial Supply
The muscular branches of the brachial artery

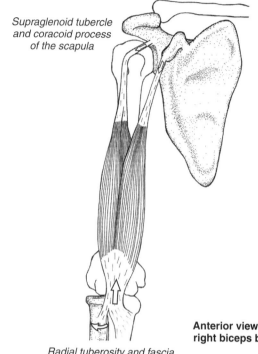

Supraglenoid tubercle and coracoid process of the scapula

Anterior view of the right biceps brachii

Radial tuberosity and fascia overlying the ulna

BRACHIALIS

bray-key-**al**-is

Action
Flexion of the forearm at the elbow joint

Innervation
The musculocutaneous nerve

Arterial Supply
Muscular branches of the brachial artery

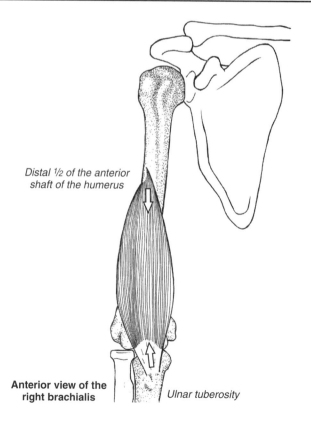

Distal ½ of the anterior shaft of the humerus

Anterior view of the right brachialis

Ulnar tuberosity

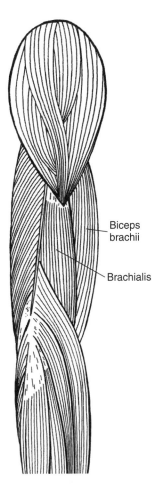

Biceps brachii

Brachialis

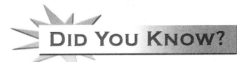

DID YOU KNOW?

The bicipital groove of the humerus is so named because the long head of the biceps brachii courses through it.

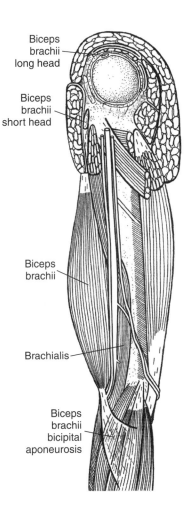

Biceps brachii long head

Biceps brachii short head

Biceps brachii

Brachialis

Biceps brachii bicipital aponeurosis

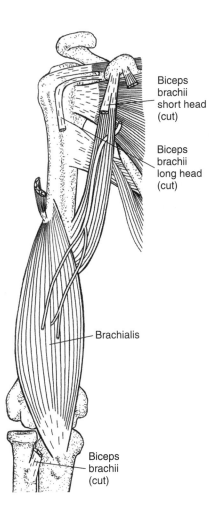

Biceps brachii short head (cut)

Biceps brachii long head (cut)

Brachialis

Biceps brachii (cut)

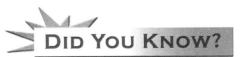

DID YOU KNOW?

The brachialis is a strong and fairly large muscle, which accounts for much of the contour of the biceps brachii being so visible. Behind every great biceps brachii is a great brachialis ☺.

TRICEPS BRACHII

try-seps **bray**-key-eye

Actions
Extension of the forearm
   at the elbow joint
   (entire muscle)
Adduction of the arm
   at the shoulder joint
   (long head)
Extension of the arm
   at the shoulder joint
   (long head)

Innervation
The radial nerve

Arterial Supply
The deep brachial artery

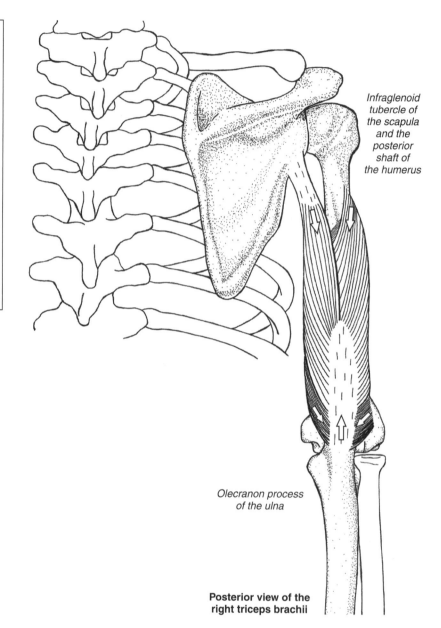

*Infraglenoid
tubercle of
the scapula
and the
posterior
shaft of
the humerus*

*Olecranon process
of the ulna*

**Posterior view of the
right triceps brachii**

Muscles of the Scapula/Arm

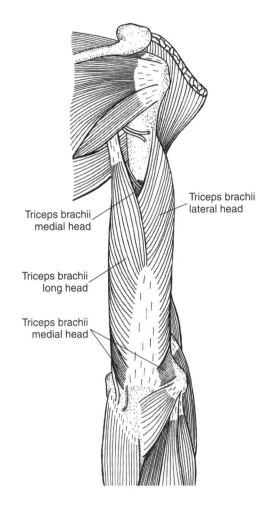

Triceps brachii
medial head

Triceps brachii
lateral head

Triceps brachii
long head

Triceps brachii
medial head

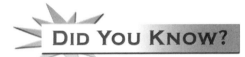

DID YOU KNOW?

*The triceps brachii has three heads,
the lateral, medial, and long heads;
only the long head crosses and
therefore can move the shoulder joint.*

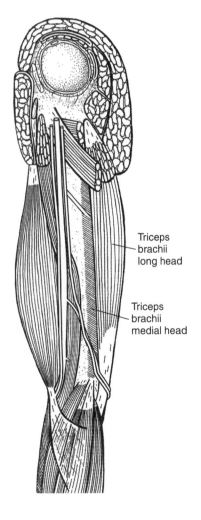

Triceps
brachii
long head

Triceps
brachii
medial head

Muscles of the Scapula/Arm

ANTERIOR VIEW OF THE RIGHT SHOULDER

SUPERIOR

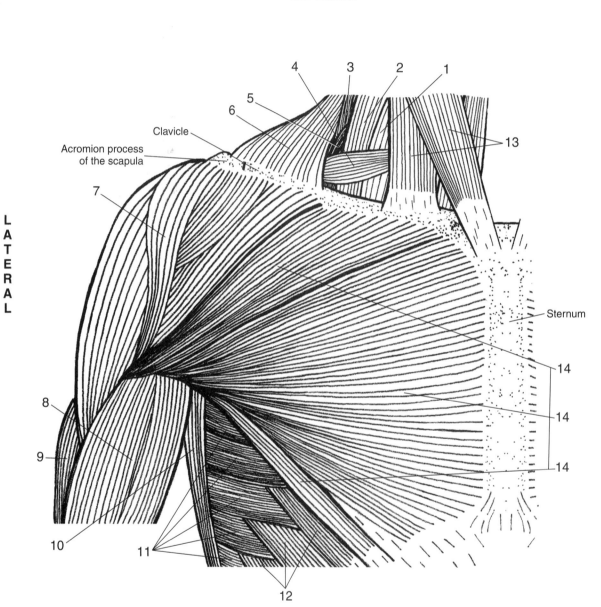

Clavicle

Acromion process
of the scapula

LATERAL

MEDIAL

Sternum

INFERIOR

POSTERIOR VIEW OF THE SHOULDERS
(SUPERFICIAL AND INTERMEDIATE)

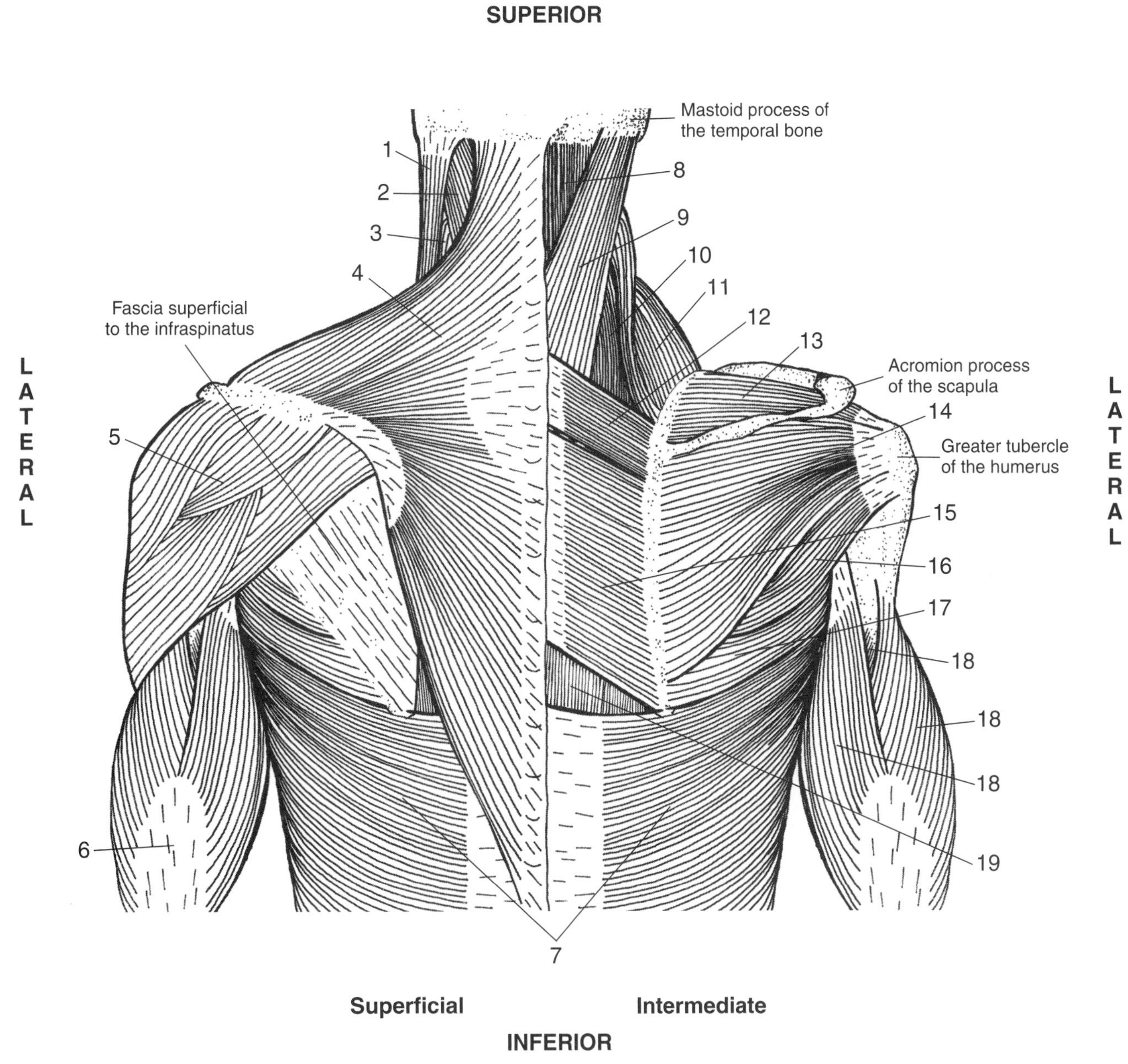

SUPERIOR

Mastoid process of
the temporal bone

1

2

3

8

4

9

10

11

Fascia superficial
to the infraspinatus

12

13

Acromion process
of the scapula

14

Greater tubercle
of the humerus

5

15

16

17

18

18

18

6

19

7

LATERAL

LATERAL

Superficial   Intermediate

INFERIOR

Muscles of the Scapula/Arm

ANTERIOR VIEW OF THE RIGHT ARM (SUPERFICIAL)

PROXIMAL

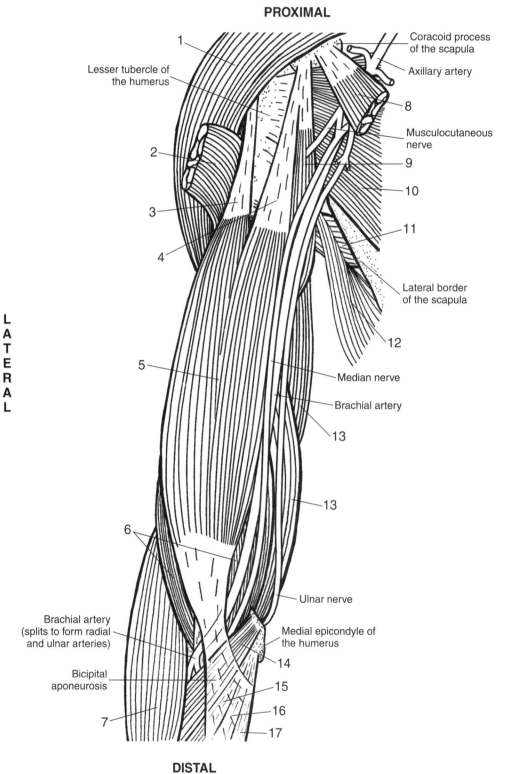

Coracoid process
of the scapula

Axillary artery

Lesser tubercle of
the humerus

Musculocutaneous
nerve

Lateral border
of the scapula

Median nerve

Brachial artery

LATERAL

MEDIAL

Ulnar nerve

Brachial artery
(splits to form radial
and ulnar arteries)

Medial epicondyle of
the humerus

Bicipital
aponeurosis

DISTAL

ANTERIOR VIEW OF THE RIGHT ARM (DEEP)

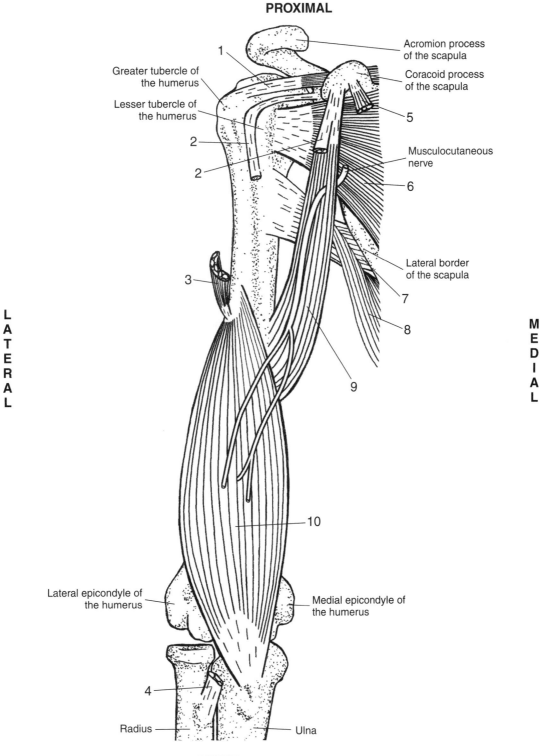

PROXIMAL

Acromion process
of the scapula

Coracoid process
of the scapula

Greater tubercle of
the humerus

Lesser tubercle of
the humerus

1

2

2

5

Musculocutaneous
nerve

6

Lateral border
of the scapula

7

8

3

9

LATERAL

MEDIAL

10

Lateral epicondyle of
the humerus

Medial epicondyle of
the humerus

4

Radius

Ulna

DISTAL

Muscles of the Scapula/Arm

MEDIAL VIEW OF THE RIGHT ARM

PROXIMAL

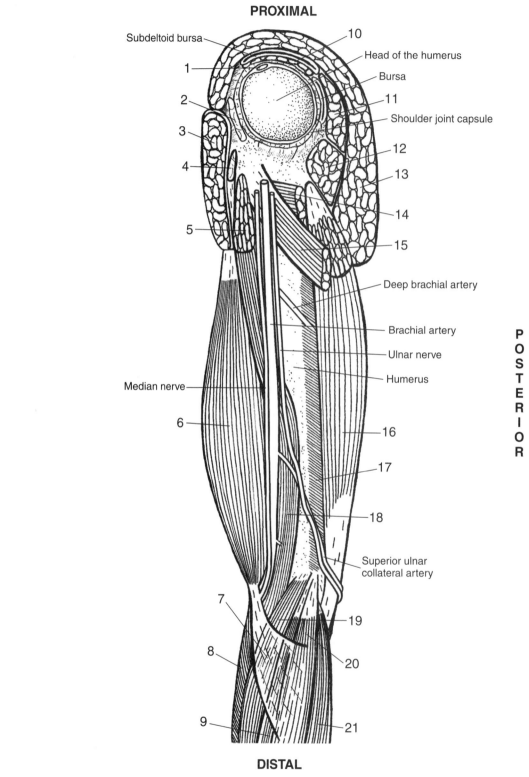

Subdeltoid bursa

10

Head of the humerus

1

Bursa

2

11

Shoulder joint capsule

3

12

4

13

14

5

15

Deep brachial artery

Brachial artery

A N T E R I O R

Ulnar nerve

Humerus

Median nerve

P O S T E R I O R

6

16

17

18

Superior ulnar collateral artery

7

19

8

20

9

21

DISTAL

LATERAL VIEW OF THE RIGHT ARM

PROXIMAL

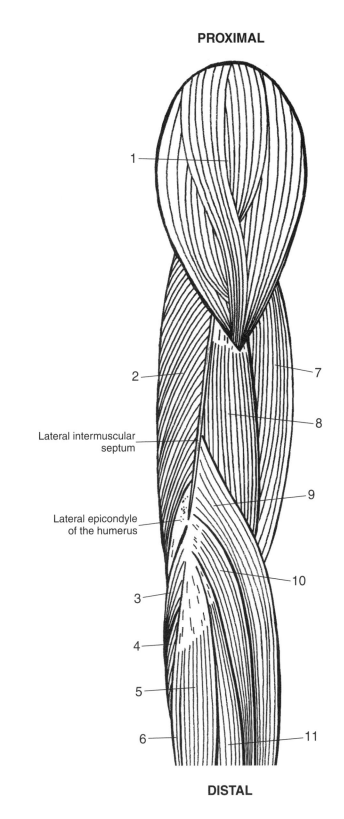

POSTERIOR

ANTERIOR

1

2

7

8

Lateral intermuscular
septum

9

Lateral epicondyle
of the humerus

3

10

4

5

6

11

DISTAL

Muscles of the Scapula/Arm

POSTERIOR VIEW OF THE RIGHT ARM

PROXIMAL

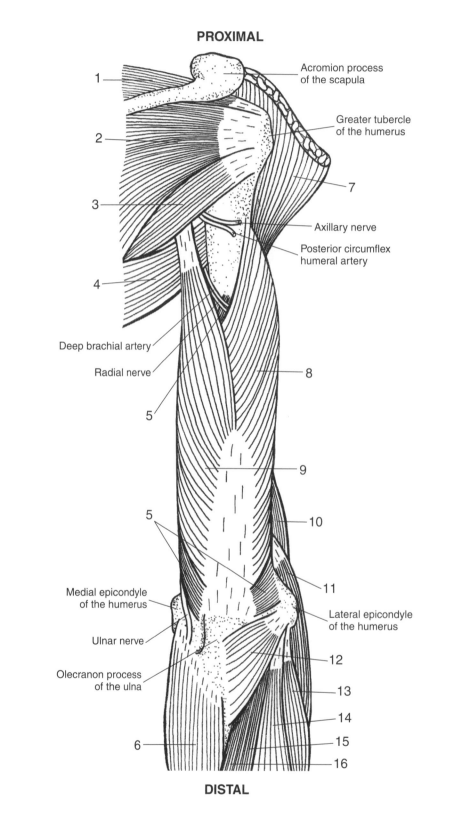

1

Acromion process
of the scapula

2

Greater tubercle
of the humerus

3

7

Axillary nerve

4

Posterior circumflex
humeral artery

MEDIAL

LATERAL

Deep brachial artery

Radial nerve

8

5

9

5

10

11

Medial epicondyle
of the humerus

Lateral epicondyle
of the humerus

Ulnar nerve

12

Olecranon process
of the ulna

13

14

6

15

16

DISTAL

ANTERIOR VIEW OF THE RIGHT GLENOHUMERAL JOINT

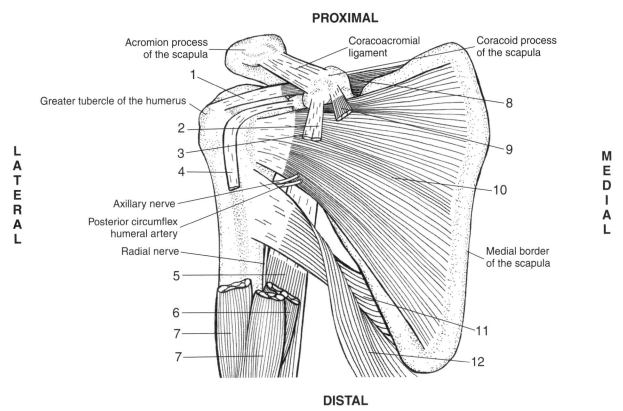

PROXIMAL

Acromion process of the scapula

Coracoacromial ligament

Coracoid process of the scapula

1

Greater tubercle of the humerus

2

3

4

8

9

10

LATERAL

Axillary nerve

Posterior circumflex humeral artery

Radial nerve

5

6

7

7

MEDIAL

Medial border of the scapula

11

12

DISTAL

POSTERIOR VIEW OF THE RIGHT GLENOHUMERAL JOINT

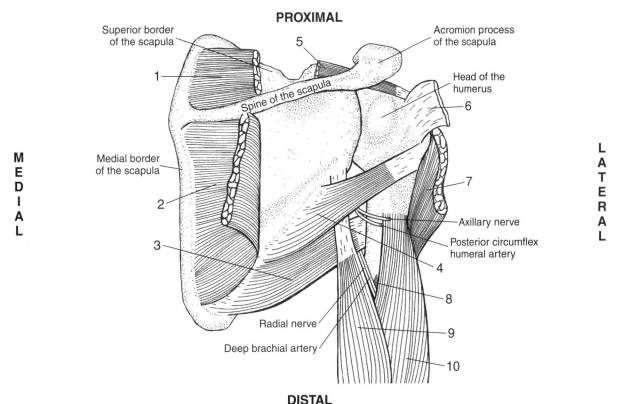

PROXIMAL

Superior border of the scapula

5

Acromion process of the scapula

1

Spine of the scapula

Head of the humerus

6

MEDIAL

Medial border of the scapula

2

3

7

Axillary nerve

Posterior circumflex humeral artery

4

8

LATERAL

Radial nerve

Deep brachial artery

9

10

DISTAL

ANTERIOR VIEW OF THE RIGHT FOREARM (SUPERFICIAL)

PROXIMAL

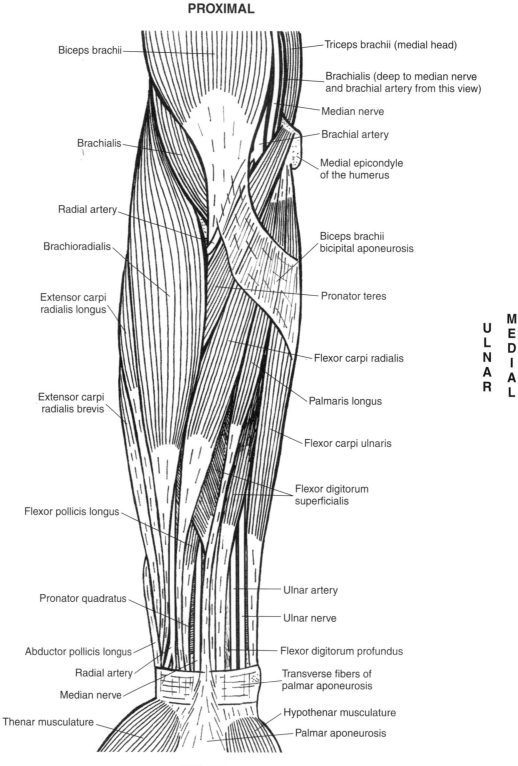

Biceps brachii

Triceps brachii (medial head)

Brachialis (deep to median nerve and brachial artery from this view)

Median nerve

Brachialis

Brachial artery

Medial epicondyle of the humerus

Radial artery

Biceps brachii bicipital aponeurosis

Brachioradialis

Pronator teres

Extensor carpi radialis longus

L A T E R A L

R A D I A L

U L N A R

M E D I A L

Flexor carpi radialis

Extensor carpi radialis brevis

Palmaris longus

Flexor carpi ulnaris

Flexor digitorum superficialis

Flexor pollicis longus

Pronator quadratus

Ulnar artery

Ulnar nerve

Abductor pollicis longus

Flexor digitorum profundus

Radial artery

Transverse fibers of palmar aponeurosis

Median nerve

Hypothenar musculature

Thenar musculature

Palmar aponeurosis

DISTAL

Muscles of the Forearm

ANTERIOR VIEW OF THE RIGHT FOREARM (INTERMEDIATE)

PROXIMAL

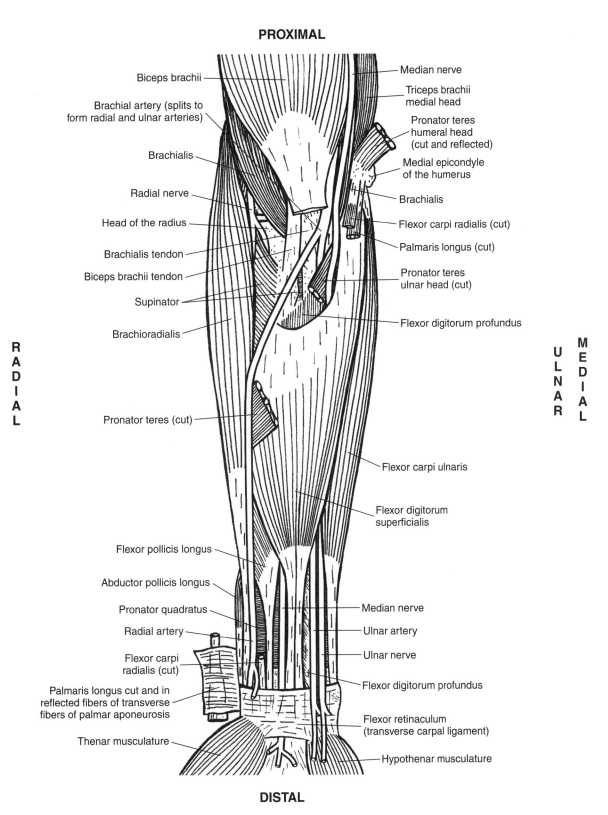

Biceps brachii

Brachial artery (splits to form radial and ulnar arteries)

Brachialis

Radial nerve

Head of the radius

Brachialis tendon

Biceps brachii tendon

Supinator

Brachioradialis

Pronator teres (cut)

Flexor pollicis longus

Abductor pollicis longus

Pronator quadratus

Radial artery

Flexor carpi radialis (cut)

Palmaris longus cut and in reflected fibers of transverse fibers of palmar aponeurosis

Thenar musculature

Median nerve

Triceps brachii medial head

Pronator teres humeral head (cut and reflected)

Medial epicondyle of the humerus

Brachialis

Flexor carpi radialis (cut)

Palmaris longus (cut)

Pronator teres ulnar head (cut)

Flexor digitorum profundus

Flexor carpi ulnaris

Flexor digitorum superficialis

Median nerve

Ulnar artery

Ulnar nerve

Flexor digitorum profundus

Flexor retinaculum (transverse carpal ligament)

Hypothenar musculature

LATERAL

RADIAL

ULNAR

MEDIAL

DISTAL

Muscles of the Forearm

ANTERIOR VIEW OF THE RIGHT FOREARM (DEEP)

PROXIMAL

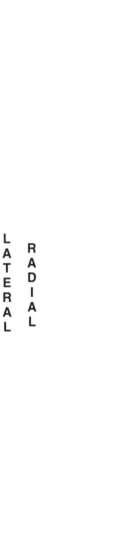

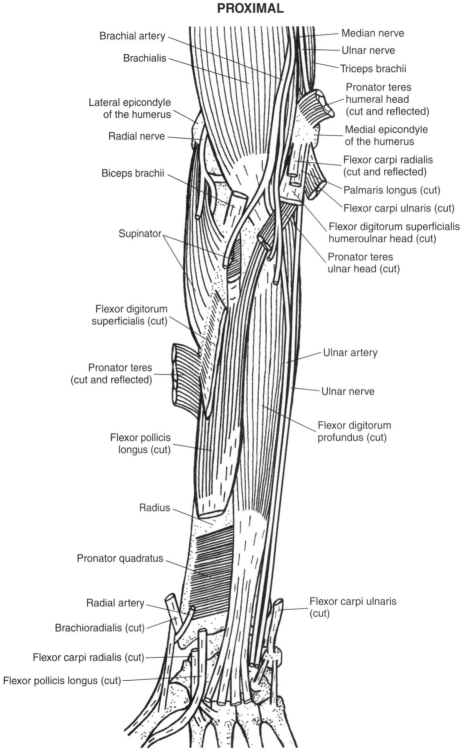

Brachial artery

Brachialis

Lateral epicondyle
of the humerus

Radial nerve

Biceps brachii

Supinator

Flexor digitorum
superficialis (cut)

Pronator teres
(cut and reflected)

Flexor pollicis
longus (cut)

Radius

Pronator quadratus

Radial artery

Brachioradialis (cut)

Flexor carpi radialis (cut)

Flexor pollicis longus (cut)

Median nerve

Ulnar nerve

Triceps brachii

Pronator teres
humeral head
(cut and reflected)

Medial epicondyle
of the humerus

Flexor carpi radialis
(cut and reflected)

Palmaris longus (cut)

Flexor carpi ulnaris (cut)

Flexor digitorum superficialis
humeroulnar head (cut)

Pronator teres
ulnar head (cut)

Ulnar artery

Ulnar nerve

Flexor digitorum
profundus (cut)

Flexor carpi ulnaris
(cut)

LATERAL RADIAL

ULNAR MEDIAL

DISTAL

Muscles of the Forearm

ANTERIOR VIEW OF THE PRONATORS AND SUPINATOR
OF THE RIGHT RADIUS

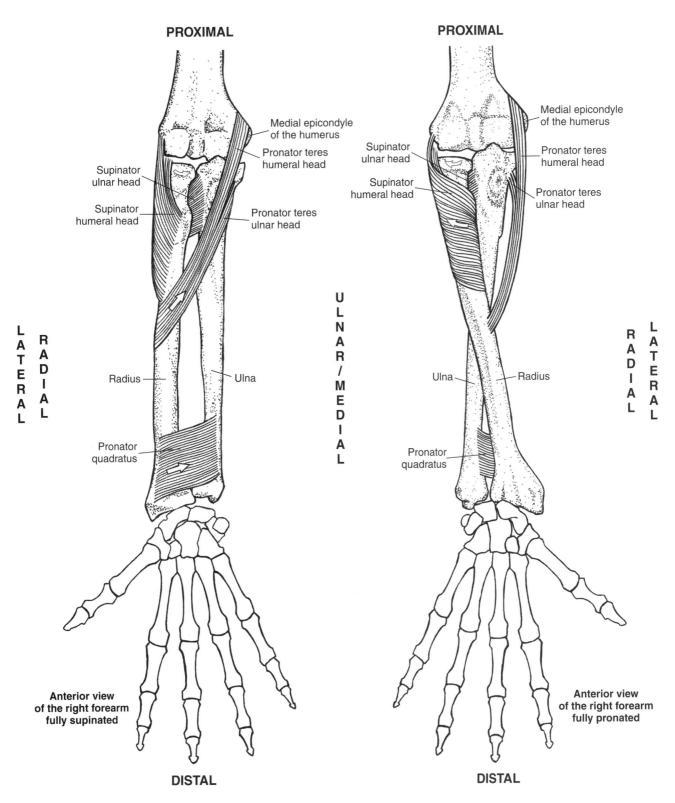

PROXIMAL

Medial epicondyle
of the humerus

Pronator teres
humeral head

Supinator
ulnar head

Supinator
humeral head

Pronator teres
ulnar head

LATERAL RADIAL

Radius

Ulna

ULNAR/MEDIAL

Pronator
quadratus

Anterior view
of the right forearm
fully supinated

DISTAL

PROXIMAL

Medial epicondyle
of the humerus

Supinator
ulnar head

Pronator teres
humeral head

Supinator
humeral head

Pronator teres
ulnar head

RADIAL LATERAL

Ulna

Radius

Pronator
quadratus

Anterior view
of the right forearm
fully pronated

DISTAL

Muscles of the Forearm

POSTERIOR VIEW OF THE RIGHT FOREARM (SUPERFICIAL)

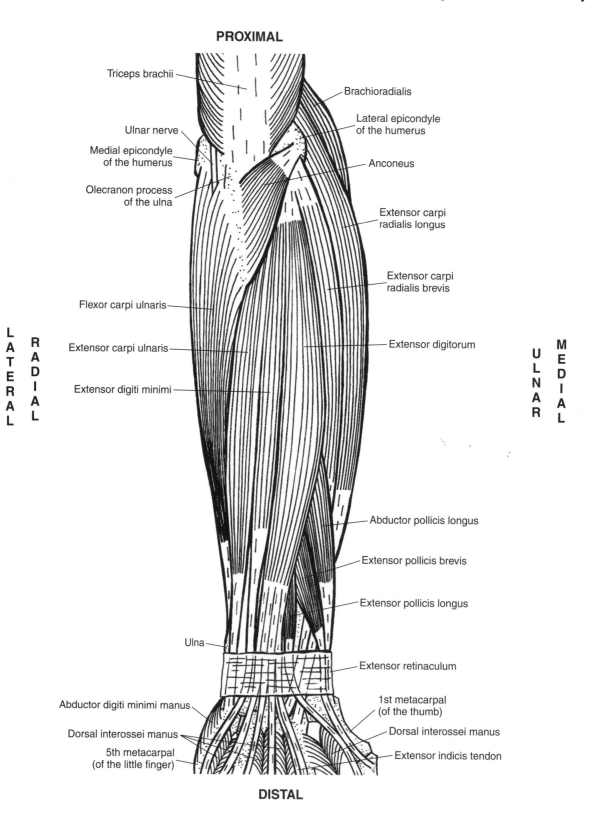

PROXIMAL

Triceps brachii

Ulnar nerve

Medial epicondyle
of the humerus

Olecranon process
of the ulna

Flexor carpi ulnaris

Extensor carpi ulnaris

Extensor digiti minimi

LATERAL

RADIAL

Brachioradialis

Lateral epicondyle
of the humerus

Anconeus

Extensor carpi
radialis longus

Extensor carpi
radialis brevis

Extensor digitorum

ULNAR

MEDIAL

Abductor pollicis longus

Extensor pollicis brevis

Extensor pollicis longus

Ulna

Extensor retinaculum

Abductor digiti minimi manus

Dorsal interossei manus

5th metacarpal
(of the little finger)

1st metacarpal
(of the thumb)

Dorsal interossei manus

Extensor indicis tendon

DISTAL

Muscles of the Forearm

POSTERIOR VIEW OF THE RIGHT FOREARM (DEEP)

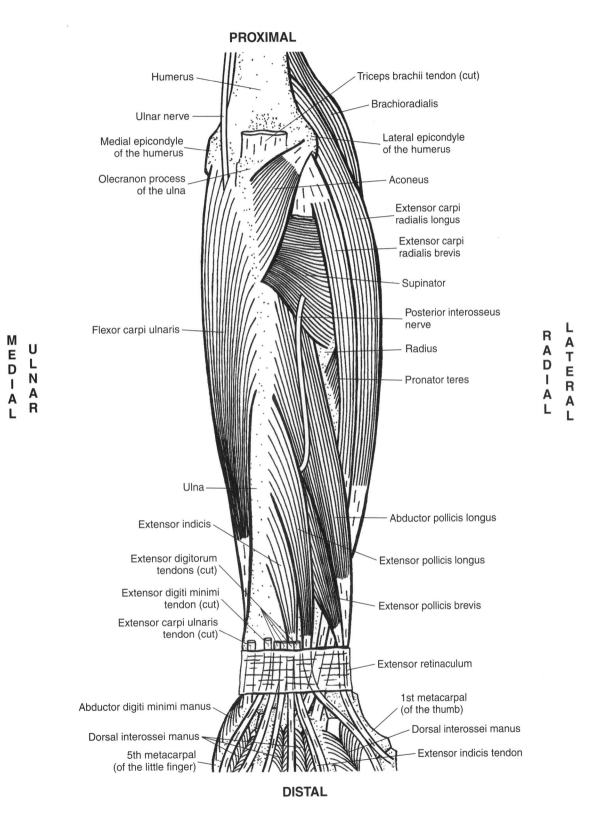

PROXIMAL

Humerus

Triceps brachii tendon (cut)

Brachioradialis

Ulnar nerve

Lateral epicondyle
of the humerus

Medial epicondyle
of the humerus

Olecranon process
of the ulna

Aconeus

Extensor carpi
radialis longus

Extensor carpi
radialis brevis

Supinator

Flexor carpi ulnaris

Posterior interosseus
nerve

Radius

Pronator teres

MEDIAL

ULNAR

RADIAL

LATERAL

Ulna

Extensor indicis

Abductor pollicis longus

Extensor digitorum
tendons (cut)

Extensor pollicis longus

Extensor digiti minimi
tendon (cut)

Extensor carpi ulnaris
tendon (cut)

Extensor pollicis brevis

Extensor retinaculum

Abductor digiti minimi manus

1st metacarpal
(of the thumb)

Dorsal interossei manus

Dorsal interossei manus

5th metacarpal
(of the little finger)

Extensor indicis tendon

DISTAL

Muscles of the Forearm

POSTERIOR VIEW OF THE RIGHT FOREARM AND HAND (SUPERFICIAL)

PROXIMAL

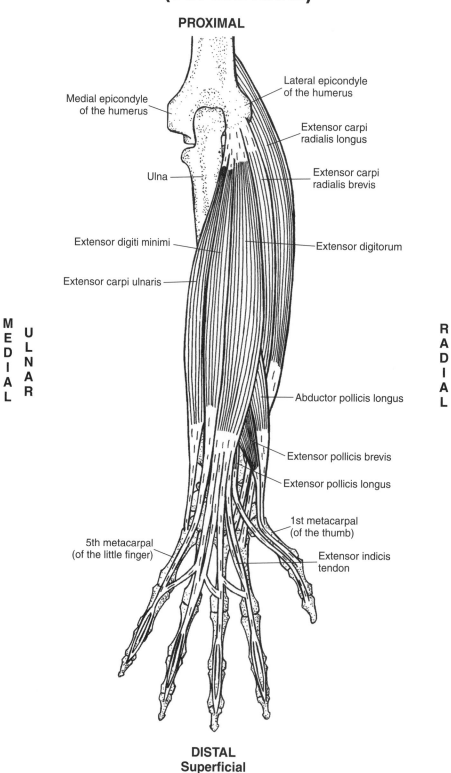

Medial epicondyle of the humerus

Ulna

Extensor digiti minimi

Extensor carpi ulnaris

Lateral epicondyle of the humerus

Extensor carpi radialis longus

Extensor carpi radialis brevis

Extensor digitorum

M E D I A L   U L N A R

R A D I A L   L A T E R A L

Abductor pollicis longus

Extensor pollicis brevis

Extensor pollicis longus

5th metacarpal (of the little finger)

1st metacarpal (of the thumb)

Extensor indicis tendon

DISTAL
Superficial

POSTERIOR VIEW OF THE RIGHT FOREARM AND HAND (DEEP)

PROXIMAL

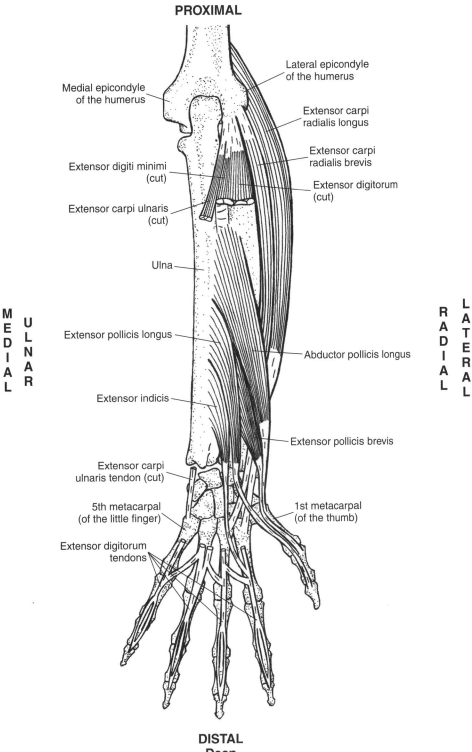

Medial epicondyle of the humerus

Lateral epicondyle of the humerus

Extensor carpi radialis longus

Extensor carpi radialis brevis

Extensor digiti minimi (cut)

Extensor digitorum (cut)

Extensor carpi ulnaris (cut)

Ulna

M E D I A L

U L N A R

R A D I A L

L A T E R A L

Extensor pollicis longus

Abductor pollicis longus

Extensor indicis

Extensor pollicis brevis

Extensor carpi ulnaris tendon (cut)

5th metacarpal (of the little finger)

1st metacarpal (of the thumb)

Extensor digitorum tendons

DISTAL
Deep

Muscles of the Forearm

PRONATOR TERES

pro-**nay**-tor **te**-reez

Actions
Pronation of the forearm at the radioulnar joints
Flexion of the forearm at the elbow joint

Innervation
The median nerve

Arterial Supply
The ulnar artery

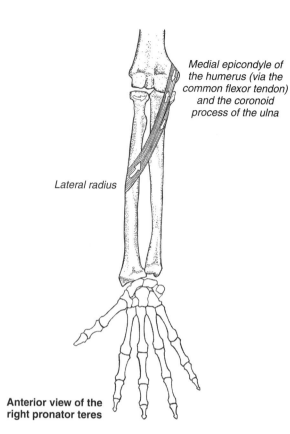

Medial epicondyle of the humerus (via the common flexor tendon) and the coronoid process of the ulna

Lateral radius

Anterior view of the right pronator teres

PRONATOR QUADRATUS

pro-**nay**-tor kwod-**ray**-tus

Action
Pronation of the forearm at the radioulnar joints

Innervation
The median nerve

Arterial Supply
The anterior interosseus artery

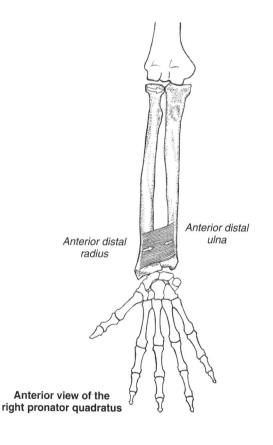

Anterior distal radius

Anterior distal ulna

Anterior view of the right pronator quadratus

Muscles of the Forearm

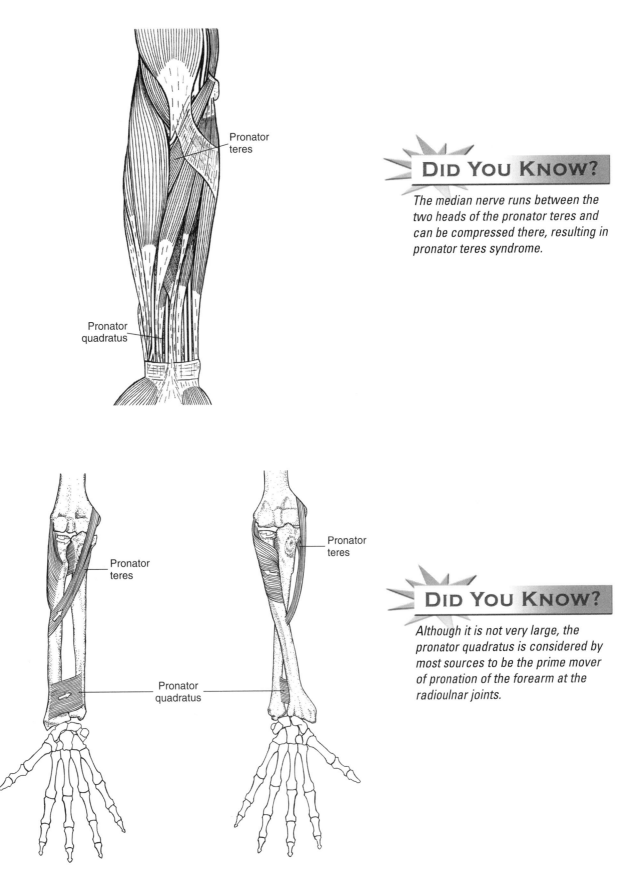

Pronator
teres

Pronator
quadratus

Pronator
teres

Pronator
teres

Pronator
quadratus

DID YOU KNOW?

The median nerve runs between the two heads of the pronator teres and can be compressed there, resulting in pronator teres syndrome.

DID YOU KNOW?

Although it is not very large, the pronator quadratus is considered by most sources to be the prime mover of pronation of the forearm at the radioulnar joints.

Muscles of the Forearm

FLEXOR CARPI RADIALIS

(OF THE WRIST FLEXOR GROUP)

fleks-or **kar**-pie **ray**-dee-a-lis

Actions
Flexion of the hand at the wrist joint

Radial deviation (abduction) of the hand at the wrist joint

Flexion of the forearm at the elbow joint

Pronation of the forearm at the radioulnar joints

Innervation
The median nerve

Arterial Supply
The ulnar and radial arteries

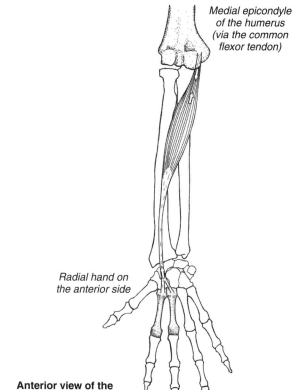

Medial epicondyle of the humerus (via the common flexor tendon)

Radial hand on the anterior side

Anterior view of the right flexor carpi radialis

PALMARIS LONGUS

(OF THE WRIST FLEXOR GROUP)

pall-**ma**-ris **long**-us

Actions
Flexion of the hand at the wrist joint

Flexion of the forearm at the elbow joint

Pronation of the forearm at the radioulnar joints

Wrinkles the skin of the palm

Innervation
The median nerve

Arterial Supply
The ulnar artery

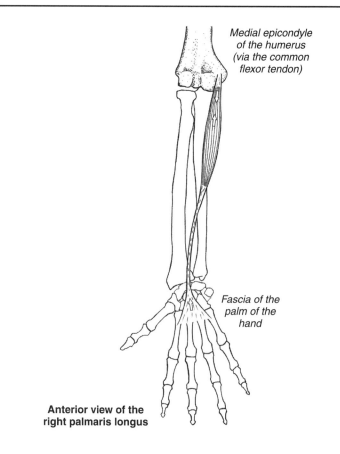

Medial epicondyle of the humerus (via the common flexor tendon)

Fascia of the palm of the hand

Anterior view of the right palmaris longus

Muscles of the Forearm

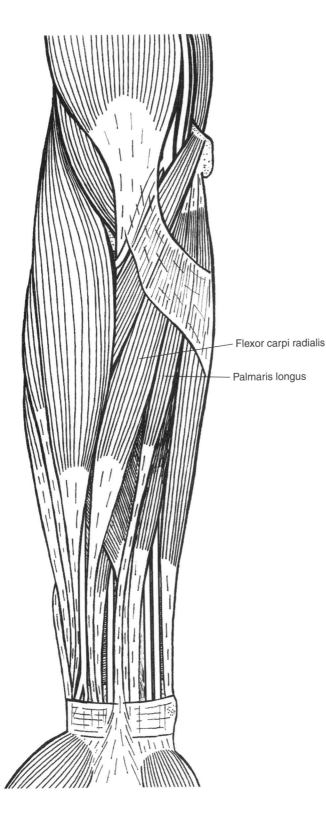

Flexor carpi radialis

Palmaris longus

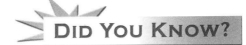

*Irritation and inflammation of the
medial epicondyle of the humerus
and/or the common flexor tendon is
known as* medial epicondylitis *and is
usually called 'golfer's elbow'.*

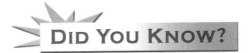

*The palmaris longus is often missing,
sometimes unilaterally, sometimes
bilaterally.*

Muscles of the Forearm

FLEXOR CARPI ULNARIS
(OF THE WRIST FLEXOR GROUP)

fleks-or kar-pie ul-na-ris

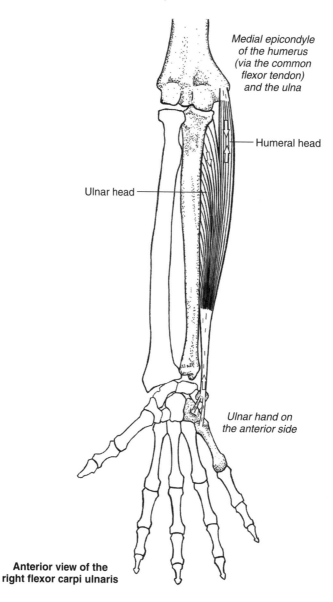

Medial epicondyle of the humerus (via the common flexor tendon) and the ulna

— Humeral head

Ulnar head —

Ulnar hand on the anterior side

Anterior view of the right flexor carpi ulnaris

Actions	Innervation	Arterial Supply
Flexion of the hand at the wrist joint Ulnar deviation (adduction) of the hand at the wrist joint Flexion of the forearm at the elbow joint	The ulnar nerve	The ulnar artery

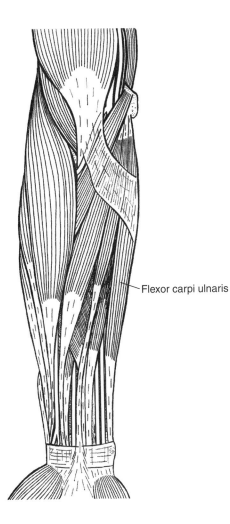

Flexor carpi ulnaris

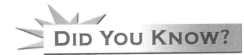

DID YOU KNOW?

All three wrist flexor group muscles (flexor carpi radialis, palmaris longus, and flexor carpi ulnaris) attach onto the medial epicondyle of the humerus via the common flexor tendon. Only the flexor carpi ulnaris has an additional proximal attachment, onto the ulna.

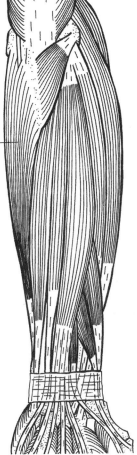

Flexor carpi ulnaris

Muscles of the Forearm

BRACHIORADIALIS
(OF THE RADIAL GROUP)

bray-key-o-**ray**-dee-**al**-is

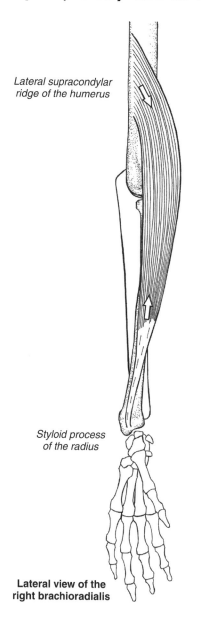

Lateral supracondylar ridge of the humerus

Styloid process of the radius

Lateral view of the right brachioradialis

Actions	**Innervation**	**Arterial Supply**
Flexion of the forearm at the elbow joint Supination of the forearm at the radioulnar joints Pronation of the forearm at the radioulnar joints	The radial nerve	Branches of the brachial artery and the radial artery

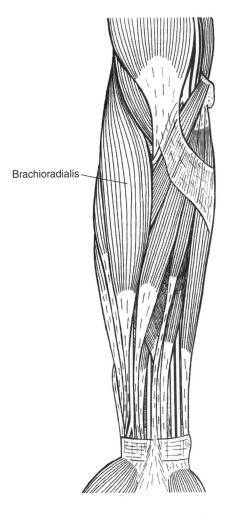

Brachioradialis

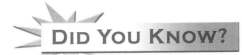

DID YOU KNOW?

The brachioradialis can both pronate and supinate the forearm at the radioulnar joints. But, it can only create these actions to a halfway position.

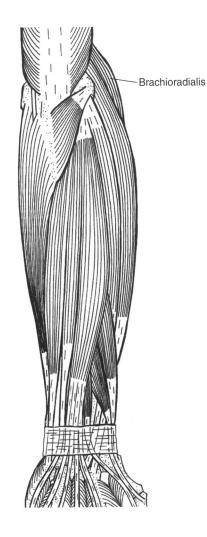

Brachioradialis

Muscles of the Forearm

FLEXOR DIGITORUM SUPERFICIALIS

fleks-or dij-i-**toe**-rum
soo-per-fish-ee-**a**-lis

Actions
Flexion of fingers #2-5 at
the metacarpophalangeal
and proximal
interphalangeal joints
Flexion of the hand at the
wrist joint
Flexion of the forearm at
the elbow joint

Innervation
The median nerve

Arterial Supply
The ulnar and radial arteries

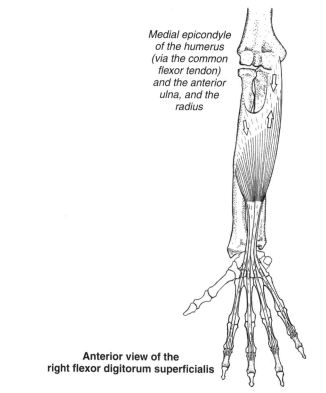

*Medial epicondyle
of the humerus
(via the common
flexor tendon)
and the anterior
ulna, and the
radius*

**Anterior view of the
right flexor digitorum superficialis**

Anterior surfaces of fingers #2-5

FLEXOR DIGITORUM PROFUNDUS

fleks-or dij-i-**toe**-rum pro-**fun**-dus

Actions
Flexion of fingers #2-5 at
the metacarpophalangeal
and proximal and distal
interphalangeal joints
Flexion of the hand at the
wrist joint

Innervation
The median and the ulnar
nerves

Arterial Supply
The ulnar and radial arteries
and the anterior
interosseus artery

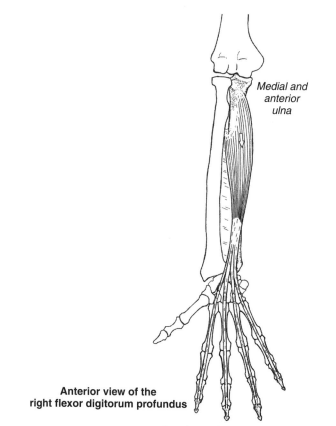

*Medial and
anterior
ulna*

**Anterior view of the
right flexor digitorum profundus**

Anterior surfaces of fingers #2-5

Muscles of the Forearm

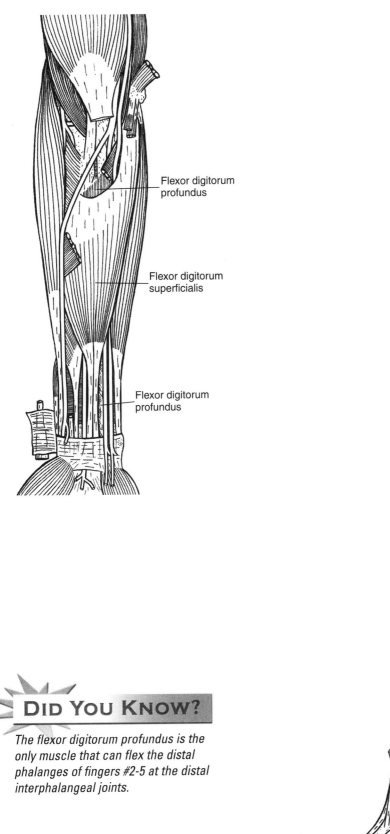

Flexor digitorum
profundus

Flexor digitorum
superficialis

Flexor digitorum
profundus

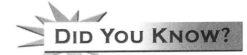

*The distal tendons of the flexor
digitorum superficialis split to allow
passage of the distal tendons of the
flexor digitorum profundus to the
distal phalanges of fingers #2-5.*

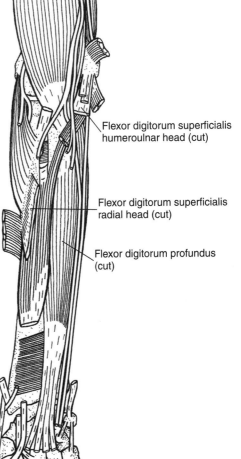

Flexor digitorum superficialis
humeroulnar head (cut)

Flexor digitorum superficialis
radial head (cut)

Flexor digitorum profundus
(cut)

*The flexor digitorum profundus is the
only muscle that can flex the distal
phalanges of fingers #2-5 at the distal
interphalangeal joints.*

Muscles of the Forearm

FLEXOR POLLICIS LONGUS

fleks-or **pol**-i-sis **long**-us

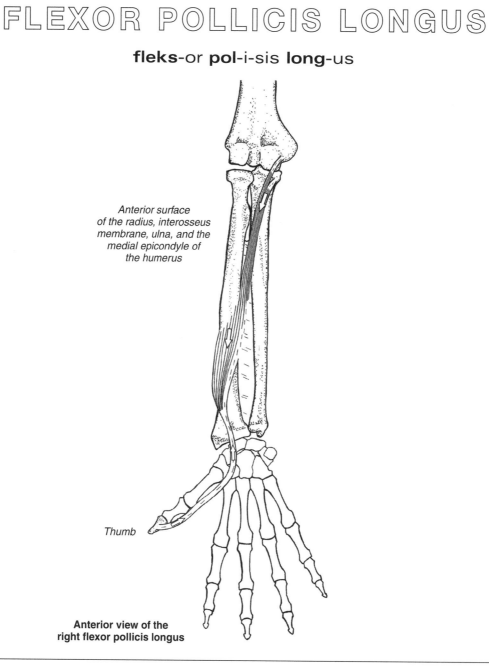

Anterior surface
of the radius, interosseus
membrane, ulna, and the
medial epicondyle of
the humerus

Thumb

**Anterior view of the
right flexor pollicis longus**

Actions	Innervation	Arterial Supply
Flexion of the thumb at the carpometacarpal, meta-carpophalangeal, and interphalangeal joints Flexion of the hand at the wrist joint Radial deviation (abduction) of the hand at the wrist joint Flexion of the forearm at the elbow joint	The median nerve	The radial artery and the anterior interosseus artery

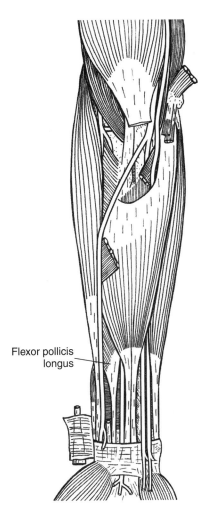

Flexor pollicis
longus

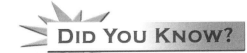

DID YOU KNOW?

The flexor pollicis longus has a common variation wherein it is missing its humeroulnar head.

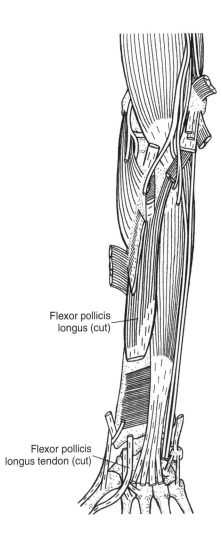

Flexor pollicis
longus (cut)

Flexor pollicis
longus tendon (cut)

Muscles of the Forearm

ANCONEUS

an-**ko**-nee-us

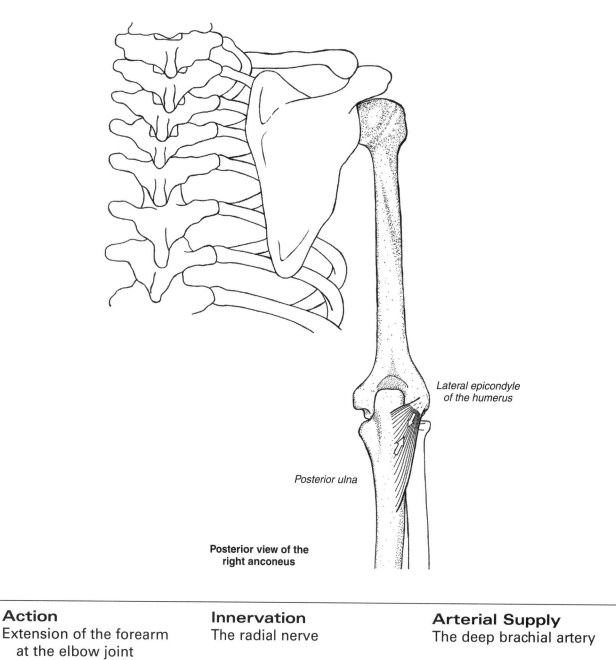

Lateral epicondyle
of the humerus

Posterior ulna

**Posterior view of the
right anconeus**

Action	**Innervation**	**Arterial Supply**
Extension of the forearm at the elbow joint	The radial nerve	The deep brachial artery

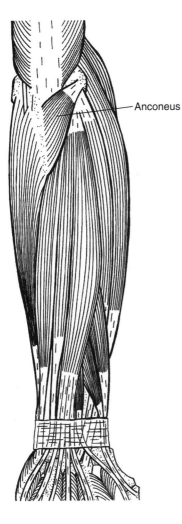

Anconeus

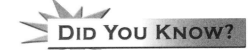

DID YOU KNOW?

The anconeus is easily palpable in the posterior proximal forearm just distal to a point that is halfway between the olecranon process of the ulna and the lateral epicondyle of the humerus.

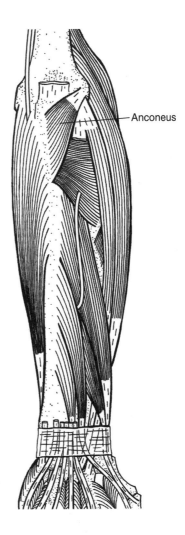

Anconeus

Muscles of the Forearm

EXTENSOR CARPI RADIALIS LONGUS

(OF THE WRIST EXTENSOR
GROUP AND THE RADIAL GROUP)

eks-**ten**-sor **kar**-pie **ray**-dee-**a**-lis **long**-us

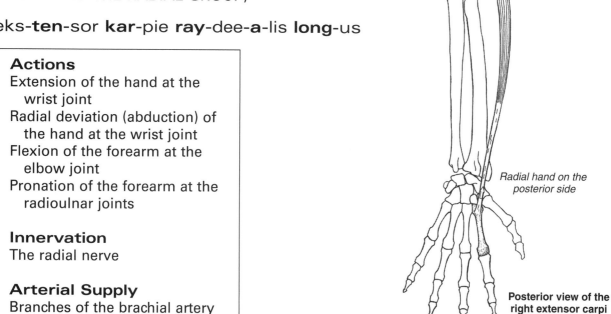

Lateral supracondylar ridge of the humerus

Radial hand on the posterior side

Posterior view of the right extensor carpi radialis longus

Actions
Extension of the hand at the
wrist joint
Radial deviation (abduction) of
the hand at the wrist joint
Flexion of the forearm at the
elbow joint
Pronation of the forearm at the
radioulnar joints

Innervation
The radial nerve

Arterial Supply
Branches of the brachial artery
and the radial artery

EXTENSOR CARPI RADIALIS BREVIS

(OF THE WRIST EXTENSOR
GROUP AND THE RADIAL GROUP)

eks-**ten**-sor **kar**-pie **ray**-dee-**a**-lis **bre**-vis

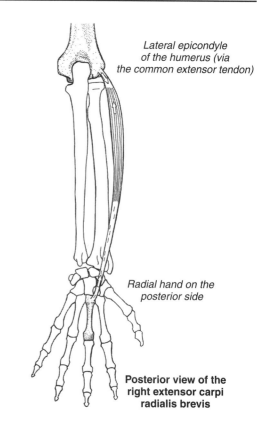

Lateral epicondyle of the humerus (via the common extensor tendon)

Radial hand on the posterior side

Posterior view of the right extensor carpi radialis brevis

Actions
Extension of the hand at the
wrist joint
Radial deviation (abduction) of
the hand at the wrist joint
Flexion of the forearm at the
elbow joint

Innervation
The radial nerve

Arterial Supply
Branches of the brachial artery
and the radial artery

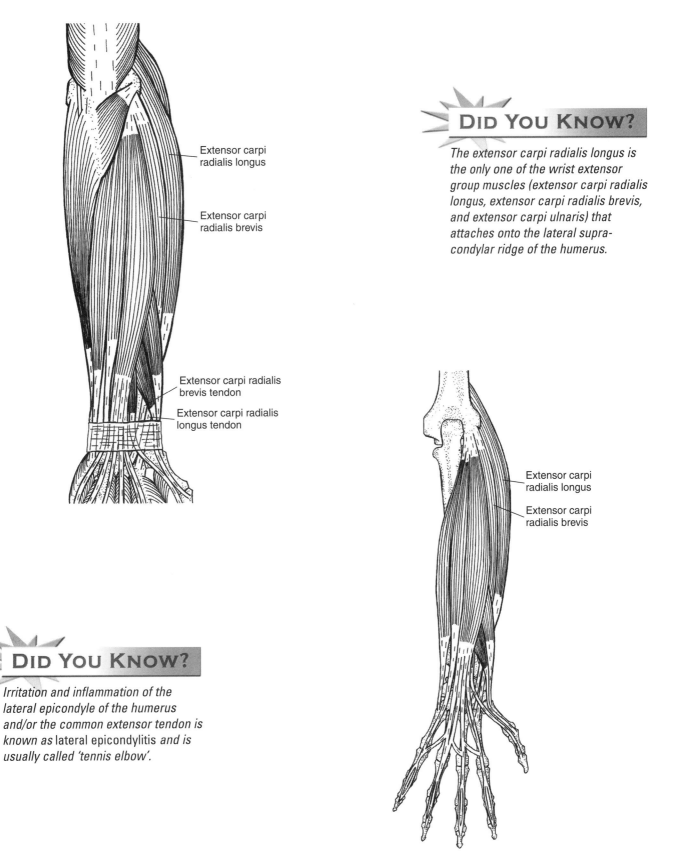

Extensor carpi
radialis longus

Extensor carpi
radialis brevis

Extensor carpi radialis
brevis tendon

Extensor carpi radialis
longus tendon

Extensor carpi
radialis longus

Extensor carpi
radialis brevis

DID YOU KNOW?

The extensor carpi radialis longus is the only one of the wrist extensor group muscles (extensor carpi radialis longus, extensor carpi radialis brevis, and extensor carpi ulnaris) that attaches onto the lateral supra-condylar ridge of the humerus.

DID YOU KNOW?

Irritation and inflammation of the lateral epicondyle of the humerus and/or the common extensor tendon is known as lateral epicondylitis *and is usually called 'tennis elbow'.*

Muscles of the Forearm

EXTENSOR CARPI ULNARIS
(OF THE WRIST EXTENSOR GROUP)

eks-**ten**-sor **kar**-pie ul-**na**-ris

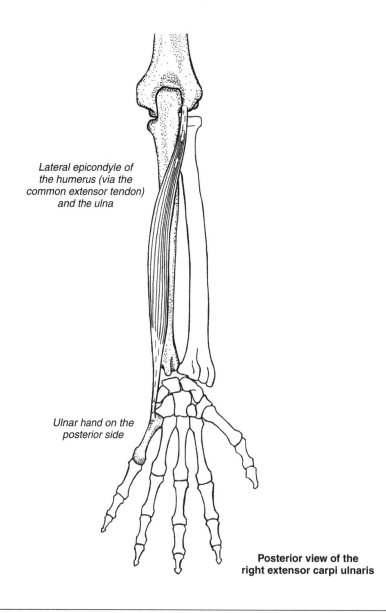

Lateral epicondyle of
the humerus (via the
common extensor tendon)
and the ulna

Ulnar hand on the
posterior side

**Posterior view of the
right extensor carpi ulnaris**

Actions	Innervation	Arterial Supply
Extension of the hand at the wrist joint Ulnar deviation (adduction) of the hand at the wrist joint Extension of the forearm at the elbow joint	The radial nerve	The posterior interosseus artery

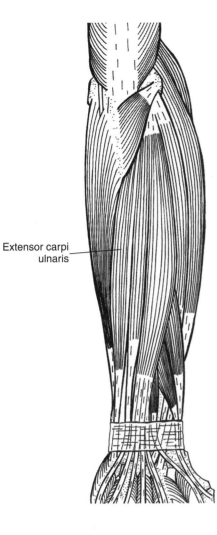

Extensor carpi
ulnaris

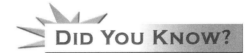

DID YOU KNOW?

The extensor carpi ulnaris is the only one of the wrist extensor group muscles (extensor carpi radialis longus, extensor carpi radialis brevis, and extensor carpi ulnaris) that has an additional proximal attachment, onto the ulna.

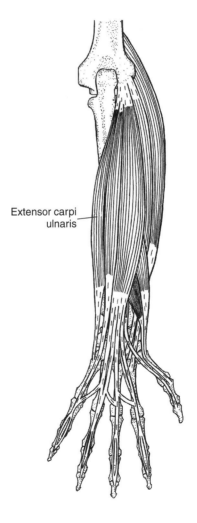

Extensor carpi
ulnaris

Muscles of the Forearm

EXTENSOR DIGITORUM

eks-**ten**-sor dij-i-**toe**-rum

Actions
Extension of fingers #2-5 at the
   metacarpophalangeal and proximal
   and distal interphalangeal joints
Extension of the hand at the wrist
   joint
Medial rotation of the little finger
   (finger #5) at the carpometacarpal
   joint
Extension of the forearm at the elbow
   joint

Innervation
The radial nerve

Arterial Supply
The posterior interosseus artery

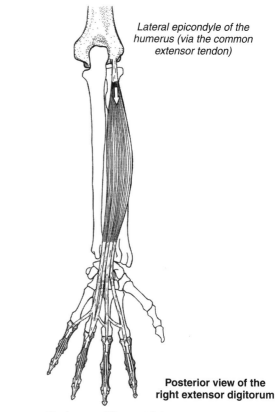

Lateral epicondyle of the
humerus (via the common
extensor tendon)

**Posterior view of the
right extensor digitorum**

Phalanges of fingers #2-5

EXTENSOR DIGITI MINIMI

eks-**ten**-sor **dij**-i-tee **min**-i-mee

Actions
Extension of the little finger (finger #5)
   at the metacarpophalangeal and
   proximal and distal interphalangeal
   joints
Extension of the hand at the wrist joint
Medial rotation of the little finger
   (finger #5) at the carpometacarpal
   joint
Extension of the forearm at the elbow
   joint

Innervation
The radial nerve

Arterial Supply
The posterior interosseus artery

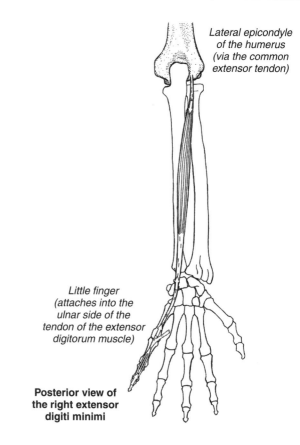

Lateral epicondyle
of the humerus
(via the common
extensor tendon)

*Little finger
(attaches into the
ulnar side of the
tendon of the extensor
digitorum muscle)*

**Posterior view of
the right extensor
digiti minimi**

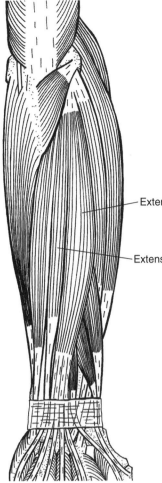

Extensor digitorum

Extensor digiti minimi

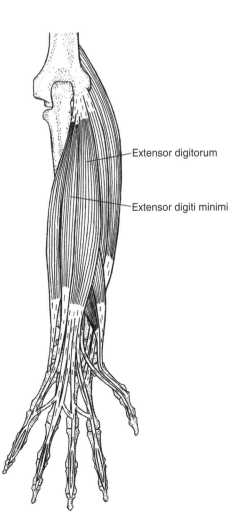

Extensor digitorum

Extensor digiti minimi

Muscles of the Forearm

SUPINATOR

sue-pin-**a**-tor

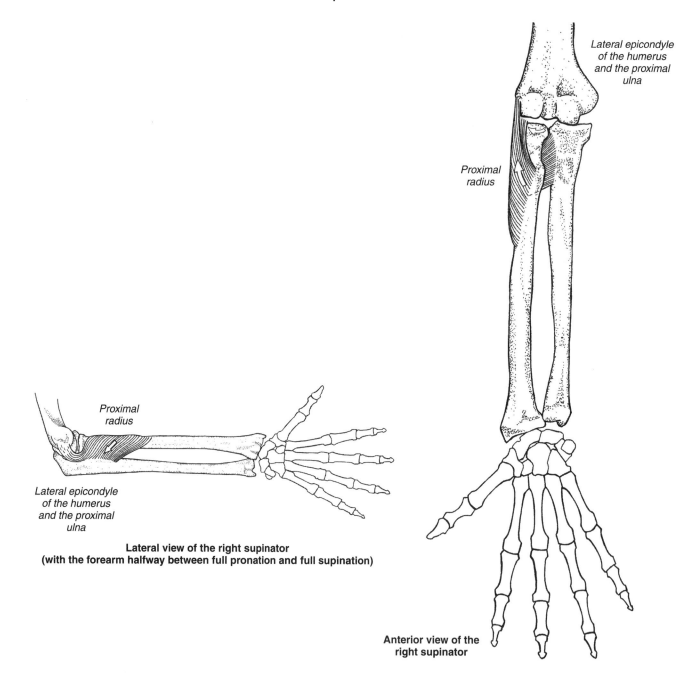

Lateral epicondyle
of the humerus
and the proximal
ulna

Proximal
radius

Proximal
radius

Lateral epicondyle
of the humerus
and the proximal
ulna

**Lateral view of the right supinator
(with the forearm halfway between full pronation and full supination)**

**Anterior view of the
right supinator**

Action	**Innervation**	**Arterial Supply**
Supination of the forearm at the radioulnar joints	The radial nerve	Branches of the radial artery and the interosseus recurrent and posterior interosseus arteries

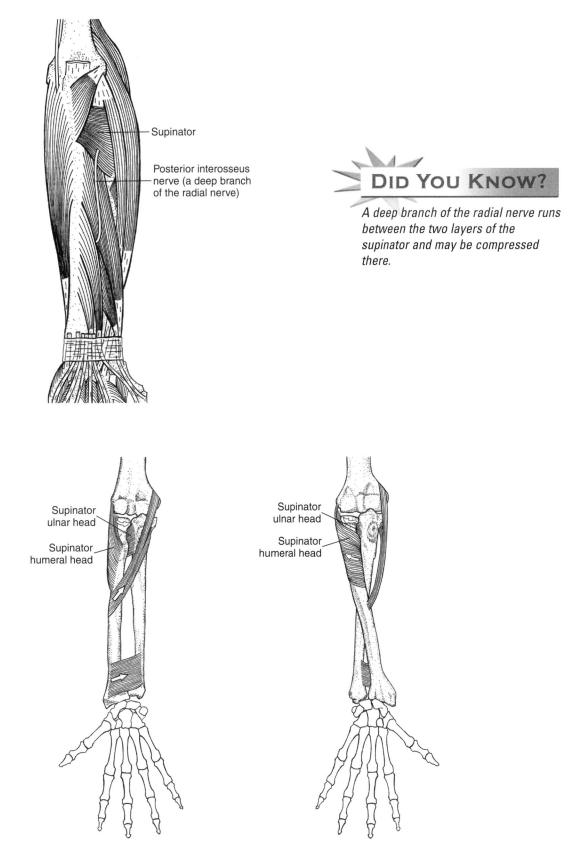

Supinator

Posterior interosseus nerve (a deep branch of the radial nerve)

DID YOU KNOW?

A deep branch of the radial nerve runs between the two layers of the supinator and may be compressed there.

Supinator ulnar head

Supinator humeral head

Supinator ulnar head

Supinator humeral head

Muscles of the Forearm

ABDUCTOR POLLICIS LONGUS

(OF THE DEEP DISTAL FOUR GROUP)

ab-**duk**-tor **pol**-i-sis **long**-us

Actions
Abduction of the thumb at the carpometacarpal joint

Extension of the thumb at the carpometacarpal joint

Lateral rotation of the thumb at the carpometacarpal joint

Radial deviation (abduction) of the hand at the wrist joint

Flexion of the hand at the wrist joint

Supination of the forearm at the radioulnar joints

Innervation
The radial nerve

Arterial Supply
The posterior interosseus artery

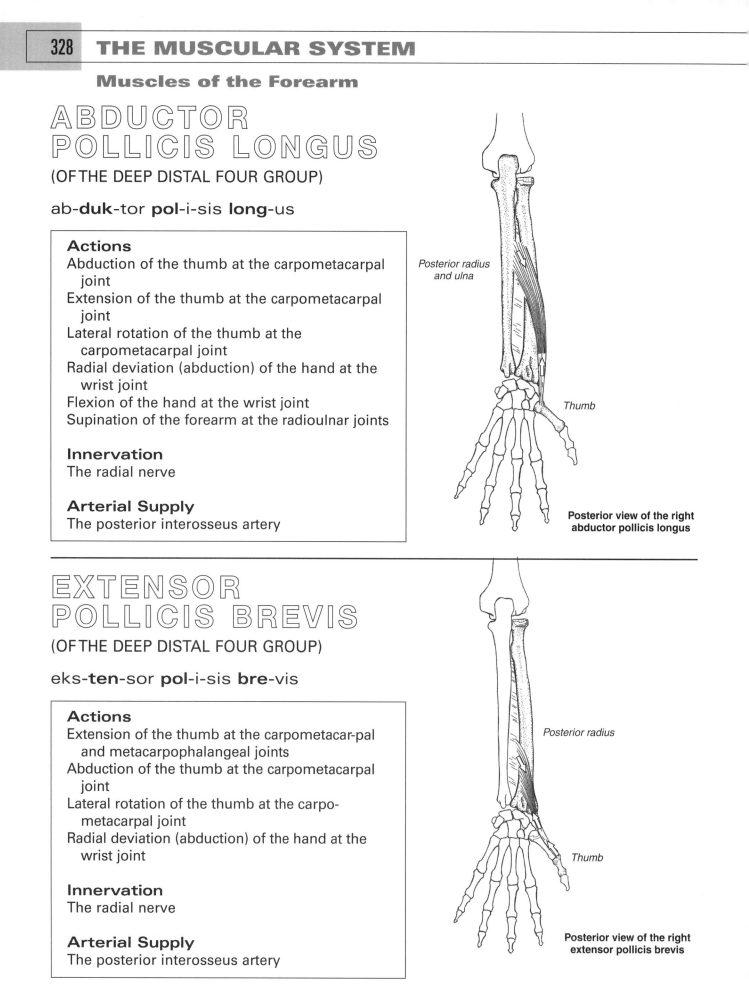

Posterior radius and ulna

Thumb

Posterior view of the right abductor pollicis longus

EXTENSOR POLLICIS BREVIS

(OF THE DEEP DISTAL FOUR GROUP)

eks-**ten**-sor **pol**-i-sis **bre**-vis

Actions
Extension of the thumb at the carpometacar-pal and metacarpophalangeal joints

Abduction of the thumb at the carpometacarpal joint

Lateral rotation of the thumb at the carpo-metacarpal joint

Radial deviation (abduction) of the hand at the wrist joint

Innervation
The radial nerve

Arterial Supply
The posterior interosseus artery

Posterior radius

Thumb

Posterior view of the right extensor pollicis brevis

Muscles of the Forearm

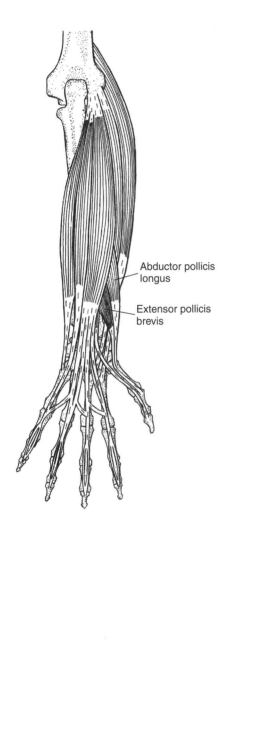

Abductor pollicis
longus

Extensor pollicis
brevis

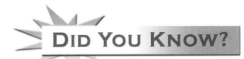

DID YOU KNOW?

*The distal tendons of these two
muscles form the lateral (radial)
border of the anatomical snuffbox.*

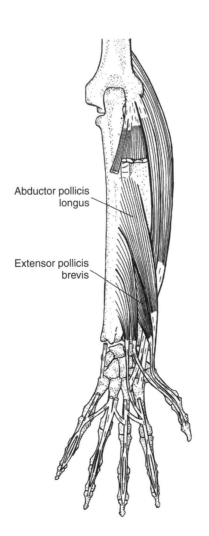

Abductor pollicis
longus

Extensor pollicis
brevis

Muscles of the Forearm

EXTENSOR POLLICIS LONGUS
(OF THE DEEP DISTAL FOUR GROUP)

eks-**ten**-sor **pol**-i-sis **long**-us

Actions
Extension of the thumb at the carpometacarpal, metacarpophalangeal, and
   interphalangeal joints
Lateral rotation of the thumb at the carpometacarpal joint
Extension of the hand at the wrist joint
Radial deviation (abduction) of the hand at
   the wrist joint
Supination of the forearm at the radioulnar
   joints

Innervation
The radial nerve

Arterial Supply
The posterior interosseus artery

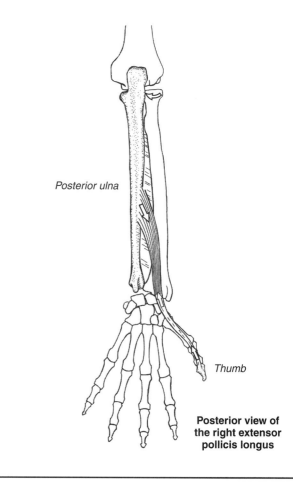

Posterior ulna

Thumb

**Posterior view of
the right extensor
pollicis longus**

EXTENSOR INDICIS
(OF THE DEEP DISTAL FOUR GROUP)

eks-**ten**-sor **in**-di-sis

Actions
Extension of the index finger (finger #2) at
   the metacarpophalangeal and proximal
   and distal interphalangeal joints
Extension of the hand at the wrist joint
Adduction of the index finger (finger #2) at
   the metacarpophalangeal joint
Supination of the forearm at the radioulnar
   joints

Innervation
The radial nerve

Arterial Supply
The posterior interosseus artery

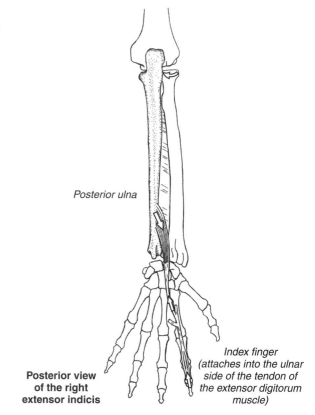

Posterior ulna

**Posterior view
of the right
extensor indicis**

*Index finger
(attaches into the ulnar
side of the tendon of
the extensor digitorum
muscle)*

Muscles of the Forearm

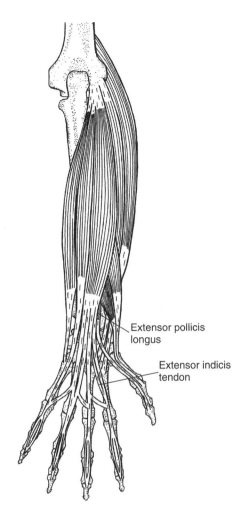

Extensor pollicis longus

Extensor indicis tendon

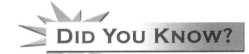

DID YOU KNOW?

The distal tendon of the extensor pollicis longus forms the medial (ulnar) border of the anatomical snuffbox.

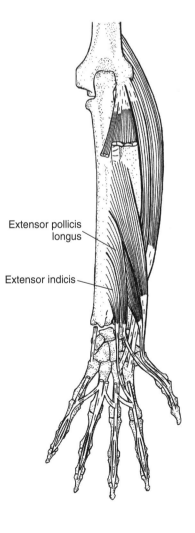

Extensor pollicis longus

Extensor indicis

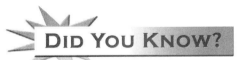

DID YOU KNOW?

The extensor indicis aids the extensor digitorum in extending the index finger, which allows us to point out, i.e., indicate things.

Muscles of the Forearm

ANTERIOR VIEW OF THE RIGHT FOREARM (SUPERFICIAL)

PROXIMAL

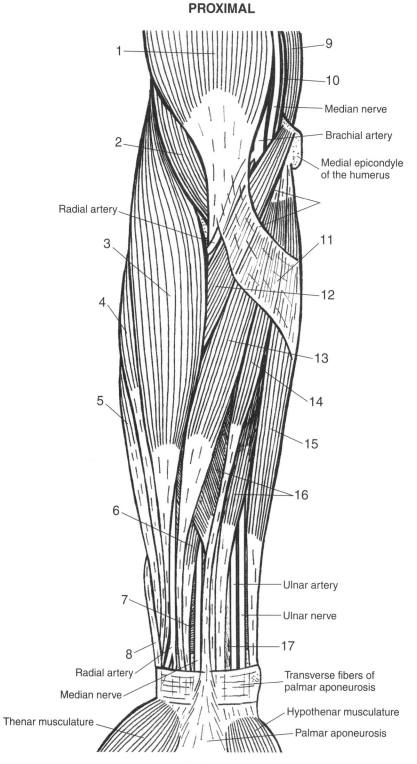

9

10

Median nerve

Brachial artery

Medial epicondyle
of the humerus

11

Radial artery

3

12

4

L A T E R A L

R A D I A L

13

14

U L N A R

M E D I A L

5

15

16

6

Ulnar artery

7

Ulnar nerve

8

17

Radial artery

Transverse fibers of
palmar aponeurosis

Median nerve

Hypothenar musculature

Thenar musculature

Palmar aponeurosis

DISTAL

ANTERIOR VIEW OF THE RIGHT FOREARM (INTERMEDIATE)

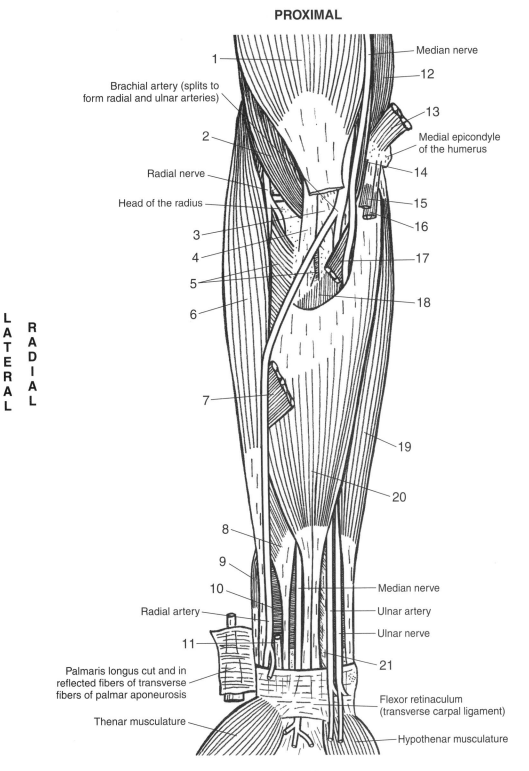

PROXIMAL

Median nerve

Brachial artery (splits to
form radial and ulnar arteries)

Radial nerve

Head of the radius

Medial epicondyle
of the humerus

1

2

3

4

5

6

7

8

9

10

11

12

13

14

15

16

17

18

19

20

21

LATERAL

RADIAL

ULNAR

MEDIAL

Radial artery

Palmaris longus cut and in
reflected fibers of transverse
fibers of palmar aponeurosis

Thenar musculature

Median nerve

Ulnar artery

Ulnar nerve

Flexor retinaculum
(transverse carpal ligament)

Hypothenar musculature

DISTAL

Muscles of the Forearm

ANTERIOR VIEW OF THE RIGHT FOREARM (DEEP)

PROXIMAL

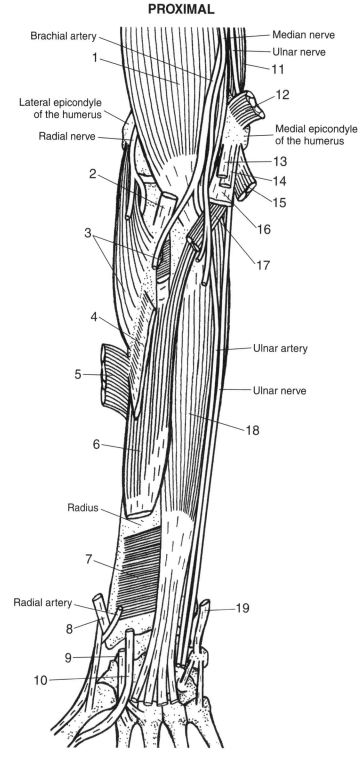

Brachial artery

Median nerve

Ulnar nerve

1

11

Lateral epicondyle
of the humerus

12

Radial nerve

Medial epicondyle
of the humerus

13

2

14

15

3

16

17

L A T E R A L

R A D I A L

4

Ulnar artery

5

Ulnar nerve

18

6

Radius

7

Radial artery

19

8

9

10

U L N A R

M E D I A L

DISTAL

ANTERIOR VIEWS OF THE PRONATORS AND SUPINATOR OF THE RIGHT RADIUS

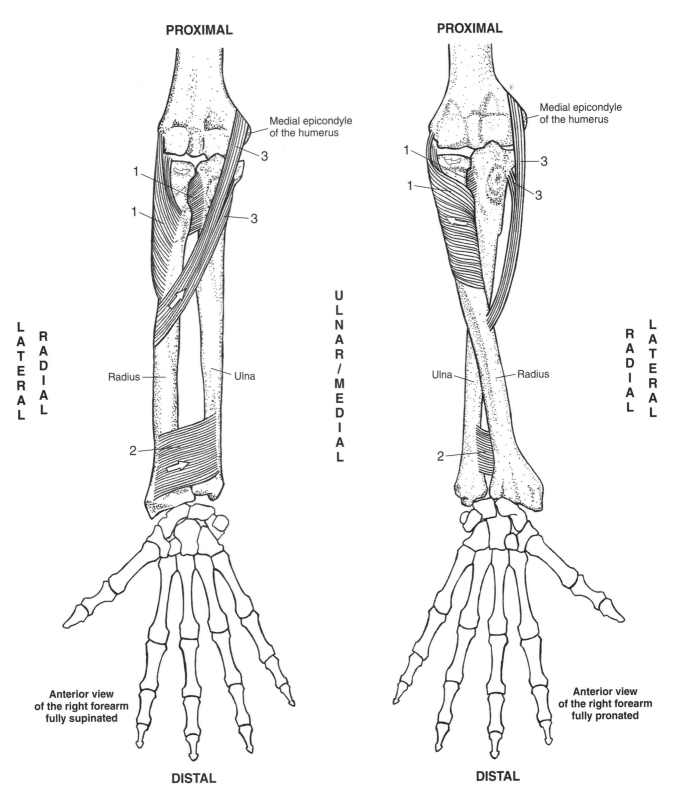

PROXIMAL

Medial epicondyle of the humerus

3

1

1

3

Radius

Ulna

LATERAL

RADIAL

ULNAR/MEDIAL

2

Anterior view of the right forearm fully supinated

DISTAL

PROXIMAL

1

Medial epicondyle of the humerus

3

3

Ulna

Radius

RADIAL

LATERAL

2

Anterior view of the right forearm fully pronated

DISTAL

Muscles of the Forearm

POSTERIOR VIEW OF THE RIGHT FOREARM (SUPERFICIAL)

PROXIMAL

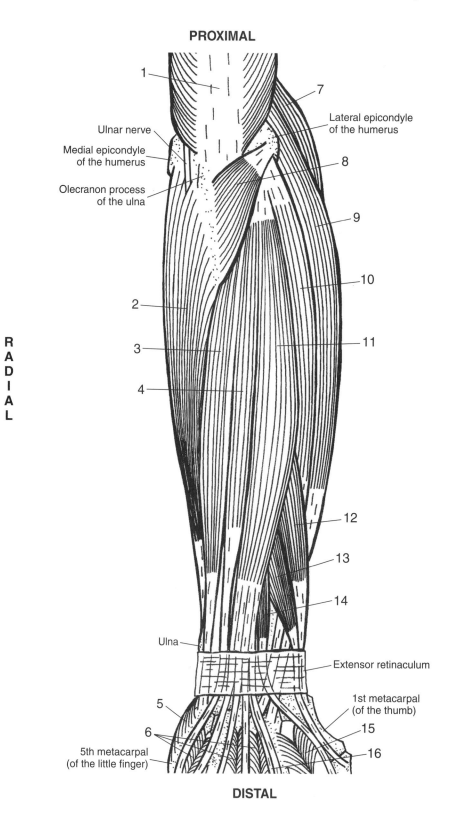

1

7

Ulnar nerve

Medial epicondyle
of the humerus

Olecranon process
of the ulna

Lateral epicondyle
of the humerus

8

9

10

11

2

3

4

L
A
T
E
R
A
L

R
A
D
I
A
L

U
L
N
A
R

M
E
D
I
A
L

12

13

14

Ulna

Extensor retinaculum

1st metacarpal
(of the thumb)

5

6

15

16

5th metacarpal
(of the little finger)

DISTAL

POSTERIOR VIEW OF THE RIGHT FOREARM (DEEP)

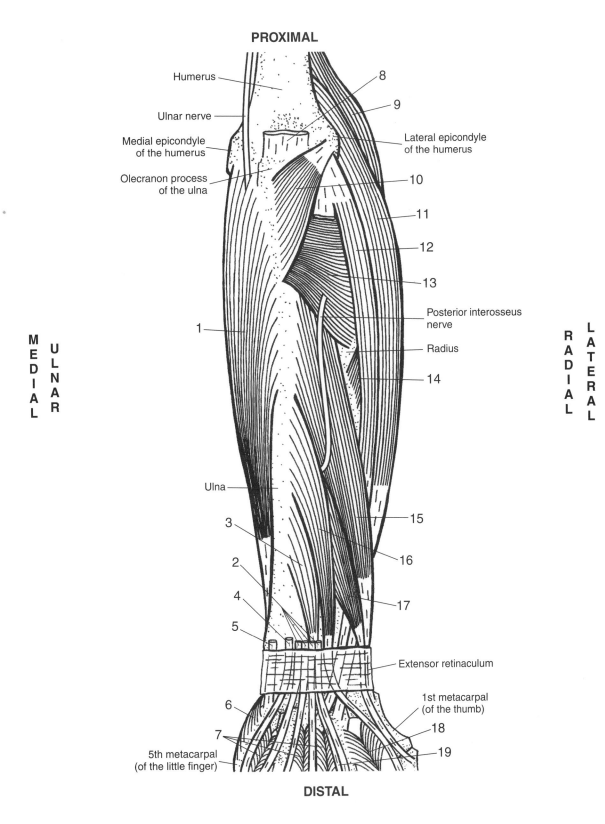

PROXIMAL

Humerus

Ulnar nerve

Medial epicondyle
of the humerus

Olecranon process
of the ulna

8

9

Lateral epicondyle
of the humerus

10

11

12

13

Posterior interosseus
nerve

Radius

14

MEDIAL ULNAR

RADIAL LATERAL

1

Ulna

3

2

4

5

15

16

17

Extensor retinaculum

1st metacarpal
(of the thumb)

6

7

18

19

5th metacarpal
(of the little finger)

DISTAL

THE MUSCULAR SYSTEM

Muscles of the Forearm

POSTERIOR VIEW OF THE RIGHT FOREARM AND HAND (SUPERFICIAL)

PROXIMAL

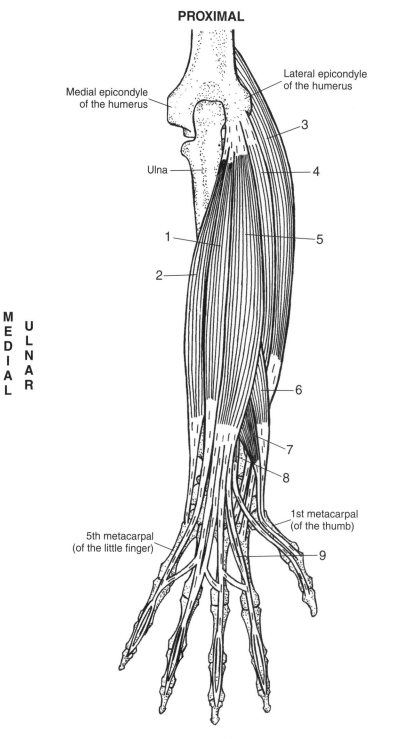

Medial epicondyle
of the humerus

Lateral epicondyle
of the humerus

Ulna

3

4

1

5

2

6

7

8

5th metacarpal
(of the little finger)

1st metacarpal
(of the thumb)

9

MEDIAL ULNAR

RADIAL LATERAL

DISTAL

POSTERIOR VIEW OF THE RIGHT FOREARM AND HAND (DEEP)

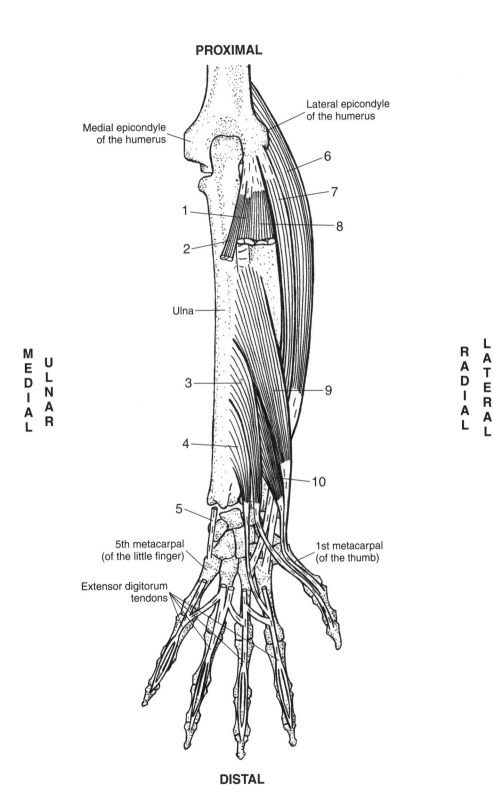

PROXIMAL

Medial epicondyle
of the humerus

Lateral epicondyle
of the humerus

6

7

1

8

2

Ulna

3

9

4

10

5

5th metacarpal
(of the little finger)

1st metacarpal
(of the thumb)

Extensor digitorum
tendons

MEDIAL   ULNAR

RADIAL   LATERAL

DISTAL

Muscles of the Hand

PALMAR VIEW OF THE RIGHT HAND (SUPERFICIAL)

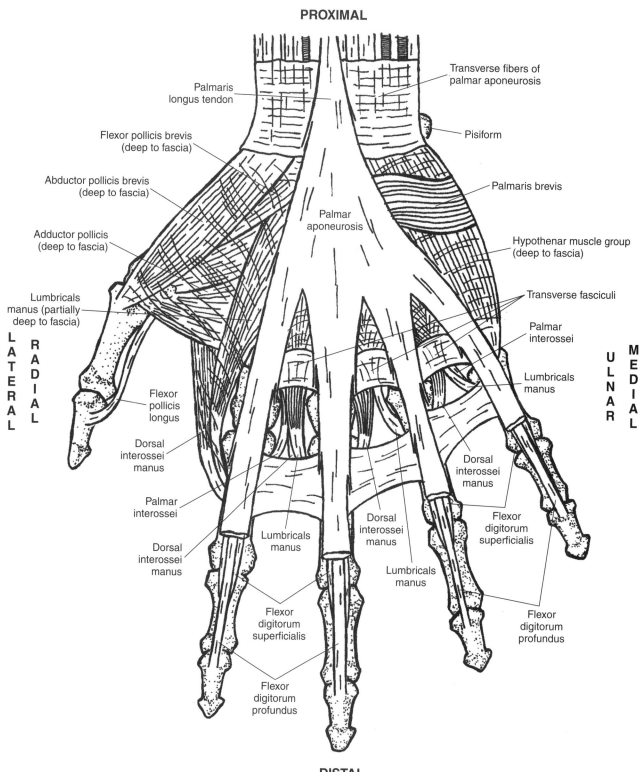

PROXIMAL

Palmaris
longus tendon

Transverse fibers of
palmar aponeurosis

Flexor pollicis brevis
(deep to fascia)

Pisiform

Abductor pollicis brevis
(deep to fascia)

Palmaris brevis

Adductor pollicis
(deep to fascia)

Palmar
aponeurosis

Hypothenar muscle group
(deep to fascia)

Lumbricals
manus (partially
deep to fascia)

Transverse fasciculi

Palmar
interossei

Lumbricals
manus

L A T E R A L   **R A D I A L**

U L N A R   **M E D I A L**

Flexor
pollicis
longus

Dorsal
interossei
manus

Dorsal
interossei
manus

Palmar
interossei

Flexor
digitorum
superficialis

Dorsal
interossei
manus

Dorsal
interossei
manus

Lumbricals
manus

Flexor
digitorum
profundus

Lumbricals
manus

Flexor
digitorum
superficialis

Flexor
digitorum
profundus

Flexor
digitorum
profundus

DISTAL

PALMAR VIEW OF THE RIGHT HAND (SUPERFICIAL MUSCULAR LAYER)

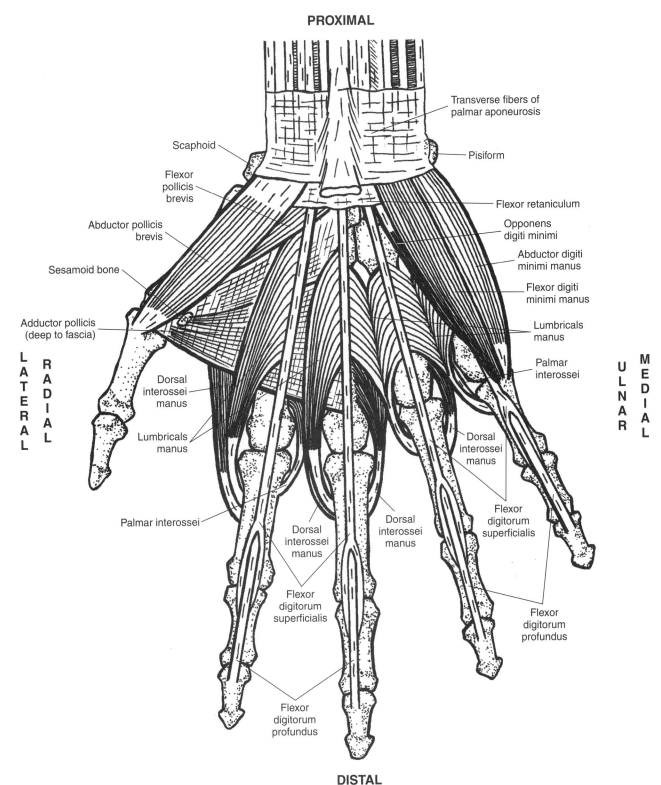

PROXIMAL

Transverse fibers of palmar aponeurosis

Scaphoid

Flexor pollicis brevis

Abductor pollicis brevis

Sesamoid bone

Adductor pollicis (deep to fascia)

Pisiform

Flexor retaniculum

Opponens digiti minimi

Abductor digiti minimi manus

Flexor digiti minimi manus

Lumbricals manus

Palmar interossei

L A T E R A L

R A D I A L

Dorsal interossei manus

Lumbricals manus

Palmar interossei

Dorsal interossei manus

Dorsal interossei manus

Flexor digitorum superficialis

Dorsal interossei manus

Dorsal interossei manus

Flexor digitorum superficialis

Flexor digitorum profundus

U L N A R

M E D I A L

Flexor digitorum profundus

DISTAL

Muscles of the Hand

PALMAR VIEW OF THE RIGHT HAND (DEEP MUSCULAR LAYER)

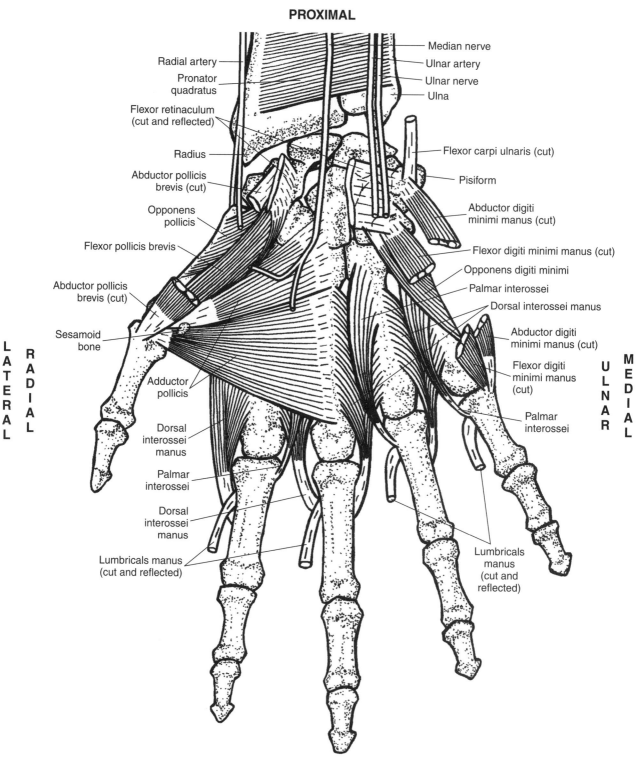

PROXIMAL

Radial artery

Pronator quadratus

Flexor retinaculum (cut and reflected)

Radius

Abductor pollicis brevis (cut)

Opponens pollicis

Flexor pollicis brevis

Abductor pollicis brevis (cut)

Sesamoid bone

Adductor pollicis

Dorsal interossei manus

Palmar interossei

Dorsal interossei manus

Lumbricals manus (cut and reflected)

Median nerve

Ulnar artery

Ulnar nerve

Ulna

Flexor carpi ulnaris (cut)

Pisiform

Abductor digiti minimi manus (cut)

Flexor digiti minimi manus (cut)

Opponens digiti minimi

Palmar interossei

Dorsal interossei manus

Abductor digiti minimi manus (cut)

Flexor digiti minimi manus (cut)

Palmar interossei

Lumbricals manus (cut and reflected)

LATERAL RADIAL

ULNAR MEDIAL

DISTAL

DORSAL VIEW OF THE RIGHT HAND

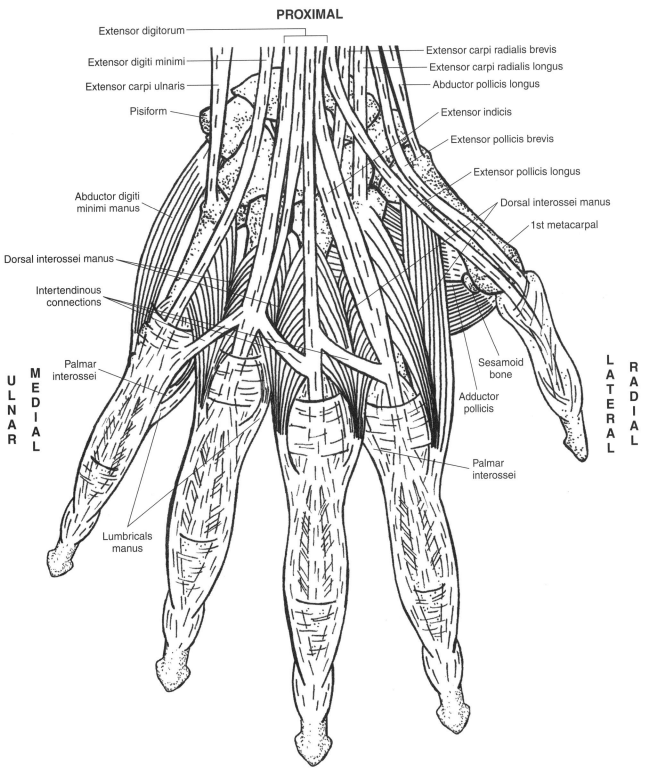

PROXIMAL

Extensor digitorum

Extensor digiti minimi

Extensor carpi ulnaris

Pisiform

Abductor digiti minimi manus

Dorsal interossei manus

Intertendinous connections

Palmar interossei

Lumbricals manus

Extensor carpi radialis brevis

Extensor carpi radialis longus

Abductor pollicis longus

Extensor indicis

Extensor pollicis brevis

Extensor pollicis longus

Dorsal interossei manus

1st metacarpal

Sesamoid bone

Adductor pollicis

Palmar interossei

ULNAR MEDIAL

LATERAL RADIAL

DISTAL

Muscles of the Hand

ABDUCTOR POLLICIS BREVIS

(OF THE THENAR EMINENCE)

ab-**duk**-tor **pol**-i-sis **bre**-vis

Actions

Abduction of the thumb at the carpometacarpal joint

Flexion of the thumb at the metacarpophalangeal joint

Extension of the thumb at the carpometacarpal and interphalangeal joints

Innervation

The median nerve

Arterial Supply

Branches of the radial artery

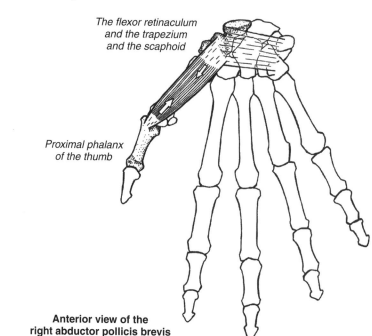

The flexor retinaculum and the trapezium and the scaphoid

Proximal phalanx of the thumb

Anterior view of the right abductor pollicis brevis

FLEXOR POLLICIS BREVIS

(OF THE THENAR EMINENCE)

fleks-or **pol**-i-sis **bre**-vis

Actions

Flexion of the thumb at the carpometacarpal and the metacarpophalangeal joints

Abduction of the thumb at the carpometacarpal joint

Innervation

The median and ulnar nerves

Arterial Supply

Branches of the radial artery

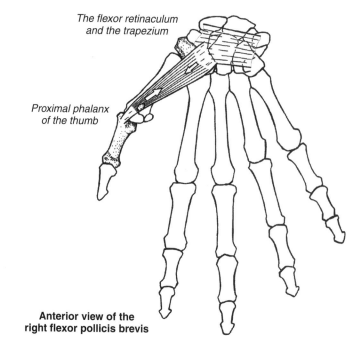

The flexor retinaculum and the trapezium

Proximal phalanx of the thumb

Anterior view of the right flexor pollicis brevis

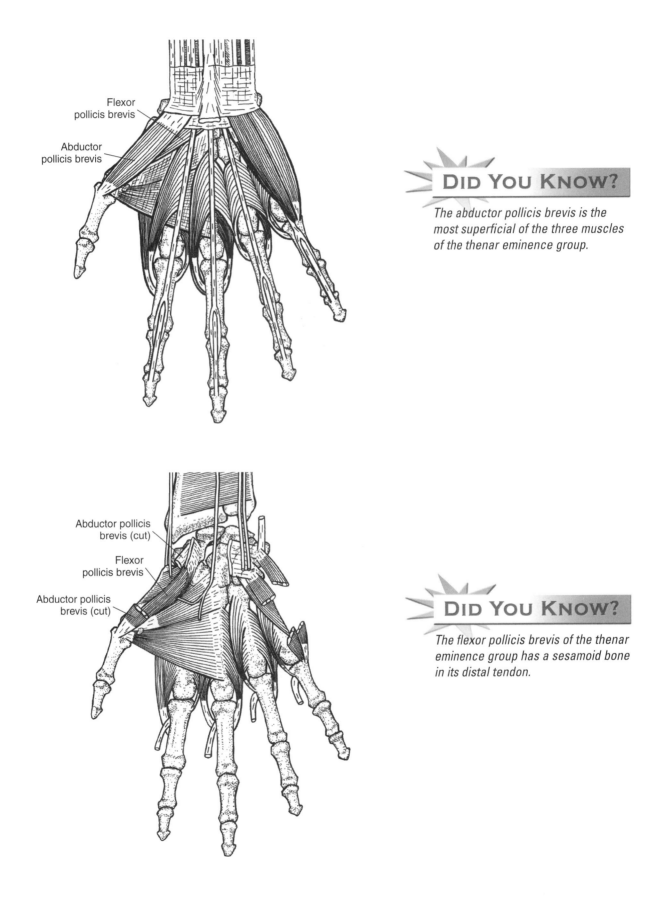

Flexor
pollicis brevis

Abductor
pollicis brevis

DID YOU KNOW?

The abductor pollicis brevis is the
most superficial of the three muscles
of the thenar eminence group.

Abductor pollicis
brevis (cut)

Flexor
pollicis brevis

Abductor pollicis
brevis (cut)

DID YOU KNOW?

The flexor pollicis brevis of the thenar
eminence group has a sesamoid bone
in its distal tendon.

Muscles of the Hand

OPPONENS POLLICIS

(OF THE THENAR EMINENCE)

op-**po**-nens **pol**-i-sis

Actions
Opposition of the thumb at
    the carpometacarpal joint
Flexion of the thumb at the
    carpometacarpal joint
Medial rotation of the thumb
    at the carpometacarpal
    joint
Abduction of the thumb at
    the carpometacarpal joint

Innervation
The median and ulnar
    nerves

Arterial Supply
Branches of the radial artery

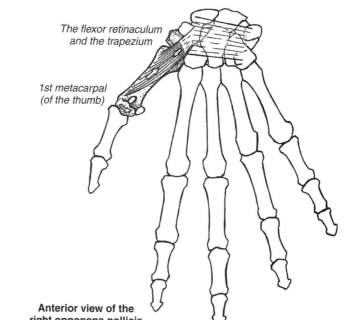

The flexor retinaculum
and the trapezium

1st metacarpal
(of the thumb)

**Anterior view of the
right opponens pollicis**

OPPONENS DIGITI MINIMI

(OF THE HYPOTHENAR EMINENCE)

op-**po**-nens **dij**-i-tee **min**-i-mee

Actions
Opposition of the little finger
    (finger #5) at the
    carpometacarpal joint
Flexion of the little finger
    (finger #5) at the
    carpometacarpal joint
Adduction of the little finger
    (finger #5) at the
    carpometacarpal joint
Lateral rotation of the little
    finger (finger #5) at the
    carpometacarpal joint

Innervation
The ulnar nerve

Arterial Supply
Branches of the ulnar artery

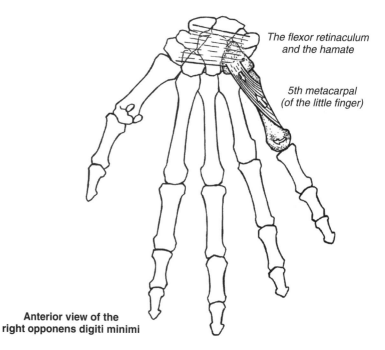

The flexor retinaculum
and the hamate

5th metacarpal
(of the little finger)

**Anterior view of the
right opponens digiti minimi**

Muscles of the Hand

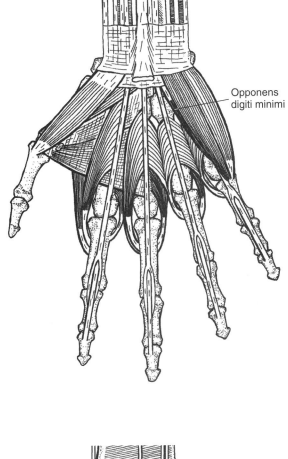

Opponens
digiti minimi

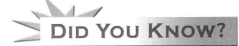

DID YOU KNOW?

The opponens pollicis is the only muscle of the thenar eminence group that attaches onto the metacarpal of the thumb instead of the proximal phalanx of the thumb.

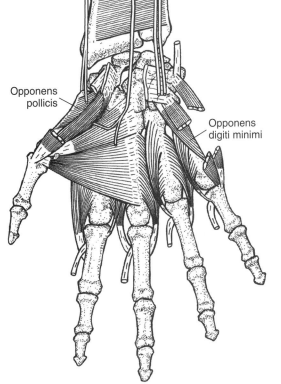

Opponens
pollicis

Opponens
digiti minimi

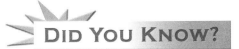

DID YOU KNOW?

The thumb is not the only opposable finger; the opponens digiti minimi of the hypothenar group opposes the little finger.

Muscles of the Hand

ABDUCTOR DIGITI MINIMI MANUS

(OF THE HYPOTHENAR EMINENCE)

ab-**duk**-tor **dij**-i-tee **min**-i-mee **man**-us

Actions
Abduction of the little finger (finger #5) at the carpometacarpal and metacarpophalangeal joints
Extension of the little finger (finger #5) at the proximal and distal interphalangeal joints

Innervation
The ulnar nerve

Arterial Supply
Branches of the ulnar artery

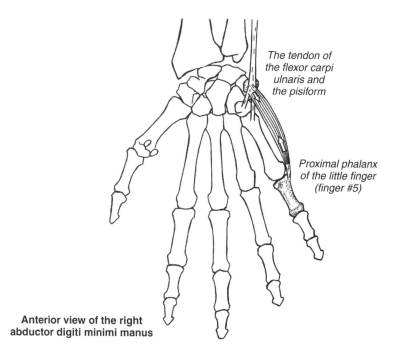

The tendon of the flexor carpi ulnaris and the pisiform

Proximal phalanx of the little finger (finger #5)

Anterior view of the right abductor digiti minimi manus

FLEXOR DIGITI MINIMI MANUS

(OF THE HYPOTHENAR EMINENCE)

fleks-or **dij**-i-tee **min**-i-mee **man**-us

Action
Flexion of the little finger (finger #5) at the meta-carpophalangeal joint

Innervation
The ulnar nerve

Arterial Supply
Branches of the ulnar artery

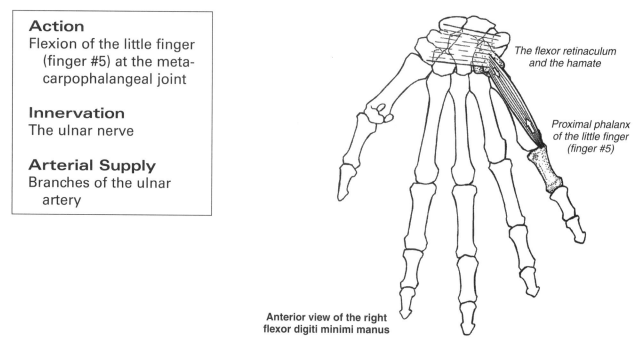

The flexor retinaculum and the hamate

Proximal phalanx of the little finger (finger #5)

Anterior view of the right flexor digiti minimi manus

Muscles of the Hand

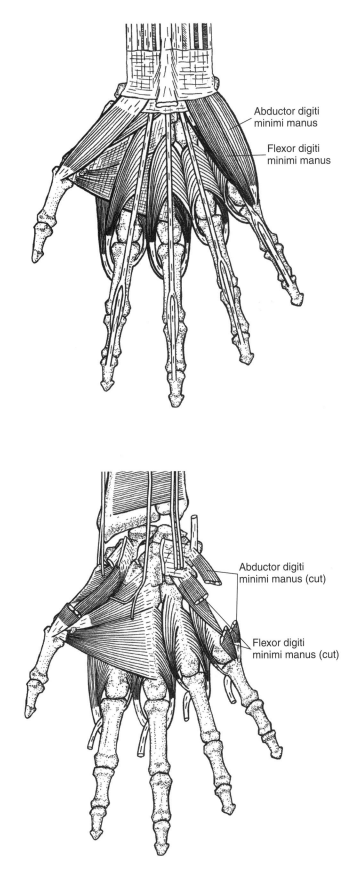

Abductor digiti
minimi manus

Flexor digiti
minimi manus

Abductor digiti
minimi manus (cut)

Flexor digiti
minimi manus (cut)

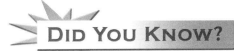

DID YOU KNOW?

The abductor digiti minimi manus is
the most superficial of the three
muscles of the hypothenar eminence
group.

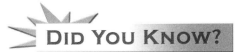

DID YOU KNOW?

The flexor digiti minimi manus of the
hypothenar eminence group is often
known simply as the flexor digiti
minimi or the flexor digiti minimi
brevis.

Muscles of the Hand

PALMARIS BREVIS

pall-**ma**-ris **bre**-vis

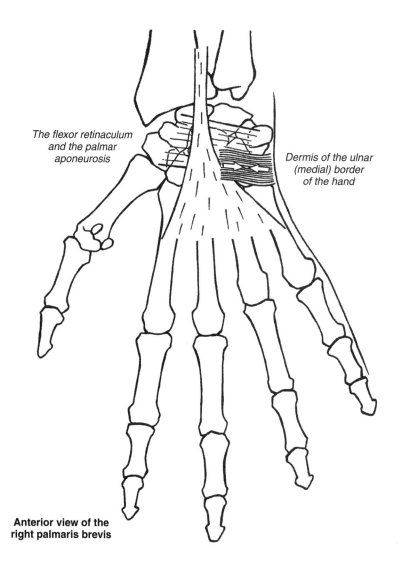

The flexor retinaculum and the palmar aponeurosis

Dermis of the ulnar (medial) border of the hand

Anterior view of the right palmaris brevis

Action	Innervation	Arterial Supply
Wrinkles the skin of the palm	The ulnar nerve	The ulnar artery and the superficial palmar branch of the radial artery

Muscles of the Hand

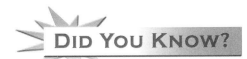

DID YOU KNOW?

The palmaris brevis' action of wrinkling the skin of the palm contributes to the strength and security of gripping an object in your hand.

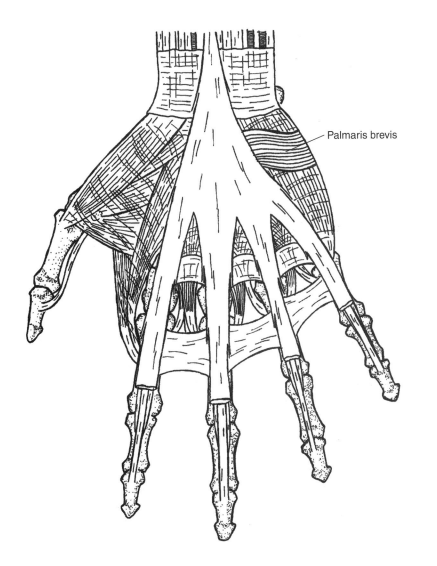

Palmaris brevis

Muscles of the Hand

ADDUCTOR POLLICIS
(OF THE CENTRAL COMPARTMENT)

ad-**duk**-tor **pol**-i-sis

Actions
Adduction of the thumb
 at the carpometa-
 carpal joint
Flexion of the thumb at
 the carpometacarpal
 and metacarpo-
 phalangeal joints
Extension of the thumb
 at the interphalangeal
 joint

Innervation
The ulnar nerve

Arterial Supply
Branches of the radial
 artery

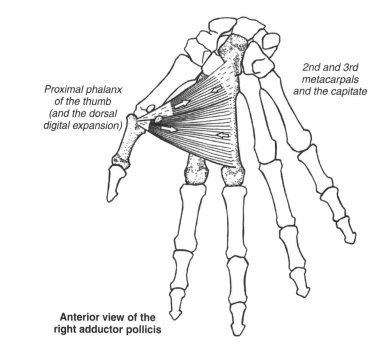

*Proximal phalanx
of the thumb
(and the dorsal
digital expansion)*

*2nd and 3rd
metacarpals
and the capitate*

**Anterior view of the
right adductor pollicis**

LUMBRICALS MANUS
(OF THE CENTRAL COMPARTMENT)
(There are four lumbrical manus muscles, named #1, #2, #3, and #4.)

lum-bri-kuls **man**-us

Actions
Extension of fingers #2-5
 at the proximal and
 distal interphalangeal
 joints
Flexion of fingers #2-5 at
 the metacarpopha-
 langeal joint

Innervation
The median and ulnar
 nerves

Arterial Supply
Branches of the radial
 and ulnar arteries

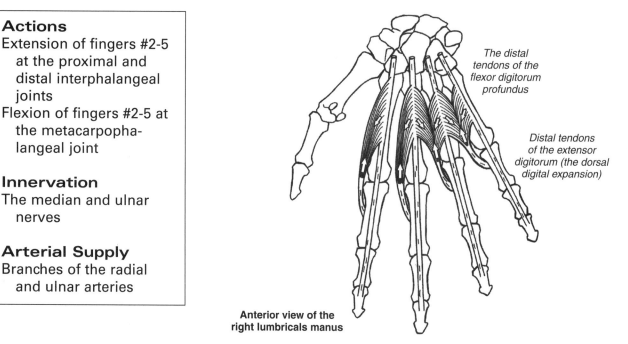

*The distal
tendons of the
flexor digitorum
profundus*

*Distal tendons
of the extensor
digitorum (the dorsal
digital expansion)*

**Anterior view of the
right lumbricals manus**

Muscles of the Hand

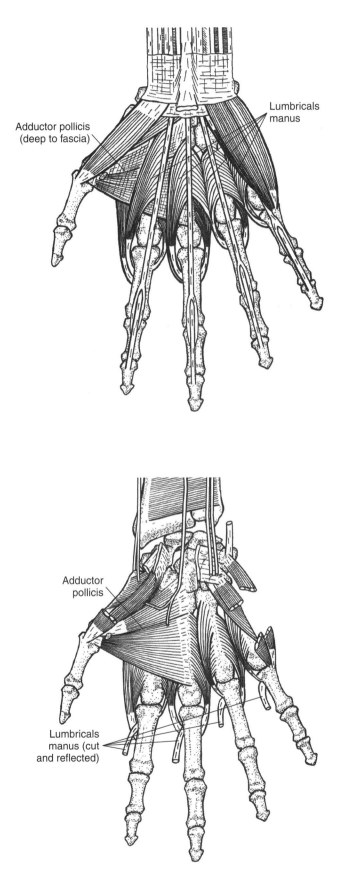

Adductor pollicis
(deep to fascia)

Lumbricals
manus

Adductor
pollicis

Lumbricals
manus (cut
and reflected)

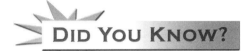

DID YOU KNOW?

There is a sesamoid bone in the distal tendon of the oblique head of the adductor pollicis.

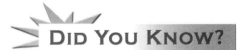

DID YOU KNOW?

The actions of the lumbricals manus (flexion of the proximal phalanges at the metacarpophalangeal joints and extension of the middle and distal phalanges at the interphalangeal joints) puts the hand in the shape of the letter 'L', as in Lumbricals ☺.

Muscles of the Hand

PALMAR INTEROSSEI
(OF THE CENTRAL COMPARTMENT)
(There are three palmar interossei, named #1, #2, and #3.)

pal-mar in-ter-oss-ee-i

Actions
Adduction of fingers #2, #4, and #5 at the metacarpophalangeal joint
Flexion of fingers #2, #4, and #5 at the metacarpophalangeal joint
Extension of fingers #2, #4, and #5 at the proximal and distal interphalangeal joints

Innervation
The ulnar nerve

Arterial Supply
Branches of the radial and ulnar arteries

The metacarpal of fingers #2, #4, and #5

Proximal phalanx of fingers #2, #4, and #5 on the "middle finger side" (and the dorsal digital expansion)

Anterior view of the right palmar interossei

DORSAL INTEROSSEI MANUS
(OF THE CENTRAL COMPARTMENT)
(There are four dorsal interossei manus muscles, named #1, #2, #3, and #4.)

dor-sul in-ter-oss-ee-i man-us

Actions
Abduction of fingers #2, #3, and #4 metacarpophalangeal joint
Flexion of fingers #2, #3, and #4 at the metacarpophalangeal joint
Extension of fingers #2, #3, and #4 at the proximal and distal interphalangeal joints

Innervation
The ulnar nerve

Arterial Supply
Branches of the radial and ulnar arteries

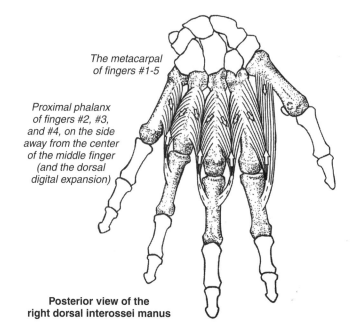

The metacarpal of fingers #1-5

Proximal phalanx of fingers #2, #3, and #4, on the side away from the center of the middle finger (and the dorsal digital expansion)

Posterior view of the right dorsal interossei manus

Muscles of the Hand

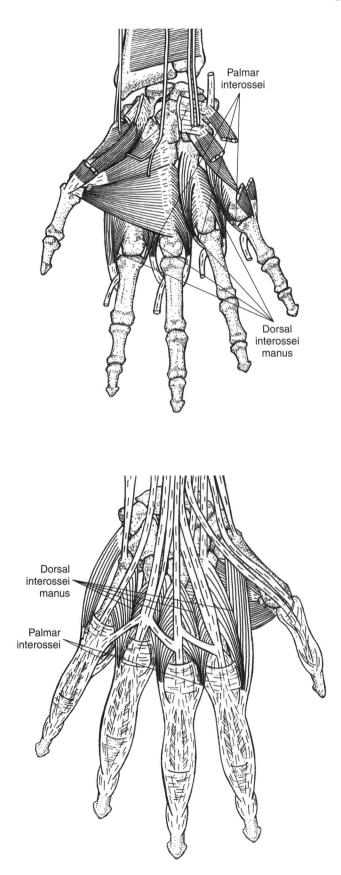

Palmar
interossei

Dorsal
interossei
manus

Dorsal
interossei
manus

Palmar
interossei

DID YOU KNOW?

*The main action of the dorsal interossei manus is abduction of the fingers at the metacarpophalangeal joints. The main action of the palmar interossei is adduction of the fingers at the metacarpophalangeal joints. The mnemonic to remember these actions is **DAB PAD; D**orsals **AB**duct, **P**almars **AD**duct.*

Muscles of the Hand

PALMAR VIEW OF THE RIGHT HAND (SUPERFICIAL)

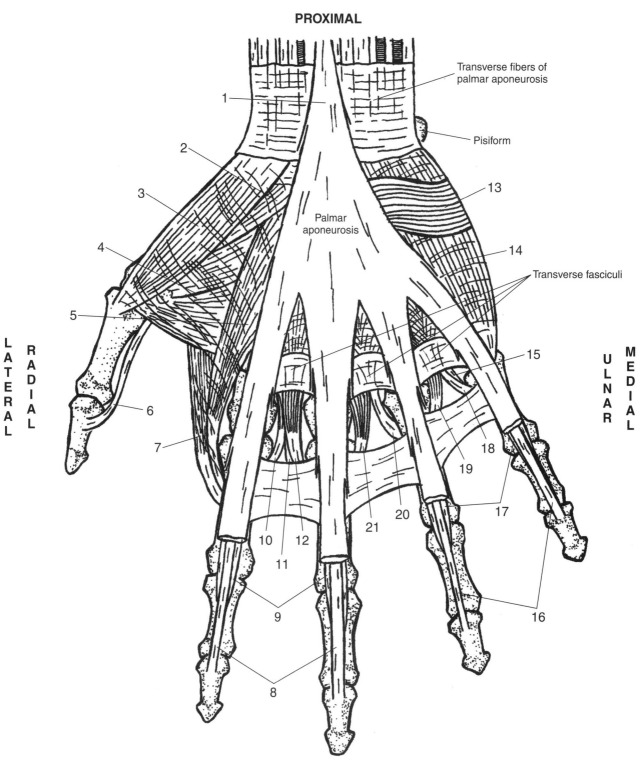

PROXIMAL

Transverse fibers of palmar aponeurosis

Pisiform

Palmar aponeurosis

Transverse fasciculi

LATERAL

RADIAL

ULNAR

MEDIAL

DISTAL

PALMAR VIEW OF THE RIGHT HAND
(SUPERFICIAL MUSCULAR LAYER)

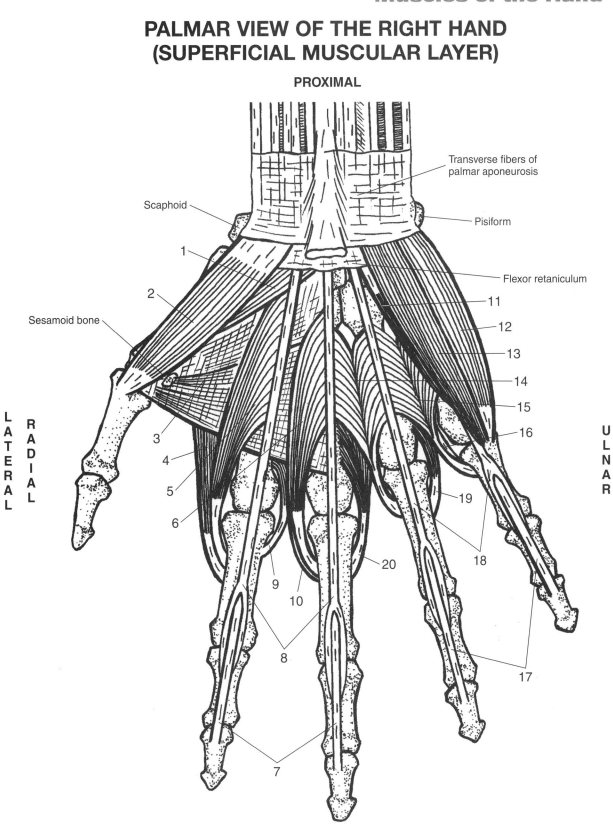

PROXIMAL

Transverse fibers of palmar aponeurosis

Scaphoid

Pisiform

1

Flexor retaniculum

2

11

Sesamoid bone

12

13

14

15

16

3

4

5

19

6

18

LATERAL

RADIAL

ULNAR

MEDIAL

9

10

20

8

17

7

DISTAL

PALMAR VIEW OF THE RIGHT HAND
(DEEP MUSCULAR LAYER)

PROXIMAL

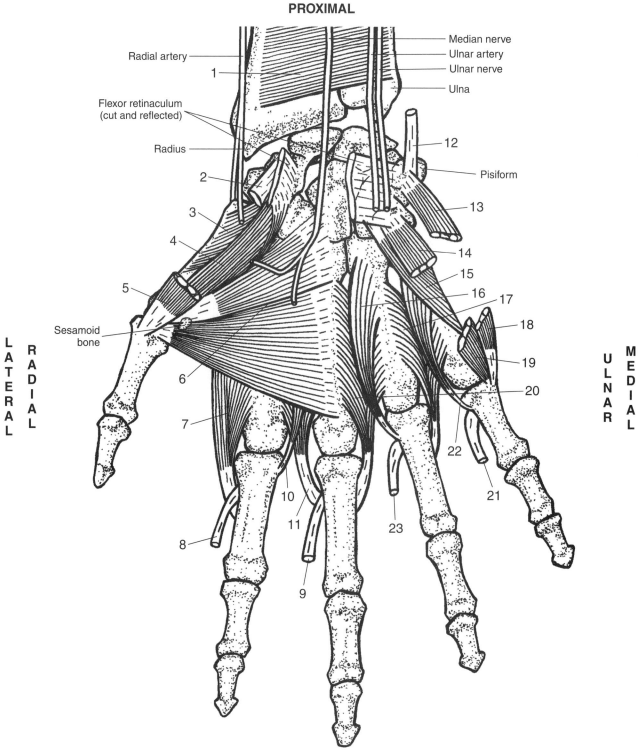

Median nerve

Ulnar artery

Ulnar nerve

Ulna

Radial artery

Flexor retinaculum
(cut and reflected)

Radius

Pisiform

Sesamoid
bone

LATERAL

RADIAL

ULNAR

MEDIAL

DISTAL

DORSAL VIEW OF THE RIGHT HAND

PROXIMAL

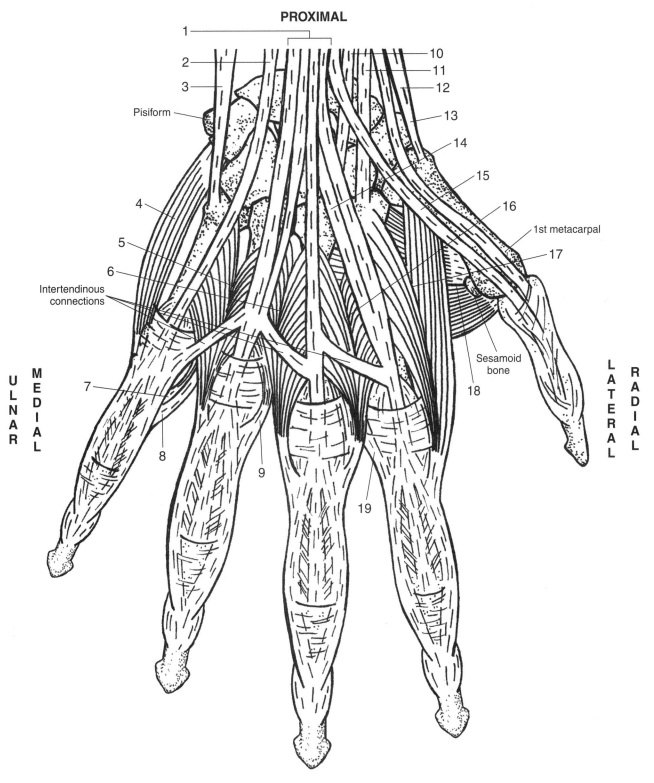

1

2

3

Pisiform

4

5

6

Intertendinous
connections

7

8

9

10

11

12

13

14

15

16

1st metacarpal

17

Sesamoid
bone

18

19

U L N A R

M E D I A L

L A T E R A L

R A D I A L

DISTAL

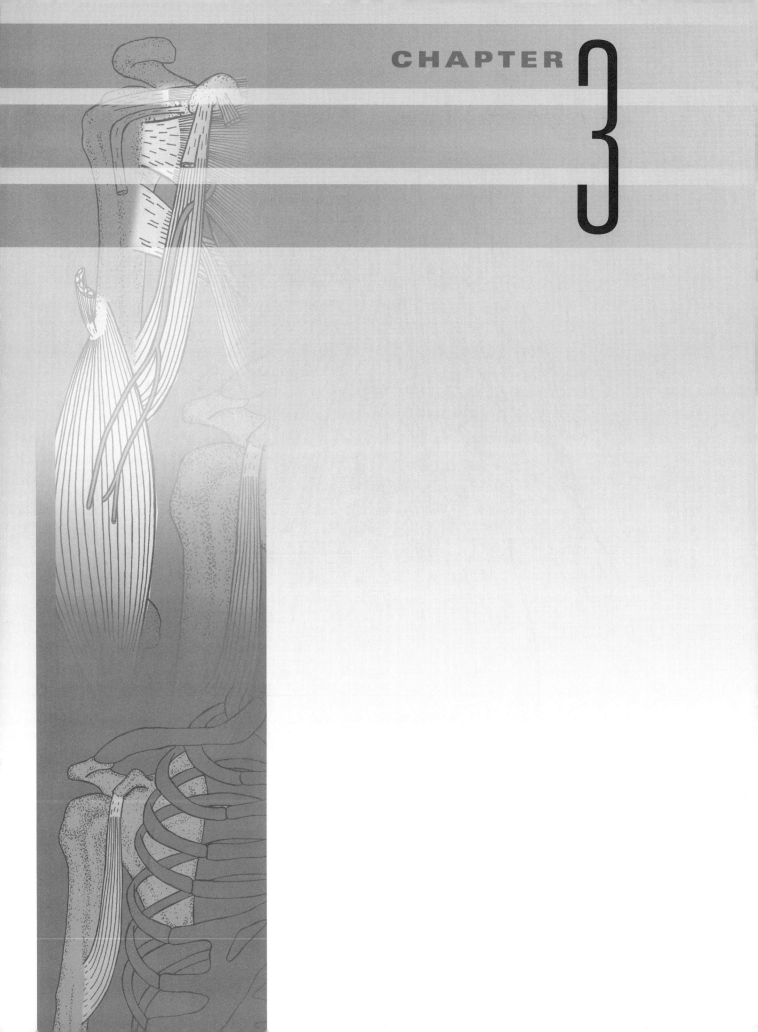

CHAPTER 3

Other Skeletal Muscles

GET READY TO EXPLORE:

Anterior Views of the Other Muscles of the Abdomen, 363

Views of the Muscles of the Perineum, 364

Views of the Muscles of the Tongue, 365

View of the Muscles of the Palate, 366

View of the Muscles of the Pharynx, 367

Views of the Muscles of the Larynx, 368

Views of the Muscles of the Larynx, 369

Views of the Extrinsic Muscles of the Right Eye, 370

View of the Muscles of the Tympanic Cavity, 371

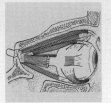

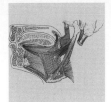

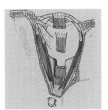

ANTERIOR VIEWS OF THE OTHER MUSCLES OF THE ABDOMEN

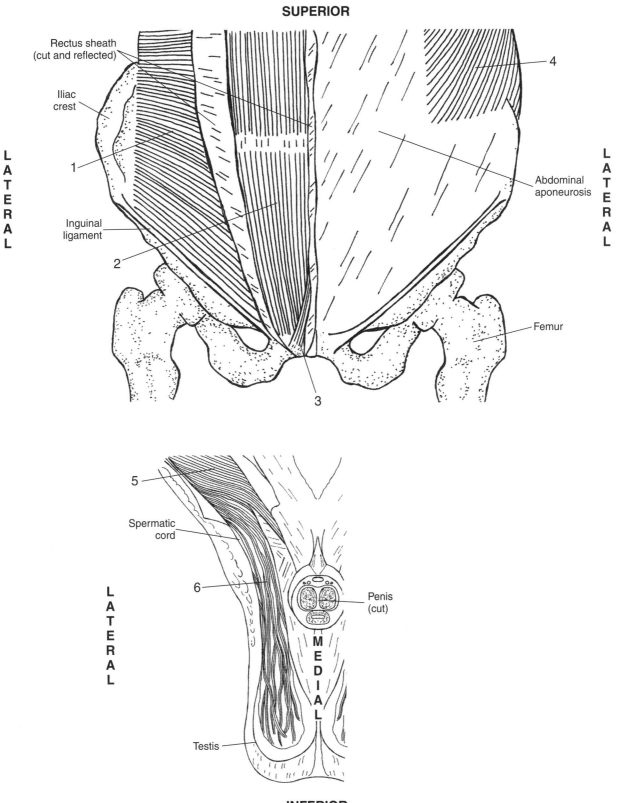

SUPERIOR

Rectus sheath
(cut and reflected)

Iliac
crest

LATERAL

1

Inguinal
ligament

2

4

Abdominal
aponeurosis

LATERAL

Femur

3

5

Spermatic
cord

6

LATERAL

Penis
(cut)

MEDIAL

Testis

INFERIOR

VIEWS OF THE MUSCLES OF THE PERINEUM

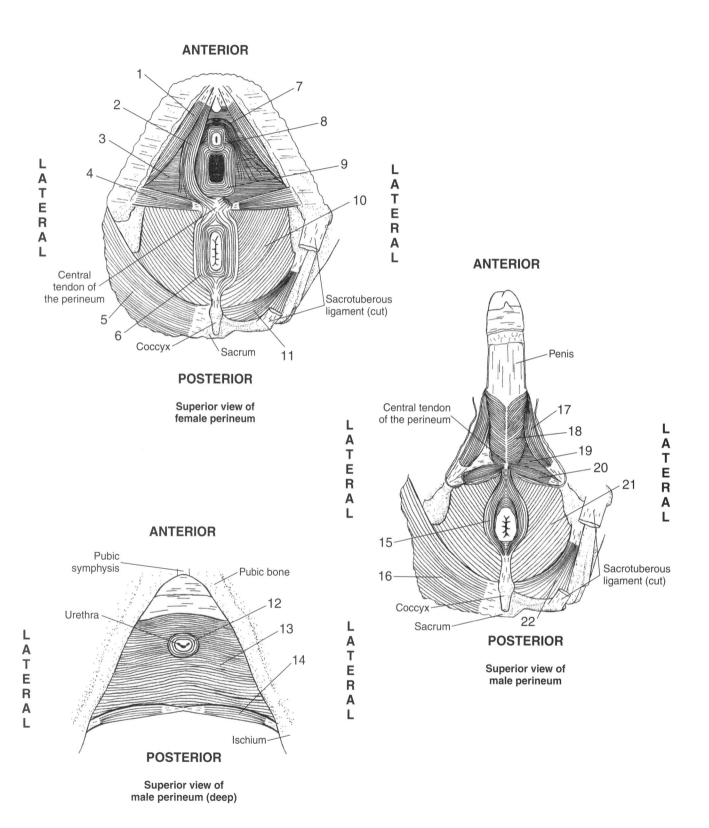

ANTERIOR

1
2
3
4
7
8
9
10

LATERAL

LATERAL

Central tendon of the perineum

5
6

Coccyx

Sacrum

Sacrotuberous ligament (cut)

11

POSTERIOR

Superior view of female perineum

ANTERIOR

Central tendon of the perineum

Penis

17
18
19
20
21

LATERAL

LATERAL

15
16

Coccyx

Sacrum

Sacrotuberous ligament (cut)

22

POSTERIOR

Superior view of male perineum

ANTERIOR

Pubic symphysis

Pubic bone

Urethra

12
13
14

LATERAL

LATERAL

Ischium

POSTERIOR

Superior view of male perineum (deep)

VIEWS OF THE MUSCLES OF THE TONGUE

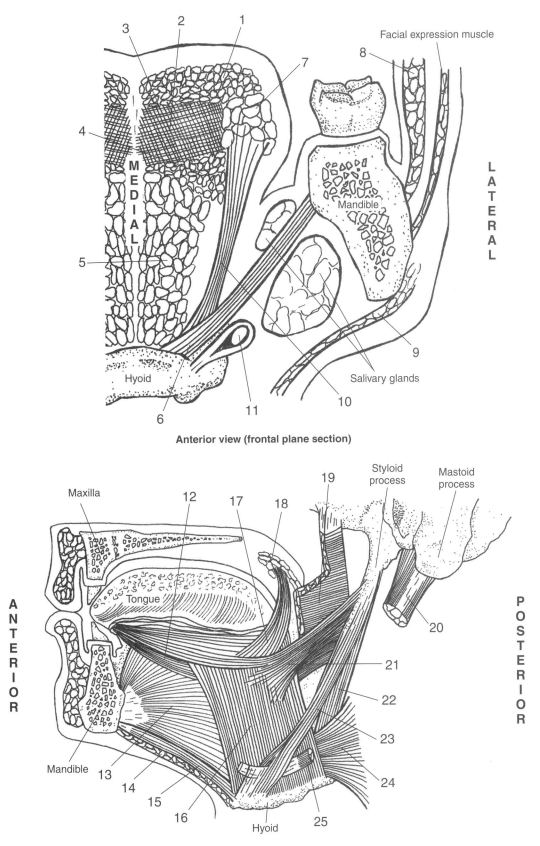

Anterior view (frontal plane section)

Lateral view (sagittal plane section)

VIEW OF THE MUSCLES OF THE PALATE

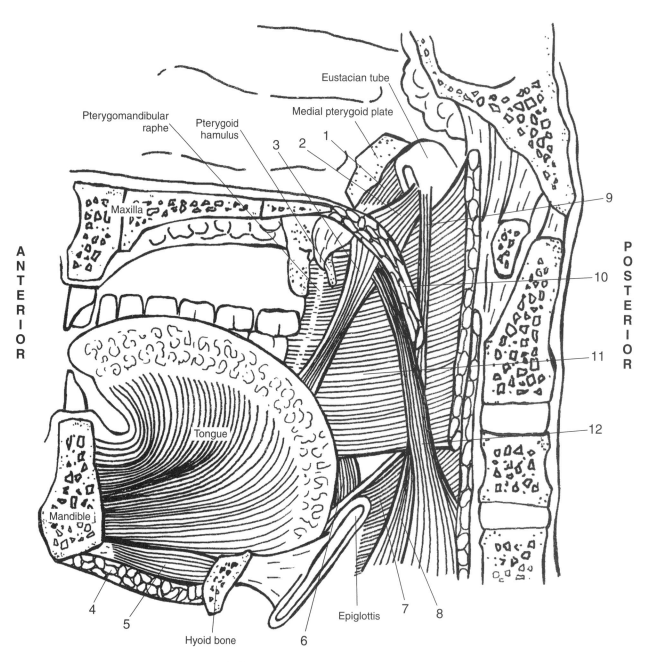

Eustacian tube

Medial pterygoid plate

Pterygomandibular raphe

Pterygoid hamulus

3 2 1

Maxilla

9

10

11

12

ANTERIOR

POSTERIOR

Tongue

Mandible

4

5

6

Hyoid bone

Epiglottis

7 8

Medial view (sagittal plane section)

VIEW OF THE MUSCLES OF THE PHARYNX

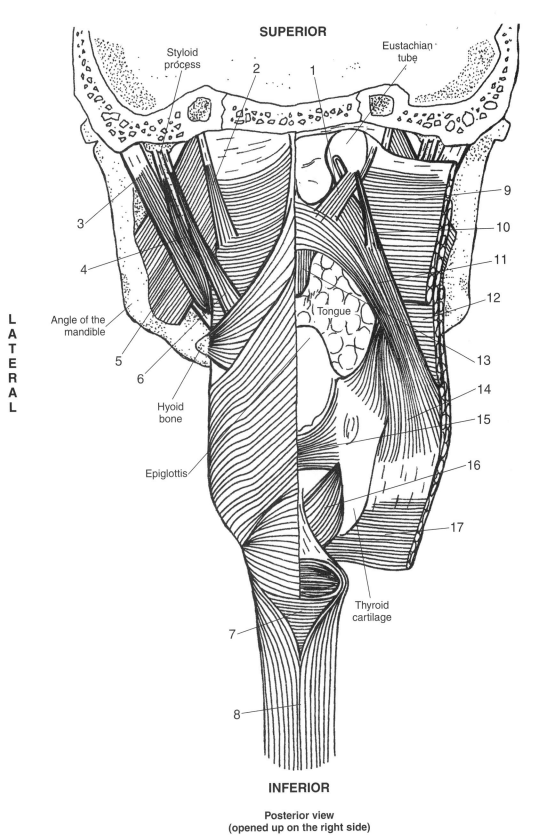

SUPERIOR

Styloid process

Eustachian tube

2   1

3

9

4

10

11

Angle of the mandible

12

5

Tongue

6

13

LATERAL

LATERAL

14

15

Hyoid bone

16

Epiglottis

17

Thyroid cartilage

7

8

INFERIOR

Posterior view
(opened up on the right side)

VIEWS OF THE MUSCLES OF THE LARYNX

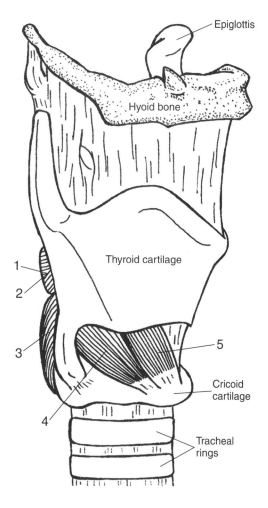

SUPERIOR

Epiglottis

Hyoid bone

Thyroid cartilage

1

2

3

4

5

Cricoid cartilage

Tracheal rings

INFERIOR

Lateral view

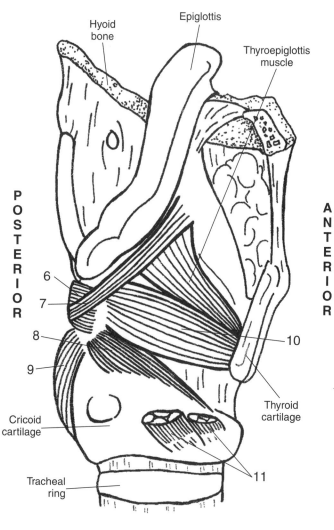

Hyoid bone

Epiglottis

Thyroepiglottis muscle

P O S T E R I O R

A N T E R I O R

6

7

8

9

10

Thyroid cartilage

Cricoid cartilage

Tracheal ring

11

Lateral view (dissected)

VIEWS OF THE MUSCLES OF THE LARYNX

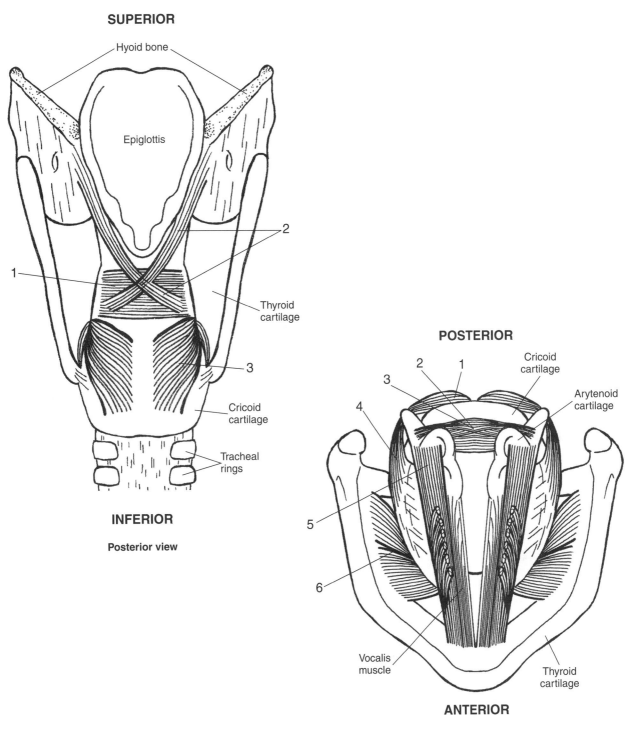

SUPERIOR

Hyoid bone

Epiglottis

2

1

Thyroid cartilage

3

Cricoid cartilage

Tracheal rings

INFERIOR

Posterior view

POSTERIOR

2 1 Cricoid cartilage

3

4

Arytenoid cartilage

5

6

Vocalis muscle

Thyroid cartilage

ANTERIOR

Superior view

VIEWS OF THE EXTRINSIC MUSCLES OF THE RIGHT EYE

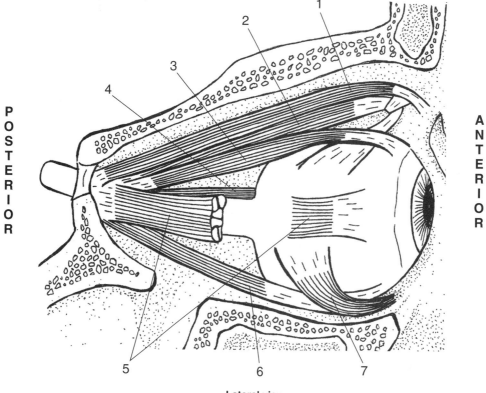

POSTERIOR

ANTERIOR

Lateral view

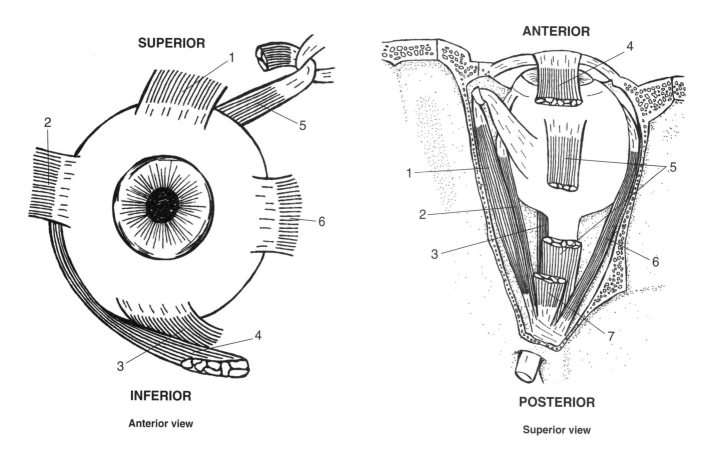

SUPERIOR

INFERIOR

Anterior view

ANTERIOR

POSTERIOR

Superior view

VIEW OF THE MUSCLES OF THE TYMPANIC CAVITY

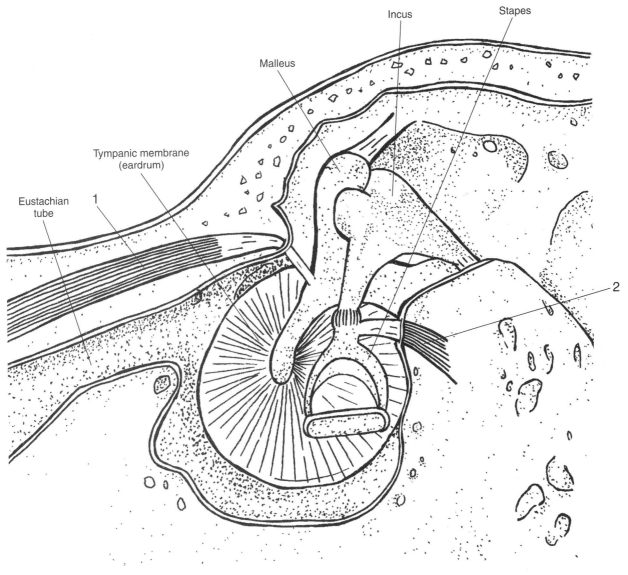

Incus

Stapes

Malleus

Tympanic membrane
(eardrum)

Eustachian
tube

1

2

Medial view (within the temporal bone)

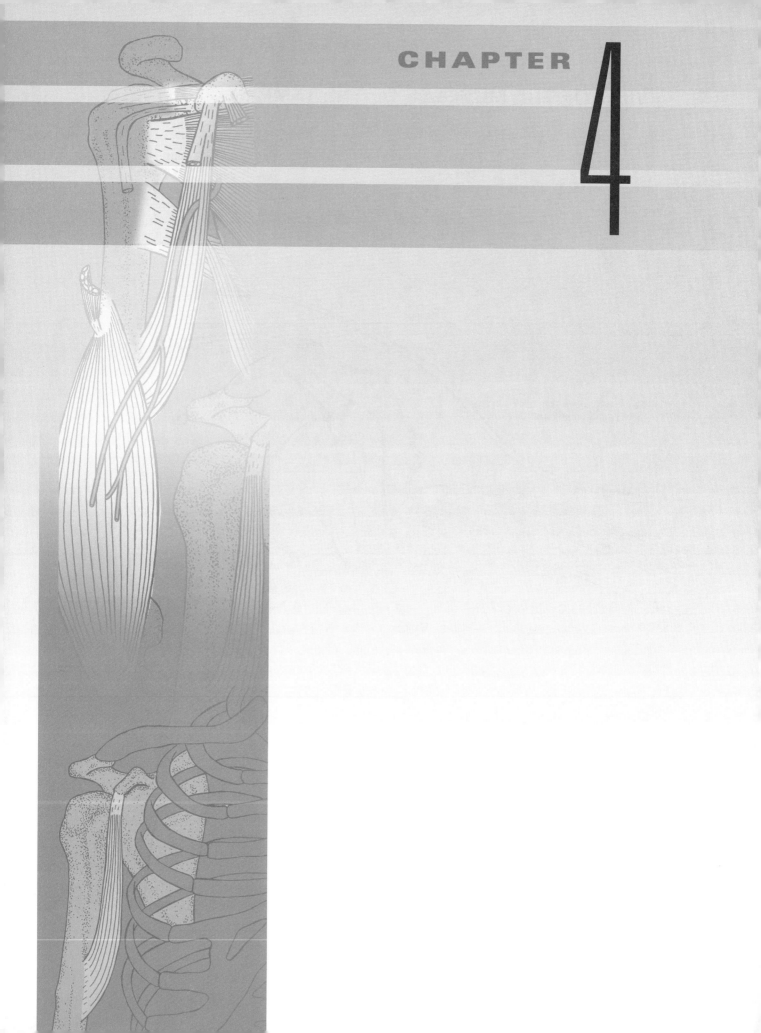

CHAPTER 4

The Nervous System

GET READY TO EXPLORE:

Cranial Nerves, 374

View of Spinal Nerve Organization, 375

View of the Cervical Plexus, 376

View of the Brachial Plexus, 377

View of the Lumbar Plexus, 378

Views of the Sacral and Coccygeal Plexuses, 379

Views of Innervation to the Right Lower Extremity, 380

Anterior View of Innervation to the Right Upper Extremity, 381

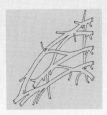

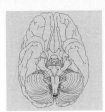

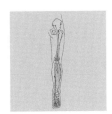

CRANIAL NERVES

ANTERIOR

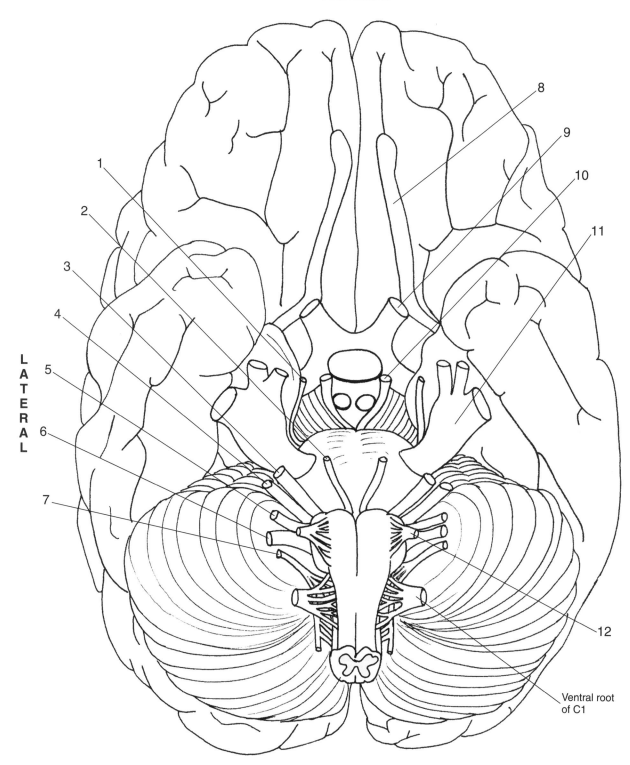

POSTERIOR

Inferior view of the brain

VIEW OF SPINAL NERVE ORGANIZATION

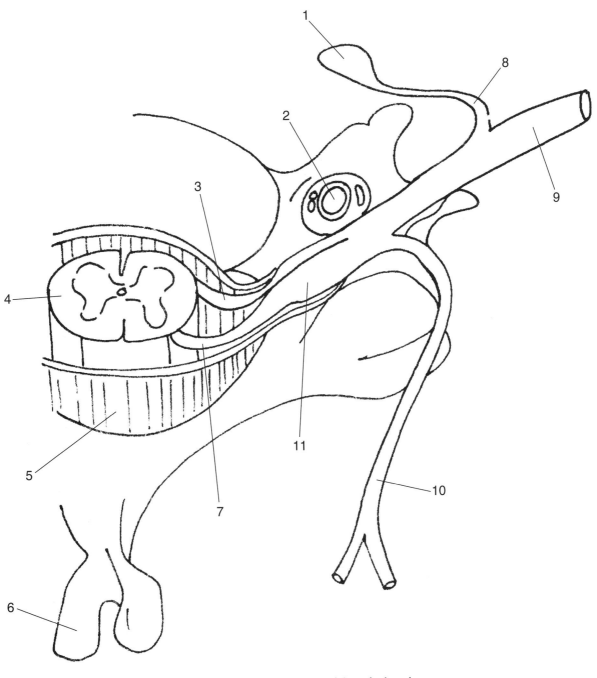

Cross section view of the spinal cord
through a cervical vertebra—spinal
nerve diagram

VIEW OF THE CERVICAL PLEXUS

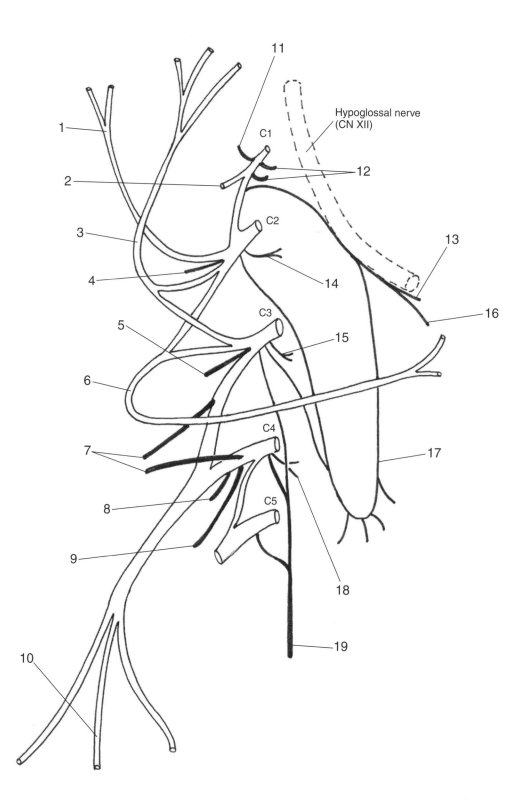

11

Hypoglossal nerve
(CN XII)

C1

1

2 ——— 12

C2

3

13

4 ——— 14

C3

5

15

6

16

C4

7

17

8

C5

9

18

10

19

VIEW OF THE BRACHIAL PLEXUS

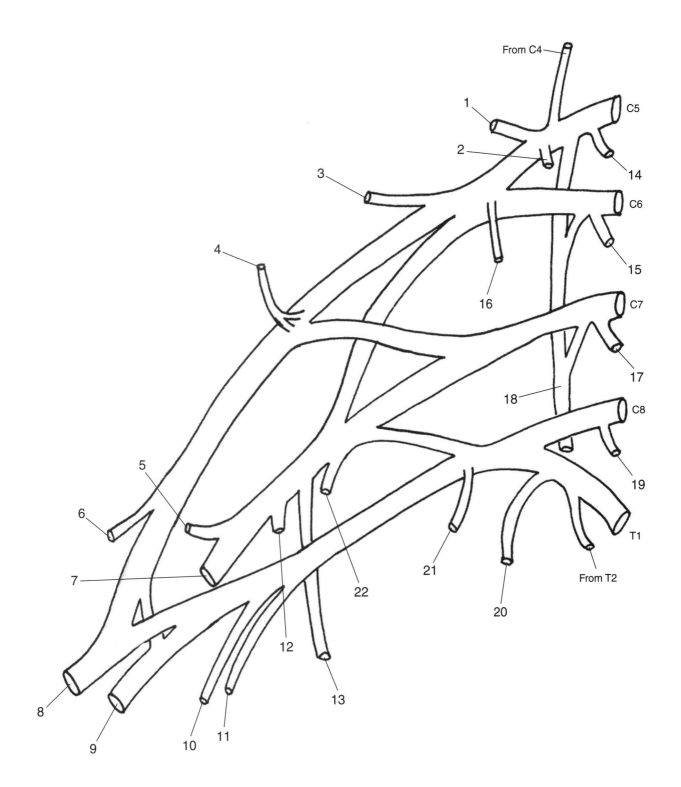

VIEW OF THE LUMBAR PLEXUS

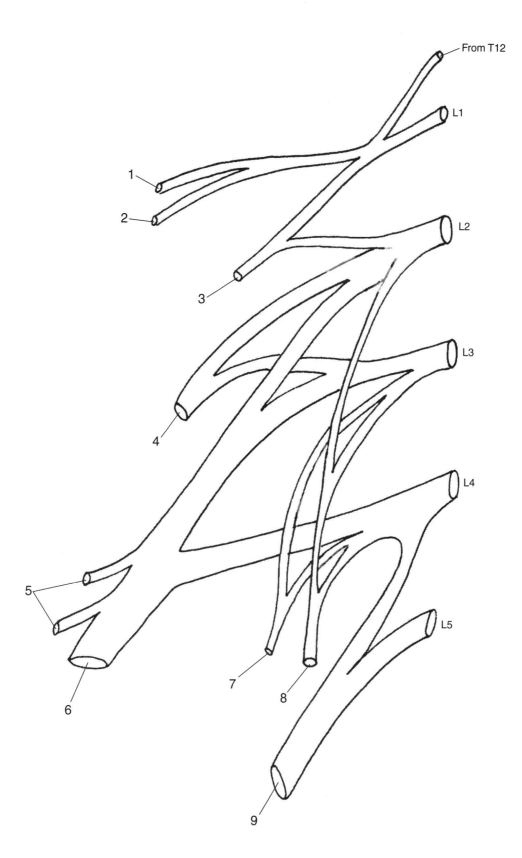

From T12

L1

L2

L3

L4

L5

1

2

3

4

5

6

7

8

9

VIEWS OF THE SACRAL AND COCCYGEAL PLEXUSES

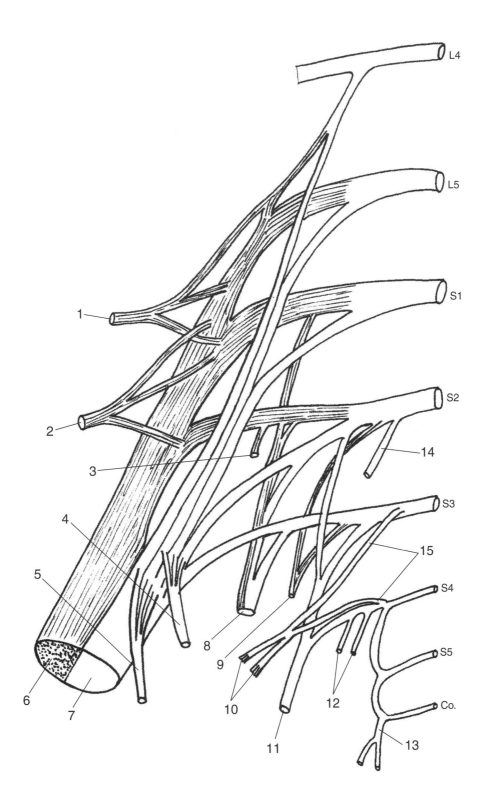

VIEWS OF INNERVATION TO THE RIGHT LOWER EXTREMITY

PROXIMAL

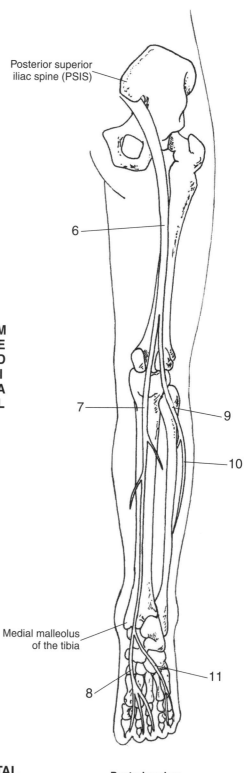

Posterior superior
iliac spine (PSIS)

Obturator
foramen

Head of
the fibula

Medial malleolus
of the tibia

L A T E R A L

M E D I A L

L A T E R A L

1

4

2

3

5

6

7

9

10

11

8

Anterior view

DISTAL

Posterior view

ANTERIOR VIEW OF INNERVATION
TO THE RIGHT UPPER EXTREMITY

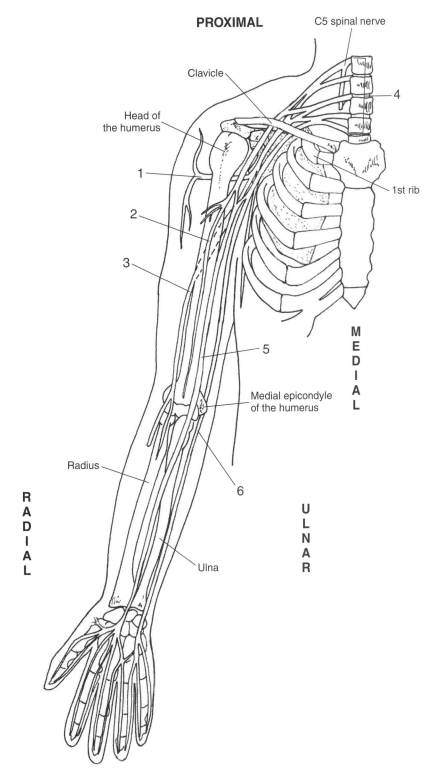

PROXIMAL

C5 spinal nerve

Clavicle

Head of
the humerus

1

2

3

4

1st rib

LATERAL

MEDIAL

5

Medial epicondyle
of the humerus

Radius

6

RADIAL

ULNAR

Ulna

DISTAL

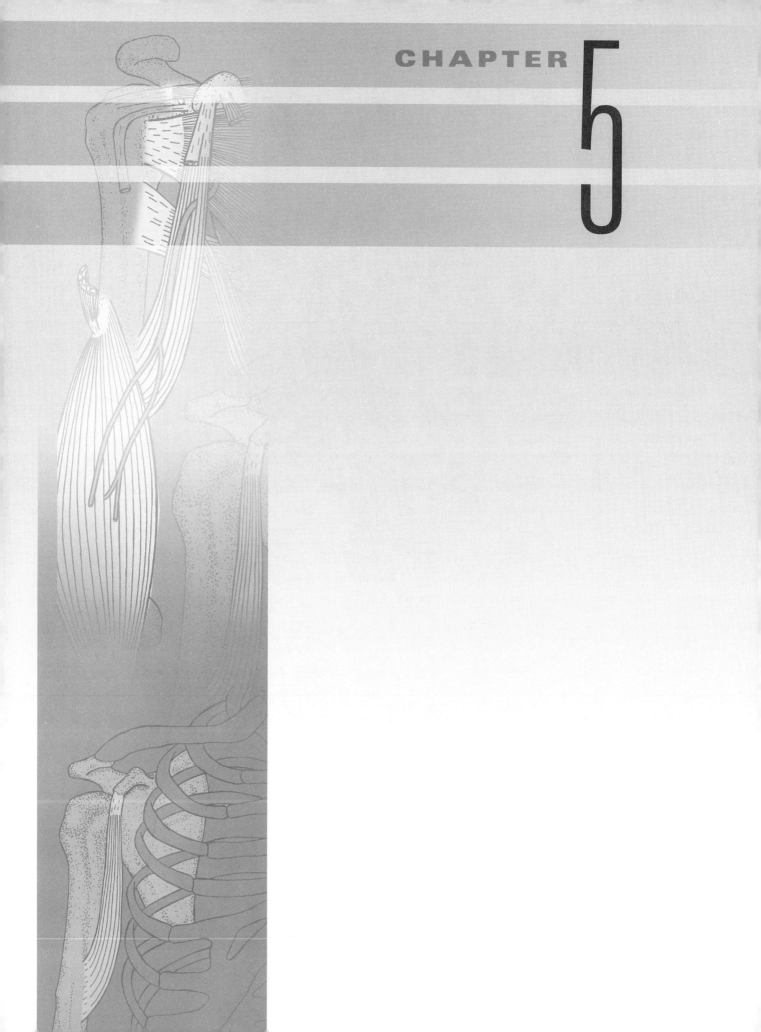

CHAPTER 5

The Arterial System

GET READY TO EXPLORE:

Lateral View of Arterial Supply to the Head and Neck, 384

Anterior View of Arterial Supply to the Trunk and Pelvis, 385

Anterior View of Arterial Supply to the Right Lower Extremity, 386

Anterior View of Arterial Supply to the Right Upper Extremity, 387

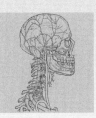

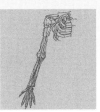

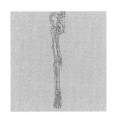

LATERAL VIEW OF ARTERIAL SUPPLY TO THE HEAD AND NECK

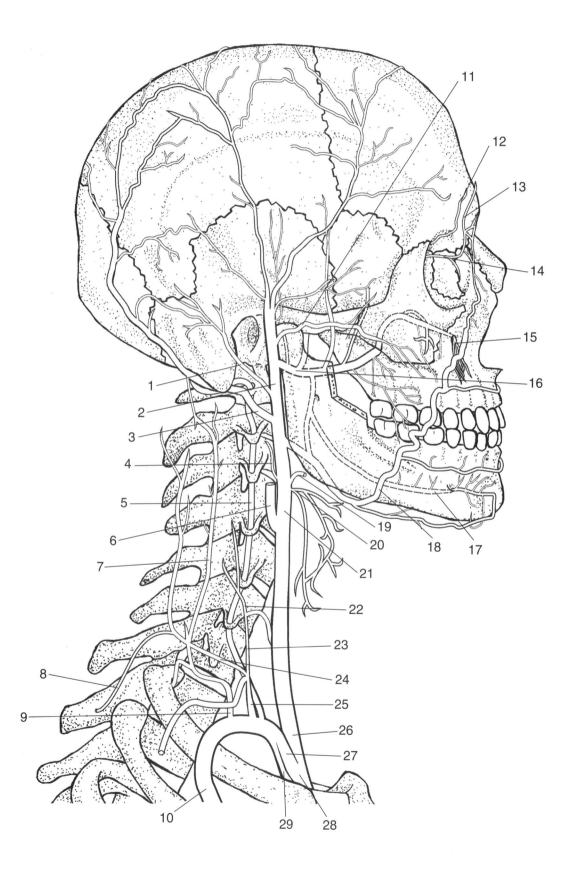

ANTERIOR VIEW OF ARTERIAL SUPPLY
TO THE TRUNK AND PELVIS

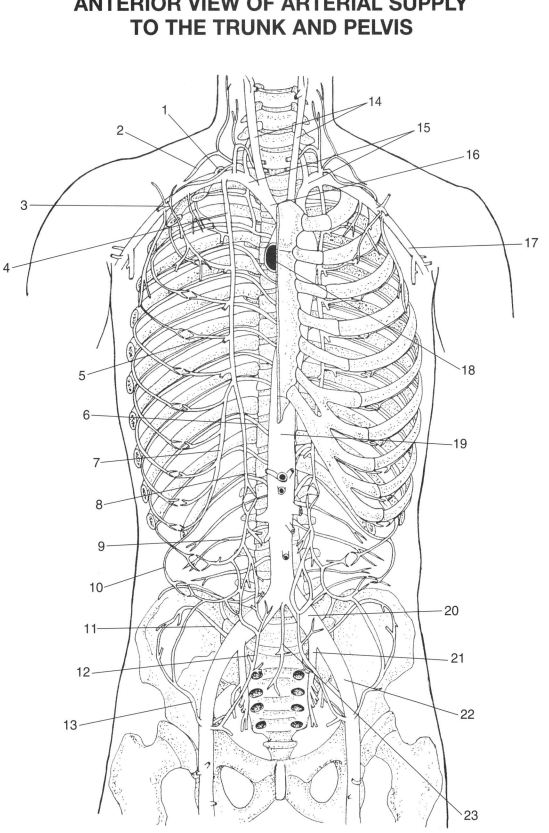

ANTERIOR VIEW OF ARTERIAL SUPPLY TO THE RIGHT LOWER EXTREMITY

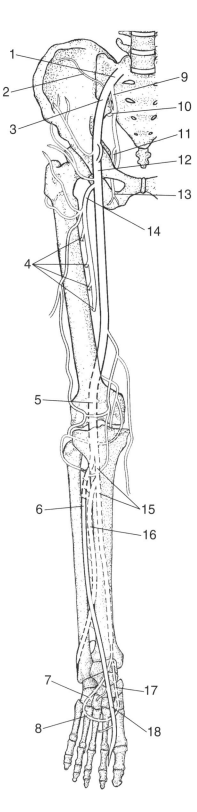

ANTERIOR VIEW OF ARTERIAL SUPPLY
TO THE RIGHT UPPER EXTREMITY

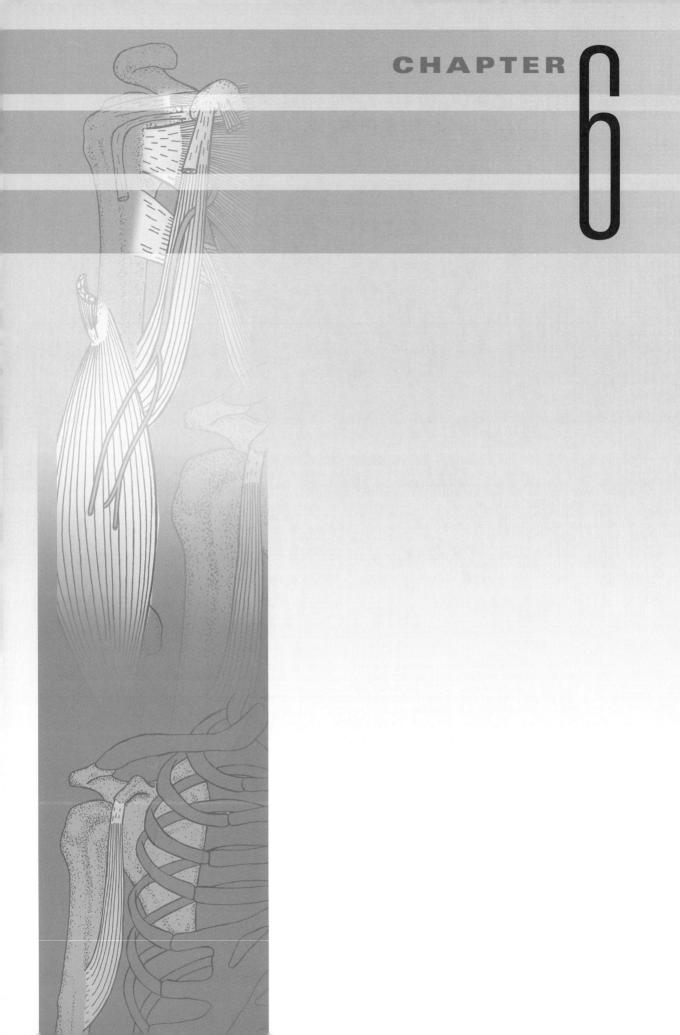

CHAPTER 6

Other Structures and Systems of the Body

GET READY TO EXPLORE:

The Cell, 390

Bone Tissue, 392

Muscle Tissue, 394

Nerve Tissue, 396

Joints, 398

Integumentary System, 400

Cardiac System, 402

Venous System, 404

Lymphatic System, 406

Respiratory System, 408

Urinary System, 410

Gastrointestinal System, 412

Immune System, 414

Endocrine System, 416

Sensory System, 418

Reproductive System, 420

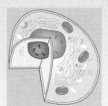

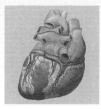

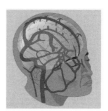

THE CELL

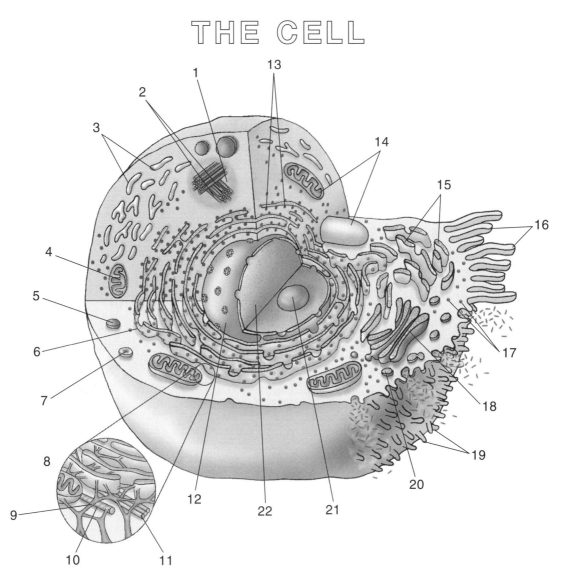

A typical cell.

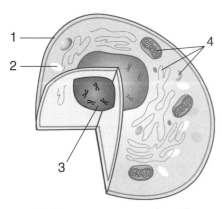

Major components of a cell.

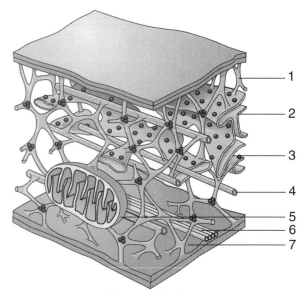

The cytoskeleton.

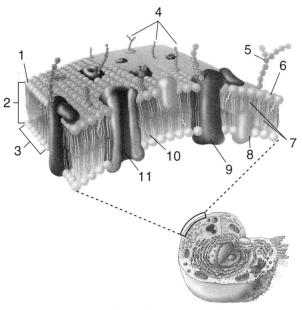

The cell membrane.

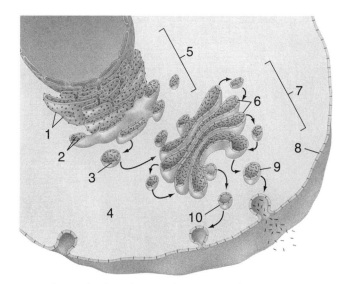

The endoplasmic reticulum and golgi apparatus.

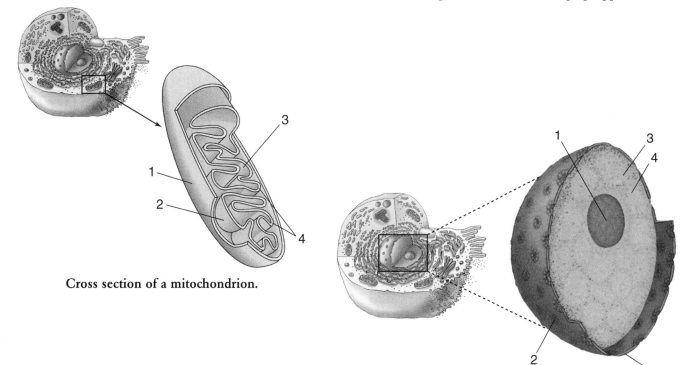

Cross section of a mitochondrion.

Cross section of the nucleus.

BONE TISSUE

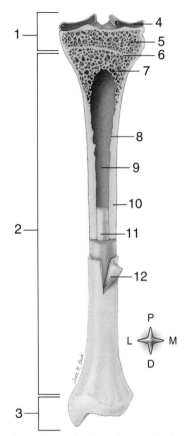

Longitudinal section of a long bone; both spongy and compact bone are illustrated.

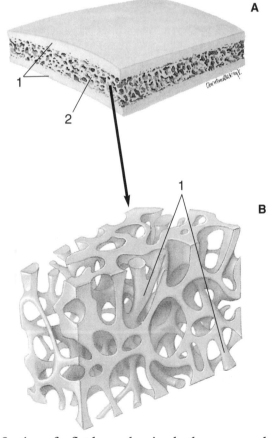

A, Section of a flat bone showing both spongy and compact bone tissue. **B,** Magnification of spongy bone tissue.

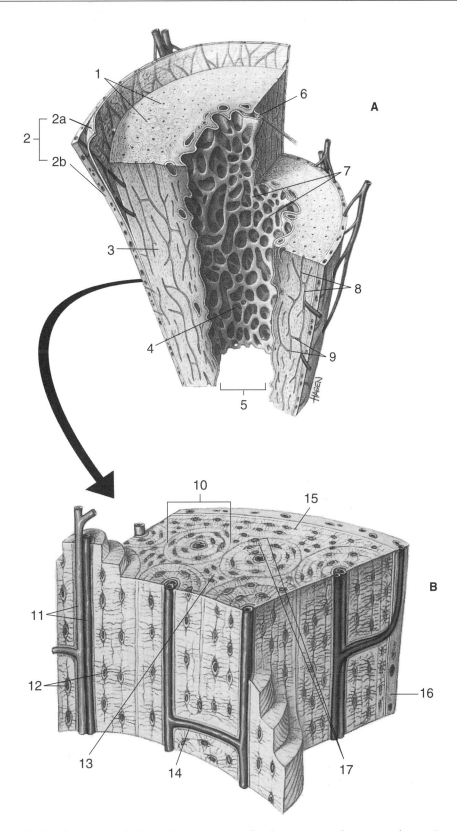

A, Longitudinal section of a long bone showing both spongy and compact bone tissue.
B, Magnification of compact bone tissue.

MUSCLE TISSUE

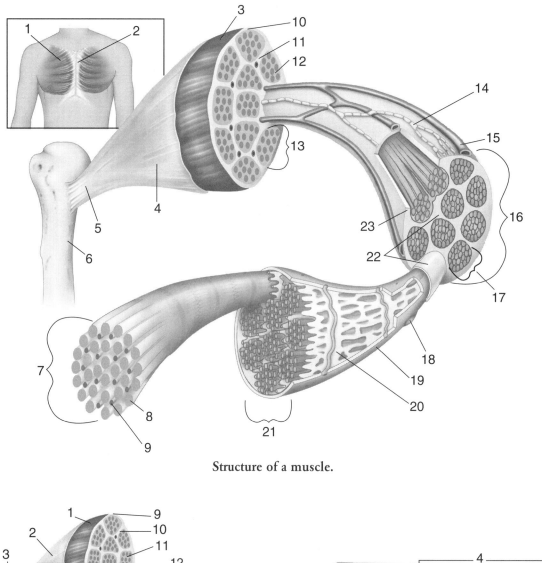

Structure of a muscle.

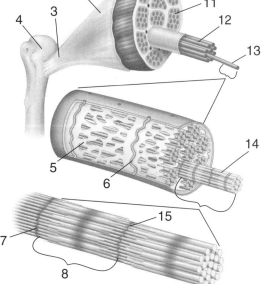

Structure of a muscle illustrating a sarcomere unit.

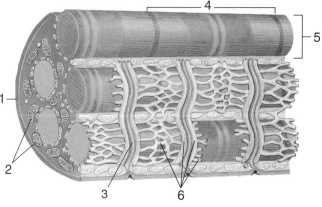

Sarcoplasmic reticulum and T tubules of a muscle fiber.

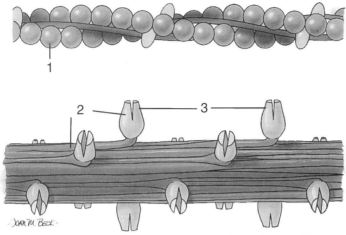
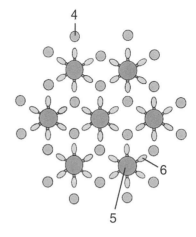

Myosin and actin filaments.

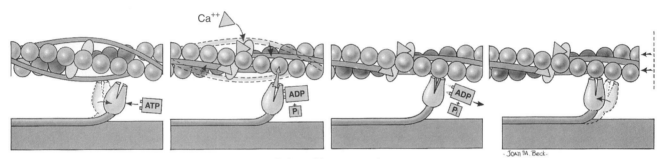

Sliding filament action.

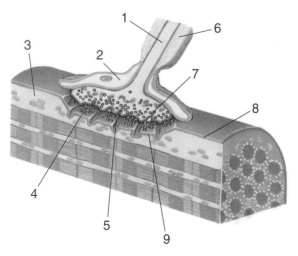

Neuromuscular junction.

NERVE TISSUE

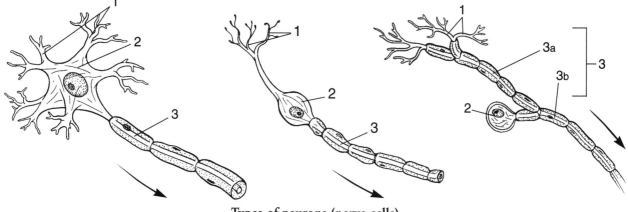

Types of neurons (nerve cells).

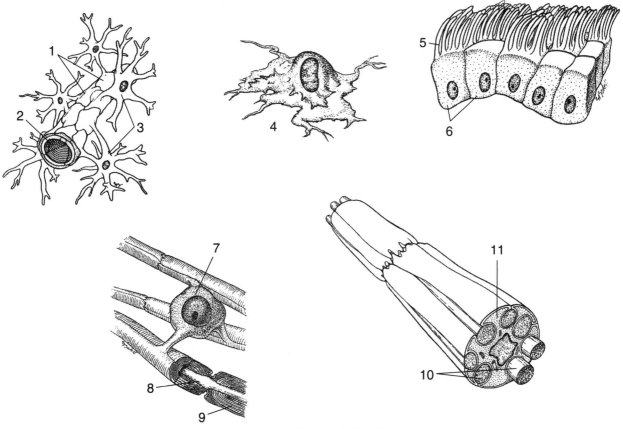

Types of neuroglial cells.

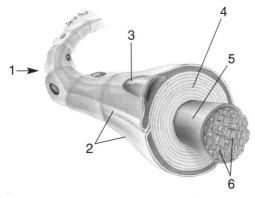

Myelinated axon of the peripheral nervous system.

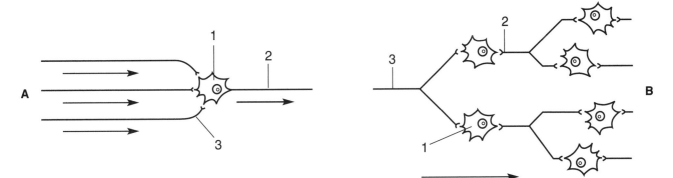

A, Convergence of neurons. **B,** Divergence of neurons.

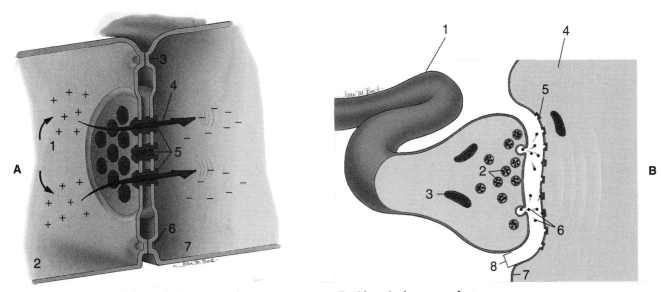

A, Electrical synapse between neurons. **B,** Chemical synapse between neurons.

JOINTS

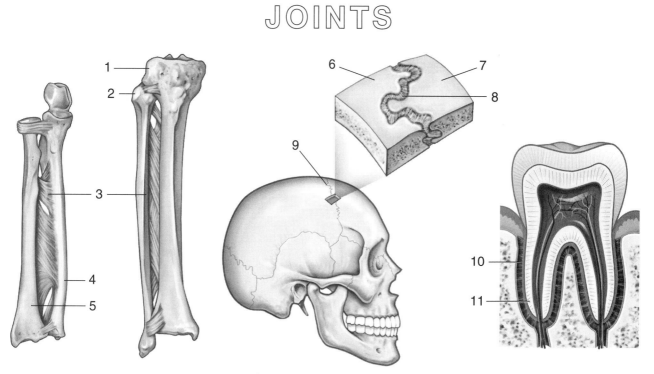

Three types of fibrous joints.

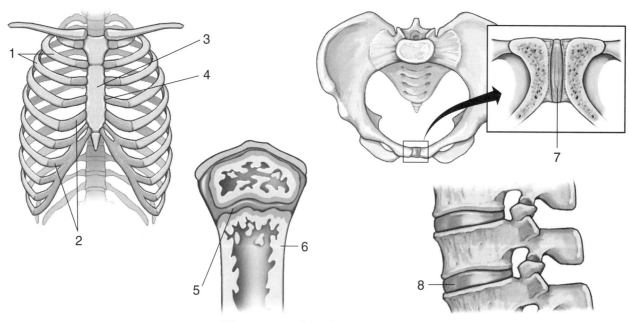

Three types of cartilaginous joints.

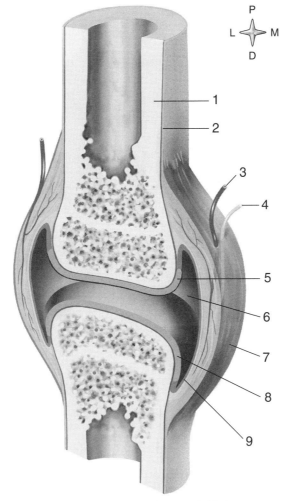

Structure of a typical synovial joint.

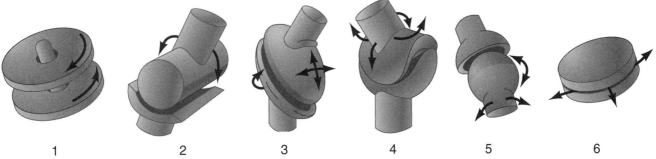

Various types of synovial joints.

INTEGUMENTARY SYSTEM

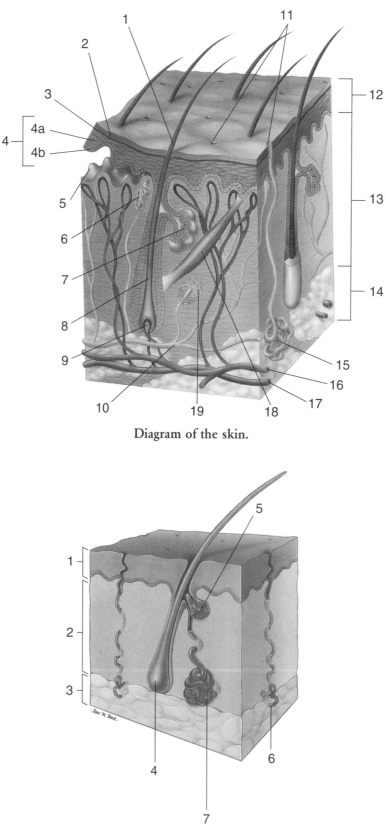

Diagram of the skin.

Glands of the skin.

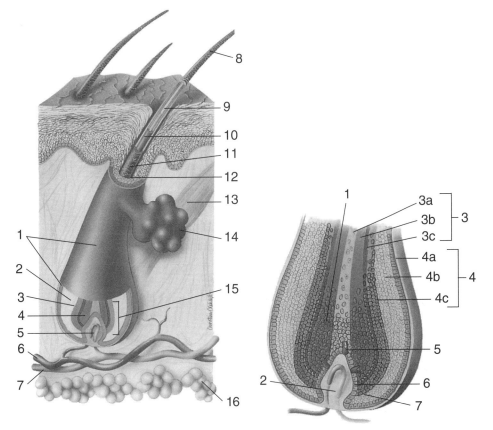

Hair follicle.

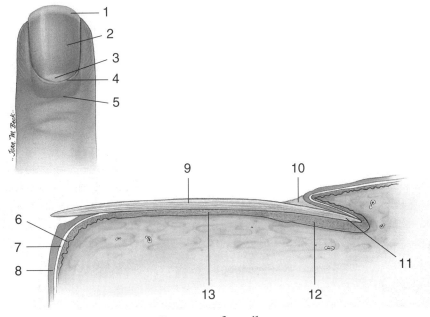

Structure of a nail.

CARDIAC SYSTEM
(THE HEART)

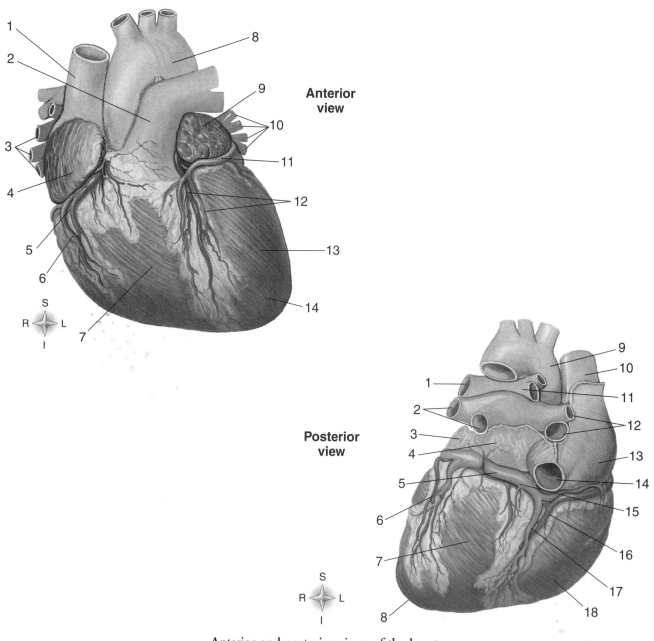

Anterior and posterior views of the heart.

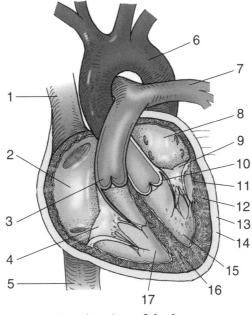

Interior view of the heart.

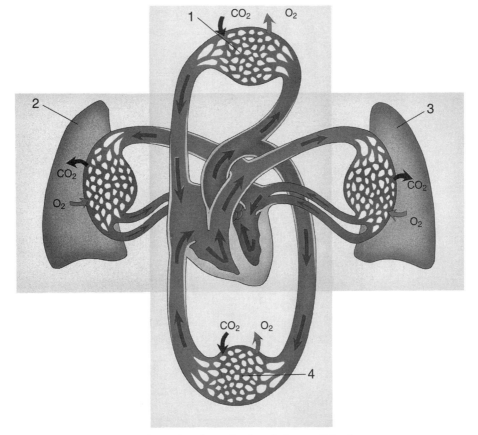

Systemic and pulmonic circulations of the heart.

VENOUS SYSTEM

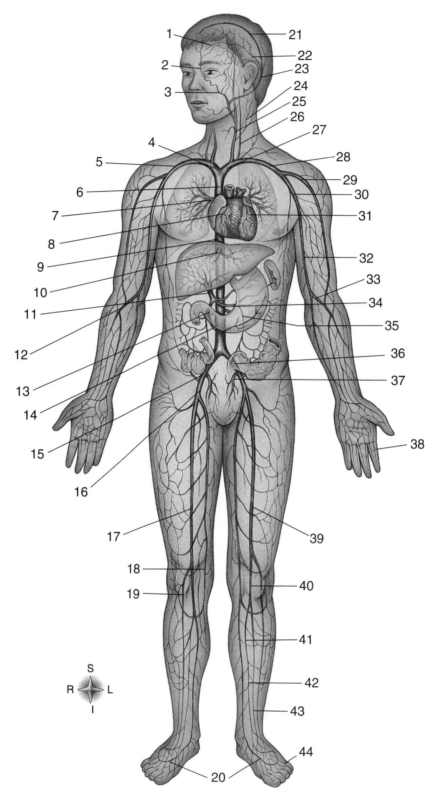

Major veins of the body.

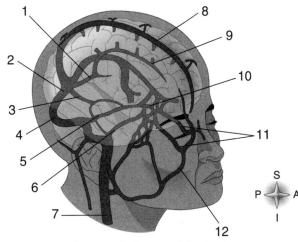

Venous drainage of the brain.

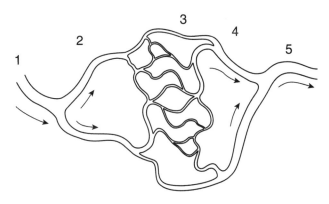

Creation of venous blood flow from capillaries.

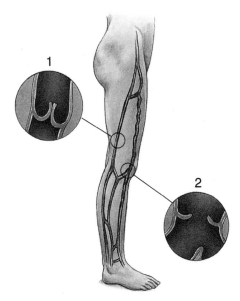

Unidirectional venous valves.

LYMPHATIC SYSTEM

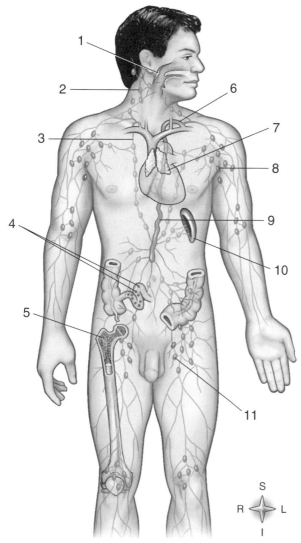

Major organs of the lymphatic system.

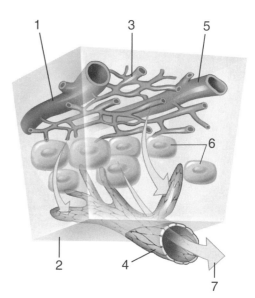

Role of lymphatic capillary in draining intercellular fluid.

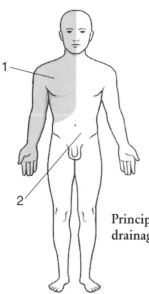

Principal lymphatic drainage of the body.

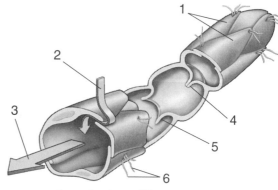

Lymphatic capillary structure.

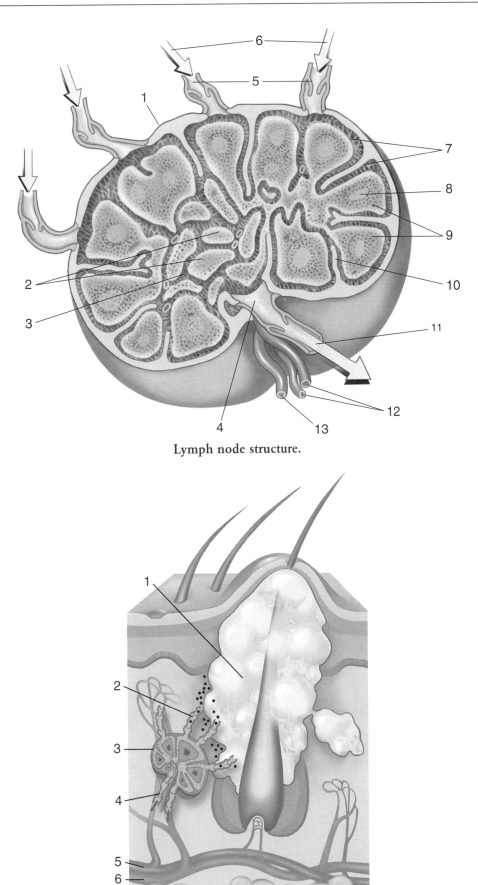

Lymph node structure.

Role of a lymph node in a skin infection.

RESPIRATORY SYSTEM

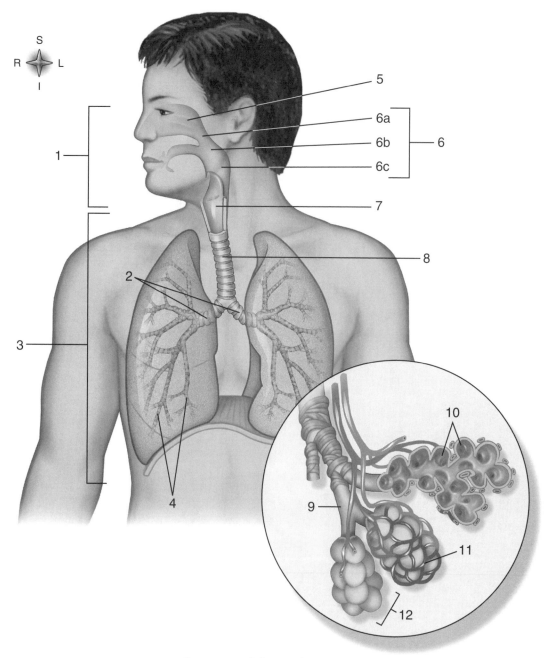

Structures of the respiratory system.

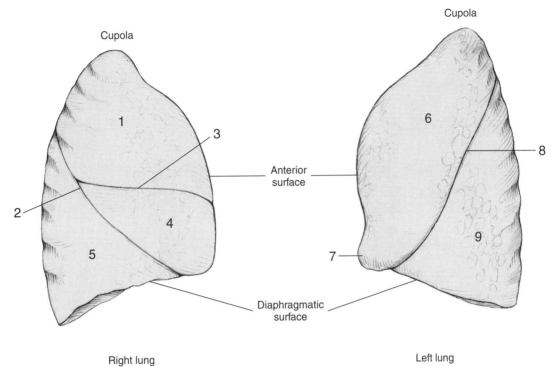

Lobes of the lungs.

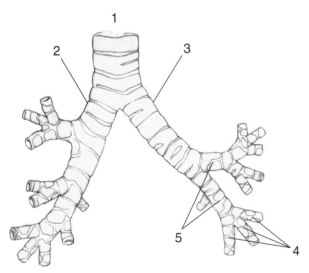

Bronchi of the lungs.

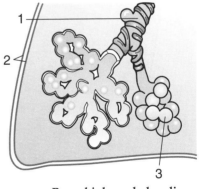

Bronchiole and alveoli.

URINARY SYSTEM

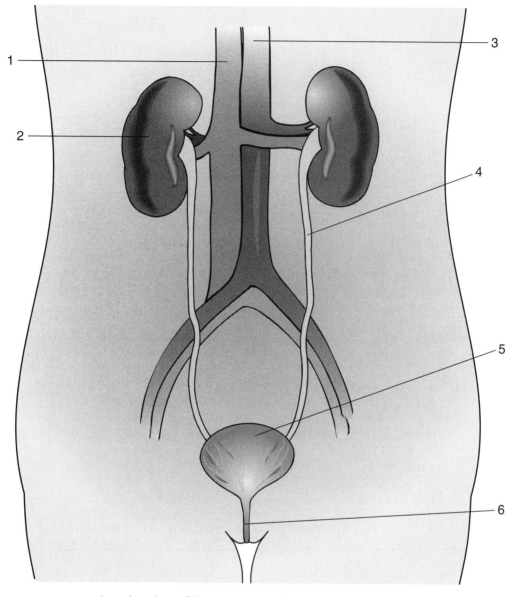

1

2

3

4

5

6

Anterior view of the structures of the urinary system.

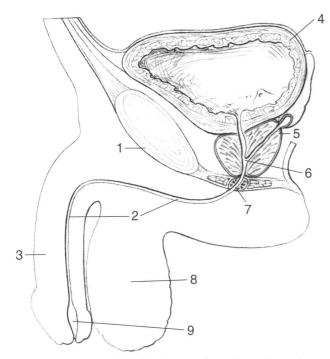

Lateral view of the bladder and urethra of a male.

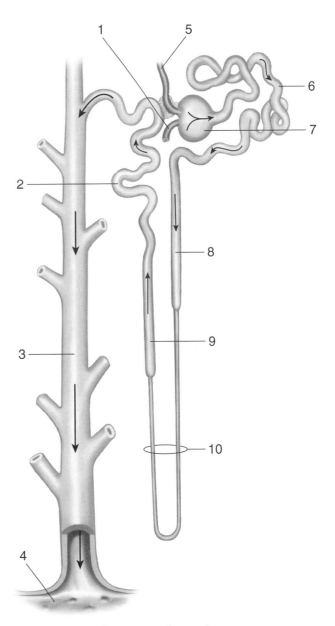

Structures of a nephron.

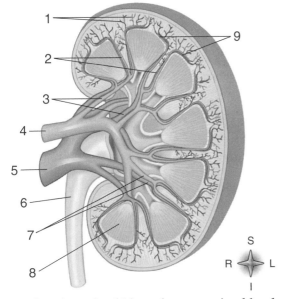

Section through a kidney demonstrating blood flow and urinary output.

GASTROINTESTINAL SYSTEM

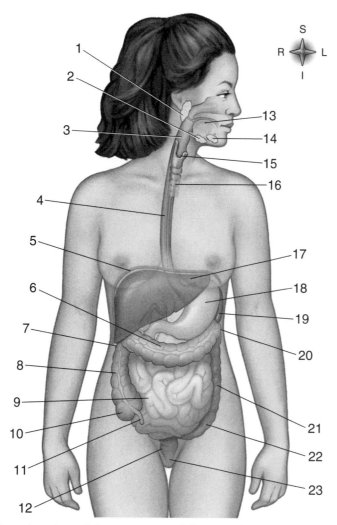

Anterior view of the structures of the gastrointestinal system.

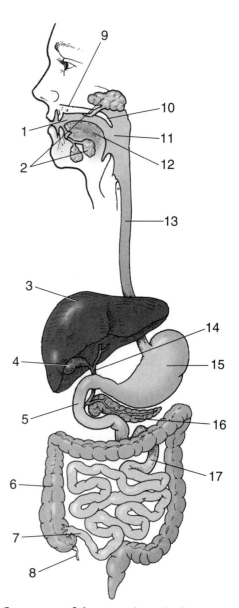

Structures of the gastrointestinal system.

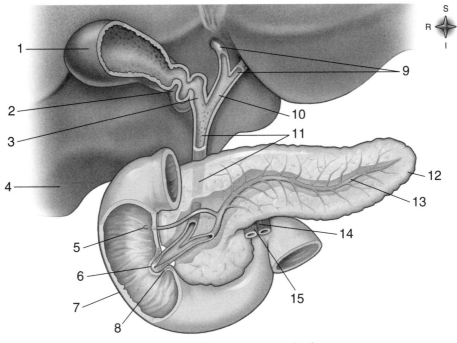

Accessory organs of the gastrointestinal system.

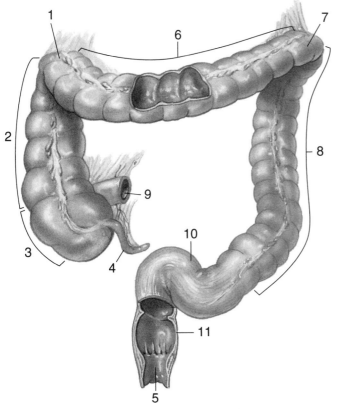

Divisions of the large intestine.

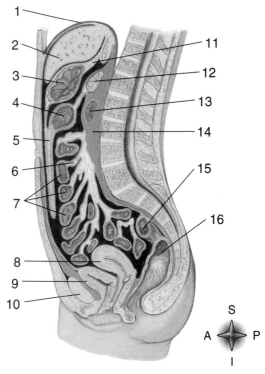

Section through the abdominopelvic cavity.

IMMUNE SYSTEM

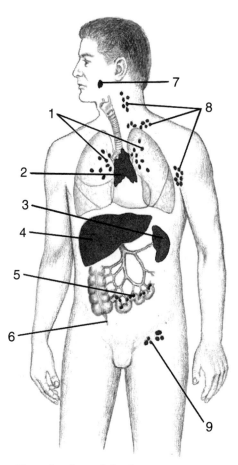

Organization of the immune system.

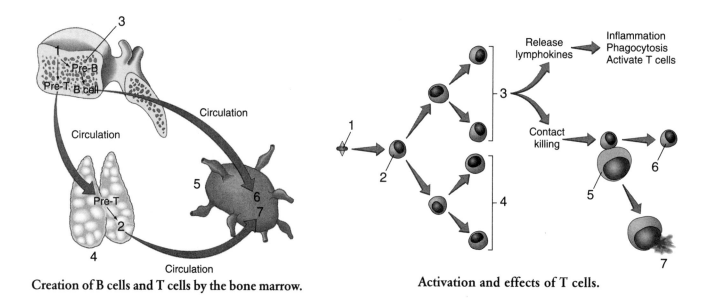

Creation of B cells and T cells by the bone marrow.

Activation and effects of T cells.

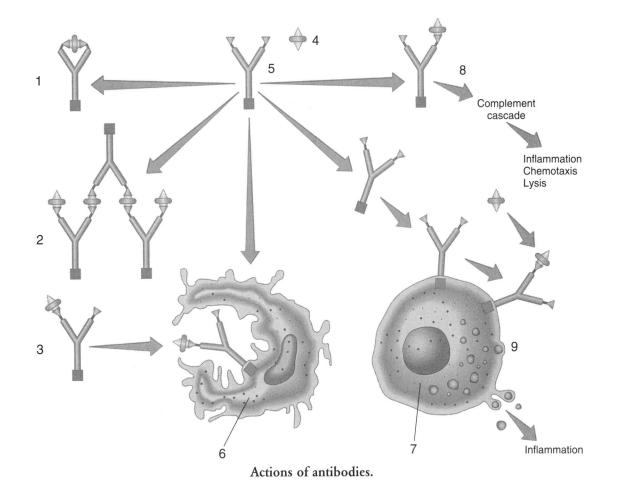

Actions of antibodies.

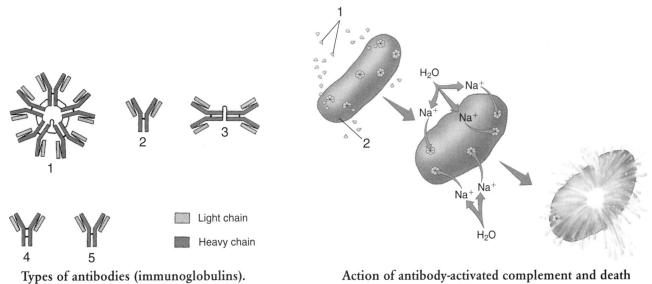

Types of antibodies (immunoglobulins).

Action of antibody-activated complement and death of bacterium.

ENDOCRINE SYSTEM

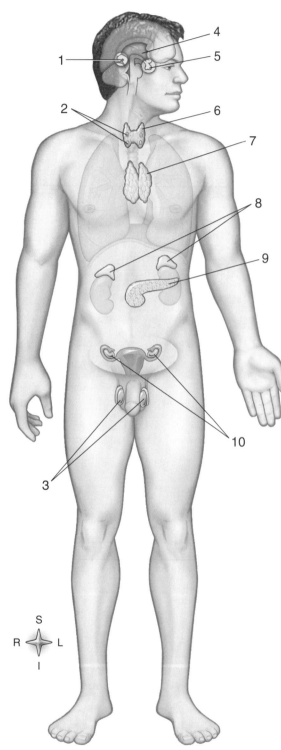

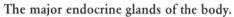

The major endocrine glands of the body.

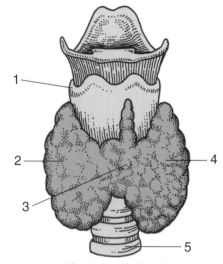

The thyroid gland.

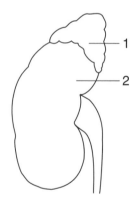

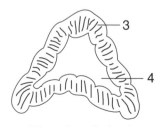

The adrenal gland.

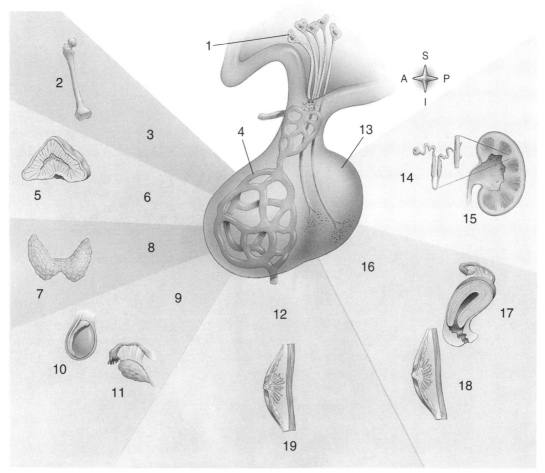

The hypothalamus and pituitary hormones.

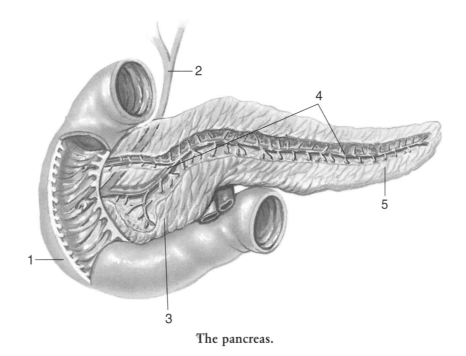

The pancreas.

SENSORY SYSTEM

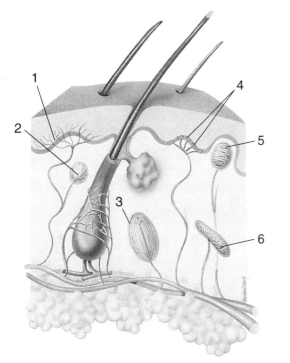

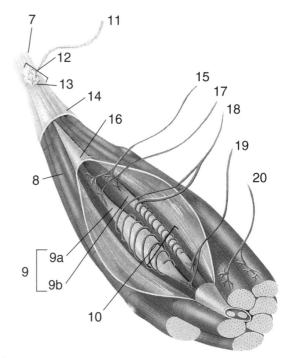

Somatic and stretch receptors.

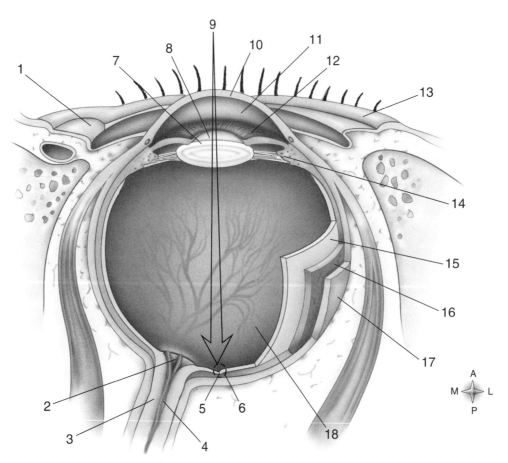

Superior view of a horizontal section of the eye.

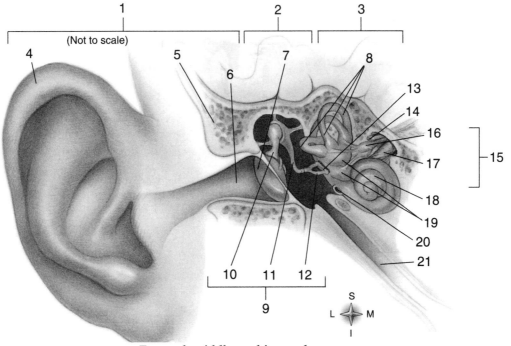

External, middle, and internal ear.

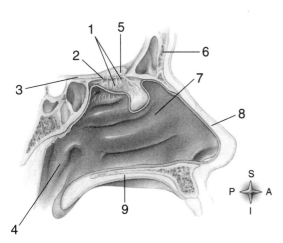

Lateral view of the internal nose.

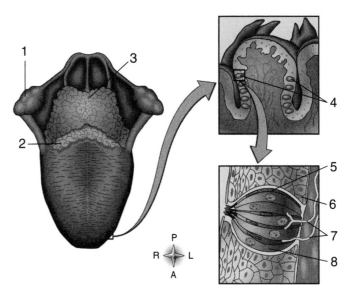

Dorsal surface of the tongue, cross section through a papilla, and a taste bud.

REPRODUCTIVE SYSTEM

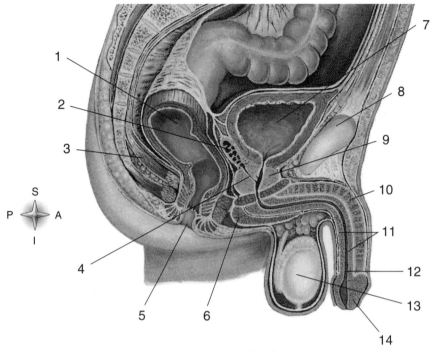

Male reproductive organs.

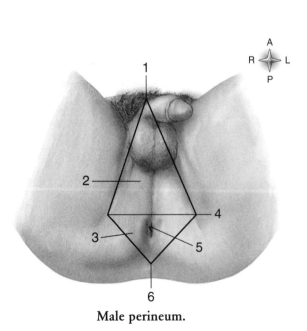

Male perineum.

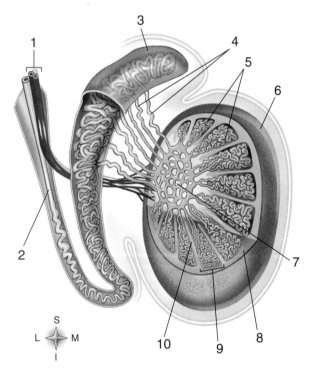

Tubules of the testis and epididymis.

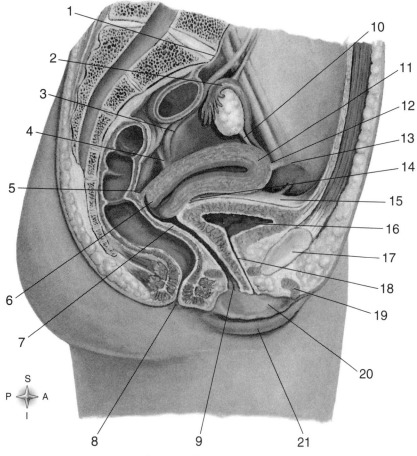

Female reproductive organs.

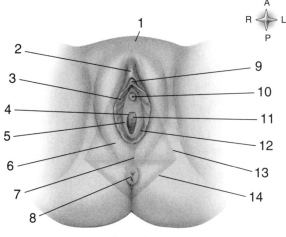

Female perineum.

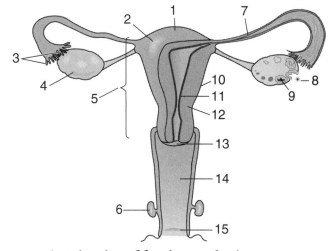

Anterior view of female reproductive organs.

Answer Key

CHAPTER 1 LABELING ANSWERS: THE SKELETAL SYSTEM

Page 3 Anterior View of the Bones and Bony Landmarks of the Head
1. Frontal bone
2. Nasal bone
3. Sphenoid bone
4. Temporal bone
5. Lacrimal bone
6. Ethmoid bone
7. Zygomatic bone
8. Zygomaticomaxillary suture
9. Maxilla
10. Vomer
11. Alveolar process of the maxilla
12. Alveolar process of the mandible
13. Mandible
14. Superciliary arch of the frontal bone
15. Parietal bone
16. Lesser wing of the sphenoid
17. Greater wing of the sphenoid
18. Palatine bone
19. Frontal process of the maxilla
20. Infraorbital foramen of the maxilla
21. Canine fossa of the maxilla
22. Incisive fossa of the maxilla
23. Ramus of the mandible
24. Incisive fossa of the mandible
25. Angle of the mandible
26. Mental foramen of the mandible
27. Oblique line of the mandible
28. Mental tubercle of the mandible
29. Symphysis menti of the mandible

Page 4 Lateral View of the Bones and Bony Landmarks of the Head
1. Temporal fossa (within dotted lines)
2. Temporomandibular joint (TMJ)
3. Highest nuchal line of the occipital bone
4. Temporal bone
5. Occipital bone
6. Mastoid process of the temporal bone
7. Zygomatic arch of the temporal bone
8. Neck of the mandible
9. Zygomaticotemporal suture
10. Coronoid process of the mandible
11. Zygomaticomaxillary suture
12. Ramus of the mandible
13. Angle of the mandible
14. Mandible
15. Oblique line of the mandible
16. Mental foramen of the mandible
17. Parietal bone
18. Frontal bone
19. Sphenoid bone
20. Superciliary arch of the frontal bone
21. Lacrimal bone
22. Nasal bone
23. Zygomatic bone
24. Frontal process of the maxilla
25. Canine fossa of the maxilla
26. Maxilla
27. Incisive fossa of the maxilla
28. Alveolar process of the maxilla
29. Alveolar process of the mandible
30. Incisive fossa of the mandible
31. Mental tubercle of the mandible

Page 5 Inferior View of the Bones and Bony Landmarks of the Head
1. Maxilla
2. Palatine bone
3. Frontal bone
4. Zygomatic bone
5. Zygomatic arch (of the temporal & zygomatic bones)
6. Parietal bone

7. Sphenoid bone
8. Temporal bone
9. Parietal bone
10. Occipital bone
11. Incisive fossa of the maxilla
12. Zygomaticomaxillary suture
13. Tuberosity of the maxilla
14. Zygomaticotemporal suture
15. Greater wing of the sphenoid
16. Medial pterygoid plate of the pterygoid process of the sphenoid bone
17. Lateral pterygoid plate of the pterygoid process of the sphenoid bone
18. Vomer
19. Styloid process of the temporal bone
20. Mastoid process of the temporal bone
21. Mastoid notch of the temporal bone
22. Jugular process of the occipital bone
23. Foramen magnum
24. Highest nuchal line of the occipital bone

Page 6 Anterior View of the Bones and Bony Landmarks of the Neck

1. Temporal bone
2. Mastoid process of the temporal bone
3. Styloid process of the temporal bone
4. Greater cornu of the hyoid bone
5. Body of the hyoid bone
6. Hyoid bone
7. Lamina of the thyroid cartilage
8. Thyroid cartilage
9. Sternoclavicular joint
10. Acromioclavicular joint
11. Shoulder joint
12. Clavicle
13. Scapula
14. Costal cartilage of the first rib
15. Manubrium of the sternum
16. Basilar part of the occiput
17. Occiput
18. Anterior arch of the atlas
19. Atlas (C1)
20. Axis (C2)
21. Vertebral body
22. Vertebral transverse process (TP)
23. Posterior tubercle of the transverse process
24. Anterior tubercle of the transverse process
25. Humerus
26. Acromion process of the scapula
27. Superior border of the scapula
28. Medial border of the scapula

Page 7 Posterior View of the Bones and Bony Landmarks of the Neck

1. External occipital protuberance (EOP)
2. Occiput
3. Superior nuchal line of the occiput
4. Inferior nuchal line of the occiput
5. Superior angle of the scapula
6. Clavicle
7. Acromioclavicular joint
8. Acromion process of the scapula
9. Scapula
10. Spine of the scapula
11. Tubercle at the root of the spine of the scapula
12. Medial border of the scapula
13. Root of the spine of the scapula
14. Temporal bone
15. Mastoid process of the temporal bone
16. Mandible
17. Atlas (C1)
18. Axis (C2)
19. Vertebral spinous process (SP)
20. Vertebral transverse process (TP)
21. C7
22. First rib
23. T3

Page 8 Anterior View of the Bones and Bony Landmarks of the Trunk

1. Clavicle
2. Coracoid process of the scapula
3. Scapula
4. Medial border of the scapula
5. Inferior angle of the scapula
6. Intercostal space
7. Costal cartilage
8. Sacro-iliac joint
9. Iliac crest
10. Pelvic bone
11. Pubic crest
12. Pubic tubercle
13. Pubic symphysis
14. Sacrum
15. Cervical transverse process
16. Body of C7
17. Humerus
18. Medial lip of the bicipital groove of the humerus
19. Lateral lip of the bicipital groove of the humerus
20. Sternum
21. Xiphoid process of the sternum
22. Intervertebral disc (L3-L4)

23. Ilium
24. Ischium
25. Pubis

Page 9 Posterior View of the Bones and Bony Landmarks of the Trunk
1. Clavicle
2. Spine of the scapula
3. Root of the spine of the scapula
4. Medial border of the scapula
5. Scapula
6. Inferior angle of the scapula
7. Vertebral transverse process (TP)
8. Vertebral lamina
9. Vertebral spinous process (SP)
10. Iliac crest
11. Posterior superior iliac spine (PSIS)
12. Pelvic bone
13. Sacrum
14. Ischium
15. Pubis
16. Pubic symphysis
17. C7
18. Tubercle (of the 5th rib)
19. Angle (of the 5th rib)
20. Intercostal space
21. Inferior articular process (of L1)
22. Superior articular process (of L2)
23. Mamillary process (of L3)
24. Ilium
25. Sacro-iliac joint
26. Medial sacral crest
27. Lateral sacral crest

Page 10 Anterior View of the Bones and Bony Landmarks of the Right Pelvis
1. Vertebral transverse process (TP)
2. Sacral ala
3. Iliac crest
4. Iliac fossa
5. Internal ilium
6. Ilium
7. Anterior inferior iliac spine (AIIS)
8. Hip joint
9. Greater trochanter of the femur
10. Lesser trochanter of the femur
11. Femur
12. Fibula
13. Intervertebral disc
14. Vertebral body (L3)
15. Sacrum
16. Iliopectineal eminence (of the ilium and the pubis)

17. Apex of the sacrum
18. Coccyx
19. Pectineal line of the pubis on the superior ramus of the pubis
20. Pubis
21. Obturator foramen
22. Ischium
23. Ischial tuberosity
24. Patella
25. Knee joint
26. Tibia

Page 11 Anterior View of the Bones and Bony Landmarks of the Right Thigh
1. Iliac crest
2. Pelvic bone
3. Anterior superior iliac spine (ASIS)
4. Anterior inferior iliac spine (AIIS)
5. Greater trochanter of the femur
6. Intertrochanteric line of the femur
7. Femur
8. Shaft of the femur
9. Lateral tibial condyle
10. Head of the fibula
11. Fibula
12. Sacrum
13. Hip joint
14. Pectineal line of the pubis on the superior ramus of the pubis
15. Body of the pubis
16. Inferior ramus of the pubis
17. Ramus of the ischium
18. Ischial tuberosity
19. Patella
20. Knee joint
21. Medial tibial condyle
22. Tibial tuberosity
23. Tibia

Page 12 Posterior View of the Bones and Bony Landmarks of the Right Pelvis
1. Vertebral transverse process (TP) (of L5)
2. Sacrum
3. Sacrotuberous ligament
4. Apex of the sacrum
5. Coccyx
6. Pectineal line of the pubis on the superior ramus of the pubis
7. Pubis
8. Obturator foramen
9. Ischium
10. Ischial tuberosity

11. Trochanteric fossa of the femur
12. Femur
13. Tibia
14. Iliac crest
15. Posterior gluteal line of the ilium
16. Anterior gluteal line of the ilium
17. Ilium
18. External ilium
19. Inferior gluteal line of the ilium
20. Anterior inferior iliac spine (AIIS)
21. Ischial spine
22. Head of the femur
23. Hip joint
24. Greater trochanter of the femur
25. Intertrochanteric crest of the femur
26. Lesser trochanter of the femur
27. Gluteal tuberosity of the femur
28. Knee joint
29. Fibula

Page 13   Posterior View of the Bones and Bony Landmarks of the Right Thigh

1. Sacrum
2. Sacrotuberous ligament
3. Body of the pubis
4. Inferior ramus of the pubis
5. Ramus of the ischium
6. Ischial tuberosity
7. Pectineal line of the femur
8. Medial lip of the linea aspera of the femur
9. Femur
10. Medial supracondylar line of the femur
11. Adductor tubercle of the femur
12. Medial tibial condyle
13. Tibia
14. Iliac crest
15. Pelvic bone
16. Anterior superior iliac spine (ASIS)
17. Anterior inferior iliac spine (AIIS)
18. Hip joint
19. Greater trochanter of the femur
20. Gluteal tuberosity of the femur
21. Linea aspera of the femur
22. Lateral lip of the linea aspera of the femur
23. Shaft of the femur
24. Lateral supracondylar line of the femur
25. Knee joint
26. Lateral tibial condyle
27. Head of the fibula
28. Fibula

Page 14   Anterior View of the Bones and Bony Landmarks of the Right Leg

1. Lateral supracondylar line of the femur
2. Lateral condyle of the femur
3. Knee joint
4. Lateral condyle of the tibia
5. Head of the fibula
6. Fibula
7. Lateral malleolus of the fibula
8. Calcaneus
9. Cuboid
10. Base of (5th) metatarsal
11. Proximal phalanx of (5th) toe
12. Middle phalanx of (5th) toe
13. Distal phalanx of (5th) toe
14. Femur
15. Medial condyle of the femur
16. Tibia
17. Interosseus membrane
18. Ankle joint
19. Medial malleolus of the tibia
20. Talus
21. Navicular
22. 1st cuneiform
23. 2nd cuneiform
24. 3rd cuneiform
25. Metatarsals #1-5
26. Proximal phalanx of the big toe
27. Distal phalanx of the big toe

Page 15   Posterior View of the Bones and Bony Landmarks of the Right Leg

1. Femur
2. Medial condyle of the femur
3. Knee joint
4. Soleal line of the tibia
5. Tibia
6. Calcaneus
7. Medial malleolus of the tibia
8. Tuberosity of the calcaneus
9. Talus
10. Navicular
11. 3rd cuneiform
12. 2nd cuneiform
13. 1st cuneiform
14. Metatarsals #1-5
15. Proximal phalanx of the big toe
16. Distal phalanx of the big toe
17. Lateral supracondylar line of the femur
18. Lateral condyle of the femur
19. Lateral condyle of the tibia
20. Head of the fibula
21. Fibula

22. Interosseus membrane
23. Lateral malleolus of the fibula
24. Cuboid
25. Base of (5th) metatarsal
26. Proximal phalanx of (5th) toe
27. Middle phalanx of (5th) toe
28. Distal phalanx of (5th) toe

Page 16   Dorsal View of the Bones and Bony Landmarks of the Right Foot
1. Cuboid
2. Metatarsals #1-5 (Numbering begins with the big toe as toe #1 and ends with the little toe as toe #5.)
3. Metatarsophalangeal joint (MTP joint)
4. Proximal phalanx of a toe
5. Proximal interphalangeal joint (PIP joint)
6. Middle phalanx of a toe
7. Distal interphalangeal joint (DIP joint)
8. Distal phalanx of a toe
9. Calcaneus
10. Talus
11. Navicular
12. 1st cuneiform
13. 2nd cuneiform
14. 3rd cuneiform
15. Base of a metatarsal
16. Head of a metatarsal
17. Base of a phalanx
18. Proximal phalanx of the big toe
19. Head of a phalanx
20. Interphalangeal joint (IP joint)
21. Distal phalanx of the big toe

Page 17   Plantar View of the Bones and Bony Landmarks of the Right Foot
1. Talus
2. Navicular
3. 3rd cuneiform
4. 2nd cuneiform
5. 1st cuneiform
6. Base of a metatarsal
7. Sesamoid bones
8. Base of a phalanx
9. Proximal phalanx of the big toe
10. Interphalangeal joint (IP joint)
11. Distal phalanx of the big toe
12. Calcaneal tuberosity
13. Calcaneus
14. Cuboid
15. Metatarsals #1-5 (Numbering begins with the big toe as toe #1 and ends with the little toe as toe #5.)

16. Metatarsophalangeal joint (MTP joint)
17. Proximal phalanx of a toe
18. Proximal interphalangeal joint (PIP joint)
19. Middle phalanx of a toe
20. Distal interphalangeal joint (DIP joint)
21. Distal phalanx of a toe
22. Base of a phalanx
23. Head of a phalanx

Page 18   Anterior View of the Bones and Bony Landmarks of the Right Scapula/Arm
1. Acromion process of the scapula
2. Supraglenoid tubercle of the scapula
3. Superior facet of the greater tubercle of the humerus
4. Greater tubercle of the humerus
5. Bicipital groove of the humerus
6. Lesser tubercle of the humerus
7. Deltoid tuberosity of the humerus
8. Humerus
9. Shaft of the humerus
10. Elbow joint
11. Radius
12. Radial tuberosity
13. Clavicle
14. Coracoid process of the scapula
15. Shoulder joint
16. Scapula
17. Subscapular fossa of the scapula
18. Infraglenoid tubercle of the scapula
19. Lateral border of the scapula
20. Coronoid process of the ulna
21. Ulna
22. Ulnar tuberosity

Page 19   Posterior View of the Bones and Bony Landmarks of the Right Scapula/Arm
1. Clavicle
2. Supraspinous fossa of the scapula
3. Shoulder joint
4. Spine of the scapula
5. Scapula
6. Infraspinous fossa of the scapula
7. Lateral border of the scapula
8. Infraglenoid tubercle of the scapula
9. Olecranon process of the ulna
10. Ulna
11. Acromion process of the scapula
12. Supraglenoid tubercle of the scapula

13. Superior facet of the greater tubercle of the humerus
14. Middle facet of the greater tubercle of the humerus
15. Greater tubercle of the humerus
16. Inferior facet of the greater tubercle of the humerus
17. Deltoid tuberosity of the humerus
18. Humerus
19. Shaft of the humerus
20. Head of the radius
21. Radius
22. Radial tuberosity

Page 20   Anterior View of the Bones and Bony Landmarks of the Right Forearm
1. Lateral supracondylar ridge of the humerus
2. Lateral epicondyle of the humerus
3. Head of the radius
4. Radial tuberosity
5. Radial shaft
6. Radius
7. Interosseus membrane
8. Wrist joint
9. Styloid process of the radius
10. Metacarpals #1-5
11. Proximal phalanx of the thumb
12. Distal phalanx of the thumb
13. Humerus
14. Medial supracondylar ridge of the humerus
15. Medial epicondyle of the humerus
16. Elbow joint
17. Coronoid process of the ulna
18. Supinator crest of the ulna
19. Ulna
20. Pisiform
21. Hook of hamate
22. Base of a metacarpal
23. Base of a phalanx
24. Proximal phalanx of a finger (the little finger)
25. Middle phalanx of a finger (the little finger)
26. Distal phalanx of a finger (the little finger)

Page 21   Posterior View of the Bones and Bony Landmarks of the Right Forearm
1. Medial supracondylar ridge of the humerus
2. Medial epicondyle of the humerus
3. Coronoid process of the ulna
4. Supinator crest of the ulna
5. Ulna

6. Interosseus membrane
7. Styloid process of the ulna
8. Pisiform
9. Base of a metacarpal
10. Base of a phalanx
11. Proximal phalanx of a finger (the little finger)
12. Middle phalanx of a finger (the little finger)
13. Distal phalanx of a finger (the little finger)
14. Humerus
15. Lateral supracondylar ridge of the humerus
16. Lateral epicondyle of the humerus
17. Olecranon process of the ulna
18. Head of the radius
19. Radial tuberosity
20. Radial shaft
21. Radius
22. Styloid process of the radius
23. Metacarpals #1-5
24. Proximal phalanx of the thumb
25. Distal phalanx of the thumb

Page 22   Palmar View of the Bones and Bony Landmarks of the Right Hand
1. Scaphoid
2. Scaphoid tubercle
3. Trapezium
4. Tubercle of trapezium
5. Trapezoid
6. Interphalangeal joint (IP joint)
7. Sesamoid bones
8. Proximal phalanx of the thumb
9. Distal phalanx of the thumb
10. Proximal phalanx of a finger (index finger)
11. Middle phalanx of a finger (index finger)
12. Distal phalanx of a finger (index finger)
13. Capitate
14. Lunate
15. Triquetrum
16. Pisiform
17. Hamate
18. Hook of hamate
19. Base of a metacarpal
20. Metacarpals #1-5 (Numbering begins with the thumb as finger #1 and ends with the little finger as finger #5.)
21. Head of a metacarpal
22. Base of a phalanx
23. Head of a phalanx
24. Proximal interphalangeal joint (PIP joint)
25. Distal interphalangeal joint (DIP joint)
26. Metacarpophalangeal joint (MCP joint)

Page 23   Dorsal View of the Bones and Bony Landmarks of the Right Hand

1. Lunate
2. Pisiform
3. Triquetrum
4. Hamate
5. Base of a metacarpal
6. Metacarpals #1-5 (Numbering begins with the thumb as finger #1 and ends with the little finger as finger #5.)
7. Head of a metacarpal
8. Metacarpophalangeal joint (MCP joint)
9. Base of a phalanx
10. Head of a phalanx
11. Proximal interphalangeal joint (PIP joint)
12. Distal interphalangeal joint (DIP joint)
13. Capitate
14. Scaphoid
15. Trapezium
16. Trapezoid
17. Proximal phalanx of the thumb
18. Interphalangeal joint (IP joint)
19. Sesamoid bone
20. Distal phalanx of the thumb
21. Proximal phalanx of a finger
22. Middle phalanx of a finger
23. Distal phalanx of a finger

CHAPTER 2.1 LABELING ANSWERS: MUSCLES OF THE HEAD

Page 54   Anterior View of the Head

1. Occipitofrontalis
2. Temporoparietalis
3. Orbicularis oculi
4. Procerus
5. Levator labii superioris alaeque nasi
6. Nasalis
7. Zygomaticus minor
8. Levator labii superioris
9. Zygomaticus major
10. Levator anguli oris
11. Masseter
12. Risorius
13. Depressor anguli oris
14. Depressor labii inferioris
15. Mentalis
16. Platysma
17. Occipitofrontalis (frontalis belly, cut)
18. Corrugator supercili
19. Orbicularis oculi (partially cut away)
20. Levator palpebrae superioris
21. Levator labii superioris alaeque nasi (cut)

22. Levator labii superioris (cut)
23. Zygomaticus minor (cut)
24. Zygomaticus major (cut)
25. Levator anguli oris (cut)
26. Depressor septi nasi
27. Buccinator
28. Orbicularis oris
29. Depressor anguli oris (cut)
30. Depressor labii inferioris (cut)

Page 55   Lateral View of the Head

1. Temporoparietalis
2. Occipitofrontalis (occipitalis belly)
3. Auricularis muscles
4. Splenius capitis
5. Sternocleidomastoid
6. Levator scapulae
7. Trapezius
8. Occipitofrontalis (frontalis belly)
9. Temporalis (deep to facia)
10. Corrugator supercilii
11. Procerus
12. Orbicularis oculi (partially cut)
13. Levator labii superioris alaeque nasi
14. Nasalis
15. Levator labii superioris
16. Lateral pterygoid
17. Depressor septi nasi
18. Zygomaticus minor
19. Levator anguli oris
20. Zygomaticus major
21. Orbicularis oris
22. Mentalis
23. Depressor labii inferioris
24. Depressor anguli oris
25. Risorius
26. Buccinator
27. Platysma

CHAPTER 2.2 LABELING ANSWERS: MUSCLES OF THE NECK

Page 92   Anterior View of the Neck (Superficial)

1. Omohyoid
2. Platysma
3. Sternothyroid
4. Digastric (anterior belly)
5. Mylohyoid
6. Stylohyoid
7. Digastric (posterior belly)
8. Thyrohyoid
9. Sternocleidomastoid

10. Sternocleidomastoid (clavicular head)
11. Levator scapulae
12. Sternohyoid
13. Middle scalene
14. Posterior scalene
15. Omohyoid (inferior belly)
16. Trapezius
17. Anterior scalene
18. Deltoid
19. Pectoralis major

Page 93   Anterior View of the Neck (Intermediate)

1. Mylohyoid
2. Sternocleidomastoid (cut)
3. Omohyoid (superior belly)
4. Omohyoid (inferior belly)
5. Sternocleidomastoid (cut)
6. Sternohyoid
7. Digastric (anterior belly)
8. Stylohyoid
9. Digastric (posterior belly)
10. Sternocleidomastoid (cut)
11. Thyrohyoid
12. Levator scapulae
13. Omohyoid (cut and reflected)
14. Sternothyroid
15. Middle scalene
16. Posterior scalene
17. Trapezius
18. Anterior scalene
19. Deltoid
20. Pectoralis major
21. Sternohyoid (cut and reflected)

Page 94   Anterior View of the Neck (Deep)

1. Rectus capitis lateralis
2. Rectus capitis anterior
3. Longus capitis
4. Longus colli
5. Middle scalene
6. Anterior scalene
7. Posterior scalene
8. Longus capitis (cut)
9. Rectus capitis anterior
10. Rectus capitis lateralis
11. Longus colli
12. Middle scalene
13. Anterior scalene (cut)
14. Posterior scalene

Page 95   Lateral View of the Neck

1. Stylohyoid
2. Digastric (posterior belly)
3. Splenius capitis
4. Longus capitis
5. Sternocleidomastoid
6. Levator scapulae
7. Anterior scalene
8. Middle scalene
9. Posterior scalene
10. Trapezius
11. Omohyoid (inferior belly)
12. Deltoid
13. Masseter (cut)
14. Mylohyoid
15. Digastric (anterior belly)
16. Thyrohyoid
17. Omohyoid (superior belly)
18. Sternohyoid
19. Sternothyroid
20. Sternocleidomastoid (sternal head)
21. Sternocleidomastoid (clavicular head)
22. Pectoralis major

Page 96   Posterior View of the Neck (Superficial and Intermediate)

1. Sternocleidomastoid
2. Splenius capitis
3. Levator scapulae
4. Trapezius
5. Deltoid
6. Triceps brachii
7. Latissimus dorsi
8. Semispinalis capitis (of transversospinalis group)
9. Splenius capitis
10. Splenius cervicis
11. Levator scapulae
12. Rhomboid minor
13. Supraspinatus
14. Infraspinatus
15. Teres minor
16. Rhomboid major
17. Teres major
18. Erector spinae
19. Latissimus dorsi

Page 97   Posterior View of the Neck (Intermediate and Deep)

1. Semispinalis capitis (of transversospinalis group)
2. Longissimus capitis (of erector spinae group)

3. Splenius capitis
4. Splenius cervicis
5. Iliocostalis cervicis (of erector spinae group)
6. Serratus posterior superior
7. Iliocostalis and longissimus (of erector spinae group)
8. Splenius cervicis
9. Rectus capitis posterior minor
10. Rectus capitis posterior major
11. Obliquus capitis superior
12. Obliquus capitis inferior
13. Interspinales
14. Rotatores (of transversospinalis group)
15. Levatores costarum
16. External intercostals

CHAPTER 2.3 LABELING ANSWERS: MUSCLES OF THE TRUNK

Page 146 Posterior View of the Trunk (Superficial and Intermediate)
1. Splenius capitis
2. Sternocleidomastoid
3. Rhomboid minor (cut)
4. Rhomboid major (cut)
5. Deltoid
6. Trapezius
7. Teres major
8. Triceps brachii
9. Latissimus dorsi
10. External abdominal oblique
11. Gluteus medius
12. Gluteus maximus
13. Semispinalis capitis (of transversospinalis group)
14. Splenius capitis
15. Splenius cervicis
16. Levator scapulae
17. Supraspinatus
18. Serratus posterior superior
19. Infraspinatus
20. Teres minor
21. Teres major
22. Longissimus (of erector spinae group)
23. Latissimus dorsi (cut)
24. Spinalis (of erector spinae group)
25. Triceps brachii
26. Iliocostalis (of erector spinae group)
27. Serratus anterior
28. Serratus posterior inferior
29. External abdominal oblique
30. Latissimus dorsi (cut and reflected)

31. Internal abdominal oblique
32. Gluteus medius
33. Gluteus maximus

Page 147 Posterior View of the Trunk (Deep Layers)
1. Semispinalis capitis (of transversospinalis group)
2. Longissimus (of erector spinae group)
3. Splenius capitis
4. Splenius cervicis
5. Iliocostalis (of erector spinae group)
6. Spinalis (of erector spinae group)
7. Longissimus (of erector spinae group)
8. Transversus abdominis
9. Internal abdominal oblique
10. External abdominal oblique (cut)
11. Iliocostalis (of erector spinae group)
12. Rectus capitis posterior minor
13. Rectus capitis posterior major
14. Obliquus capitis superior
15. Obliquus capitis inferior
16. Interspinales
17. Rotatores (of transversospinalis group)
18. Semispinalis (of transversospinalis group)
19. External intercostals
20. Levatores costarum
21. Quadratus lumborum
22. Multifidus (of transversospinalis group)
23. Intertransversarii
24. Sacrum

Page 148 Anterior View of the Trunk (Superficial and Intermediate)
1. Platysma
2. Deltoid
3. Pectoralis major
4. Triceps brachii
5. Biceps brachii
6. Latissimus dorsi
7. Serratus anterior
8. External abdominal oblique
9. Iliopsoas
10. Sartorius
11. Rectus femoris (of quadriceps femoris group)
12. Pectineus
13. Adductor longus
14. Sternocleidomastoid
15. Trapezius
16. Subclavius
17. External intercostals
18. Pectoralis minor

19. Coracobrachialis
20. Internal intercostals
21. Biceps brachii
22. External intercostals
23. Rectus abdominis
24. External abdominal oblique (cut)
25. Internal abdominal oblique
26. Gluteus medius
27. Tensor fasciae latae
28. Gracilis

Page 149 Anterior View of the Trunk (Intermediate and Deep)

1. Sternocleidomastoid
2. Trapezius
3. Subclavius
4. External intercostals
5. Pectoralis minor
6. Coracobrachialis
7. Internal intercostals
8. Biceps brachii
9. External intercostals
10. Rectus abdominis
11. External abdominal oblique (cut)
12. Internal abdominal oblique
13. Gracilis
14. Internal intercostals
15. Rectus abdominis
16. External abdominal oblique (cut)
17. Transversus abdominis
18. Internal abdominal oblique (cut)
19. Gluteus medius
20. Iliopsoas
21. Tensor fasciae latae
22. Sartorius
23. Rectus femoris (of quadriceps femoris group)
24. Pectineus
25. Adductor longus

Page 150 Lateral View of the Trunk

1. Trapezius
2. Supraspinatus (cut)
3. Biceps brachii (cut)
4. Subscapularis (cut)
5. Infraspinatus (cut)
6. Teres minor (cut)
7. Triceps brachii (cut)
8. Teres major (cut)
9. Serratus anterior
10. Erector spinae
11. External intercostals
12. Serratus posterior inferior

13. Internal abdominal oblique
14. Gluteus medius
15. Gluteus maximus
16. Vastus lateralis (of quadriceps femoris group)
17. Sternocleidomastoid
18. Subclavius
19. External intercostals
20. Internal intercostals
21. Pectoralis minor
22. External abdominal oblique
23. Tensor fasciae latae
24. Sartorius
25. Rectus femoris (of quadriceps femoris group)
26. Vastus lateralis (of quadriceps femoris group)

Page 151 Cross Section Views of the Trunk (Thoracic)

1. Transversus thoracis
2. Internal intercostals
3. Erector spinae and transversospinalis groups
4. Rhomboid major
5. Trapezius
6. Infraspinatus
7. Teres major
8. Subscapularis
9. Latissimus dorsi
10. Serratus anterior
11. External intercostals

Page 151 Cross Section Views of the Trunk (Lumbar)

1. Diaphragm
2. Psoas major
3. Quadratus lumborum
4. Transversus abdominis
5. Erector spinae and transversospinalis groups
6. Serratus posterior inferior
7. Latissimus dorsi
8. Internal abdominal oblique
9. External abdominal oblique

CHAPTER 2.4 LABELING ANSWERS: MUSCLES OF THE PELVIS

Page 178 Anterior View of the Right Pelvis

1. Transversus abdominis (cut)
2. Quadratus lumborum
3. Psoas major
4. Iliacus
5. Psoas minor

Page 179 Lateral View of the Right Pelvis

1. Gluteus medius
2. Gluteus maximus
3. Vastus lateralis
4. Biceps femoris
5. Semimembranosus
6. Plantaris
7. Gastrocnemius (lateral head)
8. Soleus
9. Fibularis longus
10. Tensor fasciae latae
11. Sartorius
12. Rectus femoris
13. Vastus lateralis
14. Tibialis anterior
15. Extensor digitorum longus

Page 180 Posterior View of the Right Pelvis (Superficial)

1. Gluteus maximus
2. Adductor magnus
3. Semitendinosus
4. Gracilis
5. Semimembranosus
6. Sartorius
7. Gluteus medius
8. Tensor fasciae latae
9. Biceps femoris

Page 181 Posterior View of the Right Pelvis (Deep)

1. Piriformis
2. Superior gemellus
3. Obturator internus
4. Inferior gemellus
5. Semitendinosus (cut)
6. Biceps femoris (long head, cut)
7. Gracilis
8. Adductor magnus
9. Semimembranosus
10. Gluteus medius (cut)
11. Gluteus minimus
12. Tensor fasciae latae
13. Gluteus medius (cut and reflected)
14. Quadratus femoris
15. Gluteus maximus (cut and reflected)
16. Pectineus
17. Adductor magnus

CHAPTER 2.5 LABELING ANSWERS: MUSCLES OF THE THIGH

Page 210 Anterior View of the Right Thigh (Superficial)

1. Iliacus
2. Gluteus medius
3. Tensor fasciae latae
4. Rectus femoris
5. Vastus lateralis
6. Tibialis anterior
7. Gastrocnemius
8. Fibularis longus
9. Psoas major
10. Pectineus
11. Adductor longus
12. Gracilis
13. Adductor magnus
14. Sartorius
15. Vastus medialis
16. Gastrocnemius

Page 211 Anterior View of the Right Thigh (Deep)

1. Iliopsoas (cut)
2. Quadratus femoris
3. Pectineus (cut and reflected)
4. Vastus intermedius
5. Adductor longus (cut and reflected)
6. Vastus lateralis (cut)
7. Rectus femoris (cut)
8. Vastus medialis (cut)
9. Pectineus (cut and reflected)
10. Adductor longus (cut and reflected)
11. Obturator externus
12. Gracilis (cut)
13. Adductor brevis
14. Adductor magnus
15. Gracilis (cut)
16. Sartorius (cut)
17. Semitendinosus

Page 212 Posterior View of the Right Thigh (Superficial)

1. Gluteus maximus
2. Adductor magnus
3. Gracilis
4. Semitendinosus
5. Semimembranosus
6. Sartorius
7. Gastrocnemius (medial head)
8. Soleus

9. Gluteus medius
10. Tensor fasciae latae
11. Biceps femoris (long head)
12. Biceps femoris (short head)
13. Plantaris
14. Gastrocnemius (lateral head)
15. Soleus

Page 213 Posterior View of the Right Thigh (Deep)
1. Semitendinosus (cut and reflected)
2. Biceps femoris (long head, cut and reflected)
3. Semimembranosus
4. Semitendinosus (cut and reflected)
5. Biceps femoris (short head)
6. Biceps femoris (long head, cut and reflected)

Page 214 Lateral View of the Right Thigh
1. Gluteus medius
2. Gluteus maximus
3. Vastus lateralis
4. Biceps femoris
5. Semimembranosus
6. Plantaris
7. Gastrocnemius (lateral head)
8. Soleus
9. Fibularis longus
10. Tensor fasciae latae
11. Sartorius
12. Rectus femoris
13. Vastus lateralis
14. Tibialis anterior
15. Extensor digitorum longus

Page 215 Medial View of the Right Thigh
1. Iliacus
2. Adductor longus
3. Gracilis
4. Adductor magnus
5. Rectus femoris
6. Sartorius
7. Vastus medialis
8. Sartorius
9. Gracilis
10. Semitendinosus
11. Tibialis anterior
12. Piriformis
13. Obturator internus
14. Gluteus maximus
15. Semitendinosus
16. Semimembranosus

17. Gastrocnemius (medial head)
18. Soleus

CHAPTER 2.6 LABELING ANSWERS: MUSCLES OF THE LEG

Page 240 Anterior View of the Right Leg
1. Vastus lateralis
2. Rectus femoris
3. Biceps femoris
4. Fibularis longus
5. Tibialis anterior
6. Extensor digitorum longus
7. Fibularis brevis
8. Fibularis tertius
9. Fibularis tertius tendon
10. Extensor digitorum brevis
11. Vastus medialis
12. Sartorius
13. Gracilis
14. Semitendinosus
15. Gastrocnemius
16. Soleus
17. Extensor hallucis longus
18. Extensor hallucis brevis

Page 241 Posterior View of the Right Leg (Superficial)
1. Semimembranosus
2. Gracilis
3. Sartorius
4. Semitendinosus
5. Gastrocnemius (medial head)
6. Soleus
7. Plantaris (tendon)
8. Tibialis posterior
9. Flexor digitorum longus
10. Flexor hallucis longus
11. Biceps femoris
12. Plantaris
13. Gastrocnemius (lateral head)
14. Soleus
15. Fibularis longus
16. Fibularis brevis

Page 242 Posterior View of the Right Leg (Intermediate)
1. Gastrocnemius (medial head, cut)
2. Semimembranosus (cut)
3. Popliteus
4. Soleus
5. Gastrocnemius (medial head, cut)

6. Tibialis posterior
7. Flexor digitorum longus
8. Flexor hallucis longus
9. Plantaris
10. Gastrocnemius (lateral head, cut)
11. Biceps femoris (cut)
12. Fibularis longus
13. Gastrocnemius (lateral head, cut)
14. Fibularis brevis

Page 243   Posterior View of the Right Leg (Deep)

1. Gastrocnemius (cut)
2. Semimembranosus
3. Popliteus
4. Tibialis posterior
5. Flexor digitorum longus
6. Biceps femoris
7. Gastrocnemius (lateral head, cut)
8. Plantaris (cut and reflected)
9. Soleus (cut and reflected)
10. Fibularis longus
11. Flexor hallucis longus
12. Fibularis brevis

Page 244   Lateral View of the Right Leg

1. Biceps femoris
2. Plantaris
3. Fibularis longus
4. Gastrocnemius
5. Soleus
6. Fibularis brevis
7. Fibularis tertius
8. Extensor digitorum brevis & extensor hallucis brevis
9. Vastus lateralis
10. Rectus femoris
11. Tibialis anterior
12. Extensor digitorum longus
13. Extensor hallucis longus

Page 245   Medial View of the Right Leg

1. Gracilis
2. Rectus femoris
3. Sartorius
4. Vastus medialis
5. Sartorius (pes anserine tendon)
6. Gracilis (pes anserine tendon)
7. Semitendinosus (pes anserine tendon)
8. Tibialis anterior
9. Extensor hallucis longus
10. Extensor digitorum longus

11. Adductor magnus
12. Semitendinosus
13. Semimembranosus
14. Gastrocnemius
15. Soleus
16. Plantaris
17. Flexor digitorum longus
18. Tibialis posterior
19. Flexor hallucis longus

CHAPTER 2.7 LABELING ANSWERS: INTRINSIC MUSCLES OF THE FOOT

Page 264   Dorsal View of the Right Foot

1. Fibularis longus tendon
2. Fibularis brevis
3. Extensor digitorum longus
4. Fibularis brevis tendon
5. Fibularis tertius tendon
6. Extensor digitorum brevis
7. Abductor digiti minimi pedis
8. Dorsal interossei pedis
9. Extensor hallucis longus
10. Tibialis anterior
11. Soleus
12. Extensor hallucis brevis
13. Abductor hallucis
14. Dorsal interossei pedis

Page 265   Plantar View of the Right Foot (Superficial Muscular Layer)

1. Flexor digitorum longus tendons
2. Flexor digitorum brevis tendons
3. Adductor hallucis (transverse head)
4. Lumbricals pedis
5. Flexor digiti minimi pedis
6. Abductor digiti minimi pedis
7. Flexor hallucis longus tendon
8. Flexor hallucis brevis
9. Flexor digitorum brevis
10. Abductor hallucis

Page 266   Plantar View of the Right Foot (Intermediate Muscular Layer)

1. Flexor digitorum longus tendons
2. Flexor digitorum brevis tendons (cut)
3. Adductor hallucis (transverse head)
4. Lumbricals pedis
5. Flexor digiti minimi pedis
6. Plantar interossei
7. Abductor digiti minimi pedis (partially cut)
8. Quadratus plantae

9. Flexor digitorum brevis (cut)
10. Flexor hallucis longus tendon
11. Flexor hallucis brevis
12. Abductor hallucis (cut)
13. Tibialis posterior tendon
14. Flexor digitorum longus tendon
15. Flexor hallucis longus tendon
16. Abductor hallucis (cut)

Page 267 Plantar View of the Right Foot (Deep Muscular Layer)

1. Flexor digitorum longus tendons (cut)
2. Flexor digitorum brevis tendons (cut)
3. Lumbricals pedis (cut)
4. Adductor hallucis (transverse head)
5. Flexor digiti minimi pedis
6. Abductor digiti minimi pedis (cut)
7. Plantar interossei
8. Fibularis brevis tendon
9. Fibularis longus tendon
10. Quadratus plantae (cut)
11. Flexor digitorum brevis (cut)
12. Abductor digiti minimi pedis (cut)
13. Flexor hallucis longus tendon (cut)
14. Flexor hallucis brevis
15. Adductor hallucis (oblique head)
16. Abductor hallucis (cut)
17. Tibialis posterior tendon
18. Flexor digitorum longus tendon (cut and reflected)
19. Flexor hallucis longus tendon (cut)
20. Abductor hallucis (cut)

CHAPTER 2.8 LABELING ANSWERS: MUSCLES OF THE SCAPULA/ARM

Page 290 Anterior View of the Right Shoulder

1. Anterior scalene
2. Middle scalene
3. Levator scapulae
4. Omohyoid
5. Posterior scalene
6. Trapezius
7. Deltoid
8. Biceps brachii
9. Triceps brachii
10. Latissimus dorsi
11. Serratus anterior
12. External abdominal oblique
13. Sternocleidomastoid
14. Pectoralis major

Page 291 Posterior View of the Shoulders (Superficial and Intermediate)

1. Sternocleidomastoid
2. Splenius capitis
3. Levator scapulae
4. Trapezius
5. Deltoid
6. Triceps brachii
7. Latissimus dorsi
8. Semispinalis capitis (of transversospinalis group)
9. Splenius capitis
10. Splenius cervicis
11. Levator scapulae
12. Rhomboid minor
13. Supraspinatus
14. Infraspinatus
15. Rhomboid major
16. Teres minor
17. Teres major
18. Triceps brachii
19. Erector spinae

Page 292 Anterior View of the Right Arm (Superficial)

1. Deltoid
2. Pectoralis major (cut and reflected)
3. Biceps brachii (long head)
4. Biceps brachii (short head)
5. Biceps brachii
6. Brachialis
7. Brachioradialis
8. Pectoralis minor (cut)
9. Coracobrachialis
10. Subscapularis
11. Teres major
12. Latissimus dorsi
13. Triceps brachii
14. Pronator teres
15. Flexor carpi radialis
16. Palmaris longus
17. Flexor carpi ulnaris

Page 293 Anterior View of the Right Arm (Deep)

1. Supraspinatus
2. Biceps brachii (cut)
3. Deltoid (cut)
4. Biceps brachii (cut)
5. Pectoralis minor (cut)
6. Subscapularis

7. Teres major
8. Latissimus dorsi
9. Coracobrachialis
10. Brachialis

Page 294 Medial View of the Right Arm

1. Biceps brachii (long head, cut)
2. Subscapularis (cut)
3. Pectoralis major (cut)
4. Biceps brachii (short head, cut)
5. Coracobrachialis (cut)
6. Biceps brachii
7. Bicipital aponeurosis of the biceps brachii
8. Brachioradialis
9. Flexor carpi radialis
10. Supraspinatus (cut)
11. Infraspinatus (cut)
12. Teres minor (cut)
13. Deltoid (cut)
14. Teres major (cut)
15. Latissimus dorsi (cut)
16. Triceps brachii (long head)
17. Triceps brachii (medial head)
18. Brachialis
19. Pronator teres
20. Palmaris longus
21. Flexor carpi ulnaris

Page 295 Lateral View of the Right Arm

1. Deltoid
2. Triceps brachii
3. Anconeus
4. Extensor carpi ulnaris
5. Extensor digitorum
6. Extensor digiti minimi
7. Biceps brachii
8. Brachialis
9. Brachioradialis
10. Extensor carpi radialis longus
11. Extensor carpi radialis brevis

Page 296 Posterior View of the Right Arm

1. Supraspinatus
2. Infraspinatus
3. Teres minor
4. Teres major
5. Triceps brachii (medial head)
6. Flexor carpi ulnaris
7. Deltoid (cut and reflected)
8. Triceps brachii (lateral head)

9. Triceps brachii (long head)
10. Brachioradialis
11. Extensor carpi radialis longus
12. Anconeus
13. Extensor carpi radialis brevis
14. Extensor digitorum
15. Extensor digiti minimi
16. Extensor carpi ulnaris

Page 297 Anterior View of the Right Glenohumeral Joint

1. Supraspinatus
2. Coracobrachialis (cut)
3. Biceps brachii (short head, cut)
4. Biceps brachii (long head, cut)
5. Triceps brachii
6. Coracobrachialis (cut)
7. Biceps brachii (cut)
8. Supraspinatus
9. Pectoralis minor (cut)
10. Subscapularis
11. Teres major
12. Latissimus dorsi

Page 297 Posterior View of the Right Glenohumeral Joint

1. Supraspinatus (cut)
2. Infraspinatus (cut and reflected)
3. Teres major
4. Teres minor
5. Supraspinatus (cut)
6. Infraspinatus (cut and reflected)
7. Deltoid (cut and reflected)
8. Triceps brachii (medial head)
9. Triceps brachii (long head)
10. Triceps brachii (lateral head)

CHAPTER 2.9 LABELING ANSWERS: MUSCLES OF THE FOREARM

Page 332 Anterior View of the Right Forearm (Superficial)

1. Biceps brachii
2. Brachialis
3. Brachioradialis
4. Extensor carpi radialis longus
5. Extensor carpi radialis brevis
6. Flexor pollicis longus
7. Pronator quadratus
8. Abductor pollicis longus
9. Triceps brachii (medial head)
10. Brachialis (deep to median nerve and brachial artery from this view)

11. Bicipital aponeurosis of the biceps brachii
12. Pronator teres
13. Flexor carpi radialis
14. Palmaris longus
15. Flexor carpi ulnaris
16. Flexor digitorum superficialis
17. Flexor digitorum profundus

Page 333 Anterior View of the Right Forearm (Intermediate)

1. Biceps brachii
2. Brachialis
3. Brachialis (tendon)
4. Biceps brachii (tendon)
5. Supinator
6. Brachioradialis
7. Pronator teres (cut)
8. Flexor pollicis longus
9. Abductor pollicis longus
10. Pronator quadratus
11. Flexor carpi radialis (cut)
12. Triceps brachii (medial head)
13. Pronator teres (humeral head, cut and reflected)
14. Brachialis
15. Flexor carpi radialis (cut)
16. Palmaris longus (cut)
17. Pronator teres (ulnar head, cut and reflected)
18. Flexor digitorum profundus
19. Flexor carpi ulnaris
20. Flexor digitorum superficialis
21. Flexor digitorum profundus

Page 334 Anterior View of the Right Forearm (Deep)

1. Brachialis
2. Biceps brachii (tendon)
3. Supinator
4. Flexor digitorum superficialis (cut)
5. Pronator teres (cut and reflected)
6. Flexor pollicis longus (cut)
7. Pronator quadratus
8. Brachioradialis (cut)
9. Flexor carpi radialis (cut)
10. Flexor pollicis longus (cut)
11. Triceps brachii (medial head)
12. Pronator teres (humeral head, cut and reflected)
13. Flexor carpi radialis (cut)
14. Palmaris longus (cut)
15. Flexor carpi ulnaris (cut and reflected)
16. Flexor digitorum superficialis (cut)
17. Pronator teres (ulnar head, cut)

18. Flexor digitorum profundus (cut)
19. Flexor carpi ulnaris (cut)

Page 335 Anterior Views of the Pronators and Supinator of the Right Radius

1. Supinator: ulnar head
1. Supinator: humeral head
2. Pronator quadratus
3. Pronator teres: humeral head
3. Pronator teres: ulnar head

Page 336 Posterior View of the Right Forearm (Superficial)

1. Triceps brachii
2. Flexor carpi ulnaris
3. Extensor carpi ulnaris
4. Extensor digiti minimi
5. Abductor digiti minimi manus
6. Dorsal interossei manus
7. Brachioradialis
8. Anconeus
9. Extensor carpi radialis longus
10. Extensor carpi radialis brevis
11. Extensor digitorum
12. Abductor pollicis longus
13. Extensor pollicis brevis
14. Extensor pollicis longus
15. Dorsal interossei manus
16. Extensor indicis tendon

Page 337 Posterior View of the Right Forearm (Deep)

1. Flexor carpi ulnaris
2. Extensor digitorum tendons (cut)
3. Extensor indicis
4. Extensor digiti minimi (cut)
5. Extensor carpi ulnaris (cut)
6. Abductor digiti minimi manus
7. Dorsal interossei manus
8. Triceps brachii tendon (cut)
9. Brachioradialis
10. Anconeus
11. Extensor carpi radialis longus
12. Extensor carpi radialis brevis
13. Supinator
14. Pronator teres
15. Abductor pollicis longus
16. Extensor pollicis longus
17. Extensor pollicis brevis
18. Dorsal interossei manus
19. Extensor indicis tendon

Page 338   Posterior View of the Right Forearm and Hand (Superficial)
1. Extensor digiti minimi
2. Extensor carpi ulnaris
3. Extensor carpi radialis longus
4. Extensor carpi radialis brevis
5. Extensor digitorum
6. Abductor pollicis longus
7. Extensor pollicis brevis
8. Extensor pollicis longus
9. Extensor indicis (tendon)

Page 339   Posterior View of the Right Forearm and Hand (Deep)
1. Extensor digiti minimi (cut)
2. Extensor carpi ulnaris (cut)
3. Extensor pollicis longus
4. Extensor indicis
5. Extensor carpi ulnaris tendon (cut)
6. Extensor carpi radialis longus
7. Extensor carpi radialis brevis
8. Extensor digitorum (cut)
9. Abductor pollicis longus
10. Extensor pollicis brevis

CHAPTER 2.10 LABELING ANSWERS: MUSCLES OF THE HAND

Page 356   Palmar View of the Right Hand (Superficial)
1. Palmaris longus
2. Flexor pollicis brevis (deep to fascia)
3. Abductor pollicis brevis (deep to fascia)
4. Adductor pollicis (deep to fascia)
5. Lumbricals manus (partially deep to fascia)
6. Flexor pollicis longus
7. Dorsal interossei manus
8. Flexor digitorum profundus
9. Flexor digitorum superficialis
10. Palmar interossei
11. Dorsal interossei manus
12. Lumbricals manus
13. Palmaris brevis
14. Hypothenar muscle group (deep to fascia)
15. Palmar interossei
16. Flexor digitorum profundus
17. Flexor digitorum superficialis
18. Lumbricals manus
19. Dorsal interossei manus
20. Lumbricals manus
21. Dorsal interossei manus

Page 357   Palmar View of the Right Hand (Superficial Muscular Layer)
1. Flexor pollicis brevis
2. Abductor pollicis brevis
3. Adductor pollicis (deep to fascia)
4. Dorsal interossei manus
5. Lumbricals manus
6. Lumbricals manus
7. Flexor digitorum profundus
8. Flexor digitorum superficialis
9. Palmar interossei
10. Dorsal interossei manus
11. Opponens digiti minimi
12. Abductor digiti minimi manus
13. Flexor digiti minimi manus
14. Lumbricals manus
15. Lumbricals manus
16. Palmar interossei
17. Flexor digitorum profundus
18. Flexor digitorum superficialis
19. Dorsal interossei manus
20. Dorsal interossei manus

Page 358   Palmar View of the Right Hand (Deep Muscular Layer)
1. Pronator quadratus
2. Abductor pollicis brevis (cut)
3. Opponens pollicis
4. Flexor pollicis brevis
5. Abductor pollicis brevis (cut)
6. Adductor pollicis
7. Dorsal interossei manus
8. Lumbricals manus (cut and reflected)
9. Lumbricals manus (cut and reflected)
10. Palmar interossei
11. Dorsal interossei manus
12. Flexor carpi ulnaris
13. Abductor digiti minimi manus (cut)
14. Flexor digiti minimi manus (cut)
15. Opponens digiti minimi
16. Palmar interossei
17. Dorsal interossei manus
18. Abductor digiti minimi manus (cut)
19. Flexor digiti minimi manus (cut)
20. Dorsal interossei manus
21. Lumbricals manus (cut and reflected)
22. Palmar interossei
23. Lumbricals manus (cut and reflected)

Page 359 Dorsal View of the Right Hand
1. Extensor digitorum
2. Extensor digiti minimi
3. Extensor carpi ulnaris
4. Abductor digiti minimi manus
5. Dorsal interossei manus
6. Dorsal interossei manus
7. Palmar interossei
8. Lumbricals manus
9. Lumbricals manus
10. Extensor carpi radialis brevis
11. Extensor carpi radialis longus
12. Extensor pollicis brevis
13. Abductor pollicis longus
14. Extensor indicis
15. Extensor pollicis longus
16. Dorsal interossei manus
17. Dorsal interossei manus
18. Adductor pollicis
19. Palmar interossei

CHAPTER 3 LABELING ANSWERS: OTHER SKELETAL MUSCLES

Page 363 Anterior Views of the Other Muscles of the Abdomen
1. External abdominal oblique
2. Rectus abdominis
3. Pyramidalis
4. External abdominal oblique
5. Internal abdominal oblique
6. Cremaster

Page 364 Views of the Muscles of the Perineum
1. Ischiocavernosus
2. Bulbospongiosus
3. Deep transverse perineal
4. Superficial transverse perineal
5. Gluteus maximus
6. External anal sphincter
7. Compressor urethrae
8. Sphincter urethrae
9. Sphincter urethrovaginalis
10. Levator ani
11. Coccygeus
12. Sphincter urethrae
13. Deep transverse perineal
14. Superficial transverse perineal
15. External anal sphincter
16. Gluteus maximus
17. Ischiocavernosus
18. Bulbospongiosus
19. Deep transverse perineal
20. Superficial transverse perineal
21. Levator ani
22. Coccygeus

Page 365 Views of the Muscles of the Tongue
1. Superior longitudinal muscle
2. Vertical muscle
3. Transverse muscle
4. Inferior longitudinal muscle
5. Genioglossus
6. Stylohyoid
7. Styloglossus
8. Buccinator
9. Platysma
10. Hyoglossus
11. Digastric
12. Inferior longitudinal muscle
13. Genioglossus
14. Mylohyoid
15. Geniohyoid
16. Hyoglossus
17. Palatoglossus
18. Palatopharyngeus
19. Superior pharyngeal constrictor (partially cut)
20. Digastric (cut)
21. Styloglossus
22. Stylopharyngeus
23. Stylohyoid
24. Middle pharyngeal constrictor
25. Digastric (cut)

Page 366 Views of the Muscles of the Palate
1. Tensor veli palatini
2. Levator veli palatini
3. Palatoglossus
4. Mylohyoid
5. Geniohyoid
6. Hyoglossus
7. Middle pharyngeal constrictor
8. Stylopharyngeus
9. Salpingopharyngeus
10. Musculus uvulae
11. Superior pharyngeal constrictor
12. Palatopharyngeus

Page 367 View of the Muscles of the Pharynx
1. Levator veli palatini
2. Accessory muscle bundle from temporal bone
3. Digastric
4. Stylohyoid

5. Medial pterygoid
6. Stylopharyngeus
7. Circular esophageal muscle
8. Longitudinal esophageal muscle
9. Superior pharyngeal constrictor
10. Salpingopharyngeus
11. Palatopharyngeus
12. Middle pharyngeal constrictor
13. Musculus uvulae
14. Longitudinal pharyngeal muscle
15. Transverse and oblique arytenoids
16. Posterior cricoarytenoid
17. Inferior pharyngeal constrictor

Page 368   Views of the Muscles of the Larynx
1. Transverse arytenoid
2. Oblique arytenoid
3. Posterior cricoarytenoid
4. Cricothyroid
5. Cricothyroid
6. Transverse arytenoid
7. Oblique arytenoid
8. Lateral cricoarytenoid
9. Posterior cricoarytenoid
10. Thyroarytenoid
11. Cricothyroid (cut)

Page 369   Views of the Muscles of the Larynx: superior/inferior view
1. Transverse arytenoid
2. Oblique arytenoid
3. Posterior cricoarytenoid

Page 369   Views of the Muscles of the Larynx: posterior/anterior view
1. Posterior cricoarytenoid
2. Transverse arytenoid
3. Oblique arytenoid
4. Lateral cricoarytenoid
5. Thyroarytenoid
6. Cricothyroid

Page 370   Views of the Extrinsic Muscles of the Right Eye: top illustration
1. Levator palpebrae superioris
2. Superior oblique
3. Superior rectus
4. Medial rectus
5. Lateral rectus (cut)
6. Inferior rectus
7. Inferior oblique

Page 370   Views of the Extrinsic Muscles of the Right Eye: bottom left illustration
1. Superior rectus (cut)
2. Lateral rectus (cut)
3. Inferior rectus (cut)
4. Inferior oblique (cut)
5. Superior oblique (cut)
6. Medial rectus (cut)

Page 370   Views of the Extrinsic Muscles of the Right Eye: bottom right illustration
1. Superior oblique
2. Medial rectus
3. Inferior rectus
4. Levator palpebrae superioris
5. Superior rectus
6. Lateral rectus
7. Levator palpebrae superioris

Page 371   View of the Muscles of the Tympanic Cavity
1. Tensor tympani
2. Stapedius

CHAPTER 4 LABELING ANSWERS:
THE NERVOUS SYSTEM

Page 374   Cranial Nerves
1. CN IV (trochlear nerve)
2. CN VI (adbucens nerve)
3. CN VII (facial nerve)
4. CN VIII (acoustic nerve, also known as vestibulocochlear nerve)
5. CN IX (glossopharyngeal nerve)
6. CN X (vagus nerve)
7. CN XI (spinal accessory nerve)
8. CN I (olfactory nerve)
9. CN II (optic nerve)
10. CN III (occulomotor nerve)
11. CN V (trigeminal nerve)
12. CN XII (hypoglossal nerve)

Page 375   Cross Section View of the Spinal Cord through a Cervical Vertebra—Spinal Nerve Diagram
1. Sympathetic ganglion
2. Vertebral artery
3. Ventral nerve root
4. Spinal cord
5. Dura mater
6. Vertebral spinous process (SP)
7. Dorsal nerve root

8. Gray ramus communicans of a spinal nerve
9. Ventral ramus of a spinal nerve
10. Dorsal ramus of a spinal nerve
11. Dorsal root ganglion

Page 376   View of the Cervical Plexus
1. Lesser occipital nerve
2. to the vagus nerve
3. Greater auricular nerve
4. to sternocleidomastoid
5. to levator scapulae
6. Transverse cutaneous nerve of the neck
7. to trapezius
8. to levator scapulae
9. to middle scalene
10. Supraclavicular nerve
11. to rectus lateralis
12. to rectus capitis anterior and longus capitis
13. to geniohyoid
14. to longus capitis and longus colli
15. to longus capitis, longus colli, and middle scalene
16. to thyrohyoid
17. Ansa cervicalis
18. to longus colli
19. Phrenic nerve

Page 377   View of the Brachial Plexus
1. Dorsal scapular nerve
2. to the phrenic nerve
3. Suprascapular nerve
4. Lateral pectoral nerve
5. Axillary nerve
6. Musculocutaneous nerve
7. Radial nerve
8. Median nerve
9. Ulnar nerve
10. Medial antebrachial cutaneous nerve
11. Medial brachial cutaneous nerve
12. Lower subscapular nerve
13. Thoracodorsal nerve
14. Nerve to scalenes
15. Nerve to scalenes
16. Nerve to subclavius
17. Nerve to scalenes
18. Long thoracic nerve
19. Nerve to scalenes
20. First intercostal nerve
21. Medial pectoral nerve
22. Upper subscapular nerve

Page 378   View of the Lumbar Plexus
1. Iliohypogastric nerve
2. Ilio-inguinal
3. Genitofemoral
4. Lateral cutaneous nerve of the thigh
5. to psoas and iliacus (iliopsoas)
6. Femoral nerve
7. Accessory obturator nerve
8. Obturator nerve
9. Lumbosacral trunk

Page 379   View of the Sacral and Coccygeal Plexuses
1. Superior gluteal nerve
2. Inferior gluteal nerve
3. to piriformis
4. to superior gemellus and obturator internus
5. to inferior gemellus and quadratus femoris
6. Common fibular nerve of the sciatic nerve
7. Tibial nerve of the sciatic nerve
8. Posterior femoral cutaneous nerve
9. Perforating cutaneous nerve
10. Pelvic splanchnic nerves
11. Pudendal nerve
12. to levator ani, coccygeous, and external anal sphincter
13. Anococcygeal nerves
14. Visceral branches
15. Visceral branches

Page 380   Views of Innervation to the Right Lower Extremity
1. Femoral nerve
2. Common fibular nerve of the sciatic nerve
3. Superficial fibular nerve
4. Obturator nerve
5. Deep fibular nerve
6. Sciatic nerve
7. Tibial nerve of the sciatic nerve
8. Medial plantar nerve
9. Common fibular nerve of the sciatic nerve
10. Superficial fibular nerve
11. Lateral plantar nerve

Page 381   Anterior View of Innervation to the Right Upper Extremity
1. Axillary nerve
2. Musculocutaneous nerve
3. Radial nerve
4. Brachial plexus
5. Median nerve
6. Ulnar nerve

CHAPTER 5 LABELING ANSWERS:
THE ARTERIAL SYSTEM

Page 384 Lateral View of Arterial Supply to the Head and Neck
1. Posterior auricular artery
2. Superficial temporal artery
3. Occipital artery
4. Ascending pharyngeal artery
5. Vertebral artery
6. Internal carotid artery
7. Deep cervical artery
8. Dorsal scapular artery
9. Costocervical trunk
10. Axillary artery
11. Transverse facial artery
12. Supraorbital artery
13. Supratrochlear artery
14. Ophthalmic artery
15. Infraorbital artery
16. Maxillary artery
17. Inferior alveolar artery
18. Facial artery
19. Lingual artery
20. Superior thyroid artery
21. External carotid artery
22. Ascending cervical artery
23. Inferior thyroid artery
24. Transverse cervical artery
25. Thyrocervical trunk
26. Common carotid artery
27. Subclavian artery
28. Brachiocephalic trunk
29. Internal thoracic artery

Page 385 Anterior View of Arterial Supply to the Trunk and Pelvis
1. Costocervical trunk
2. Dorsal scapular artery
3. Thoracoacromial trunk
4. Internal thoracic artery
5. Anterior intercostal artery
6. Posterior intercostal artery
7. Musculophrenic artery
8. Superior epigastric artery
9. Lumbar artery
10. Subcostal artery
11. Iliolumbar artery
12. Inferior epigastric artery
13. Deep circumflex iliac artery
14. Common carotid artery
15. Subclavian artery
16. Brachiocephalic trunk

17. Axillary artery
18. Ascending aorta
19. Descending aorta
20. Common iliac artery
21. Internal iliac artery
22. External iliac artery
23. Median sacral artery

Page 386 Anterior View of Arterial Supply to the Right Lower Extremity
1. Common iliac artery
2. Iliolumbar artery
3. External iliac artery
4. Perforating branches of the deep femoral artery
5. Popliteal artery
6. Anterior tibial artery
7. Lateral plantar artery
8. Plantar arch
9. Internal iliac artery
10. Superior gluteal artery
11. Inferior gluteal artery
12. Femoral artery
13. Obturator artery
14. Deep femoral artery
15. Posterior tibial artery
16. Fibular artery
17. Medial plantar artery
18. Dorsalis pedis artery

Page 387 Anterior View of Arterial Supply to the Right Upper Extremity
1. Suprascapular artery
2. Thoracoacromial trunk
3. Axillary artery
4. Anterior circumflex humeral artery
5. Posterior circumflex humeral artery (posterior to the humerus)
6. Brachial artery
7. Deep brachial artery
8. Radial artery
9. Interosseus recurrent artery (posterior to the radius and humerus)
10. Posterior interosseus artery
11. Deep palmar arterial arch
12. Thyrocervical trunk
13. Subclavian artery
14. Dorsal scapular artery
15. Superior thoracic artery
16. Subscapular artery
17. Lateral thoracic artery
18. Thoracodorsal artery
19. Circumflex scapular artery

20. Ulnar artery
21. Anterior interosseus artery
22. Superficial palmar arterial arch

CHAPTER 6 LABELING ANSWERS: OTHER
STRUCTURES AND SYSTEMS OF THE BODY

The Cell
Page 390   A Typical Cell
1. Centrosome
2. Centrioles
3. Smooth endoplasmic reticulum
4. Mitochondrion
5. Lysosome
6. Rough endoplasmic reticulum
7. Peroxisome
8. Cytoskeleton
9. Intermediate filament
10. Microtubule
11. Microfilament
12. Nuclear envelope
13. Ribosomes
14. Mitochondria
15. Smooth endoplasmic reticulum
16. Cilia
17. Free ribosomes
18. Golgi apparatus
19. Microvilli
20. Vesicle
21. Nucleolus
22. Nucleus

Page 390   Major Components of a Cell
1. Cell membrane
2. Cytoplasm
3. Nucleus
4. Organelles

Page 390   The Cytoskeleton
1. Intermediate filament
2. Endoplasmic reticulum
3. Ribosome
4. Microtubule
5. Mitochondrion
6. Microfilament
7. Plasma membrane

Page 391   The Cell Membrane
1. External membrane surface
2. Phospholipid bilayer
3. Internal membrane surface
4. Carbohydrate chains
5. Glycolipid
6. Polar region of phospholipid
7. Nonpolar region of phospholipid
8. Protein
9. Glycoprotein
10. Cholesterol
11. Membrane channel protein

Page 391   The Endoplasmic Reticulum and Golgi Apparatus
1. Ribosomes
2. Proteins
3. Vesicle
4. Cytoplasm
5. Endoplasmic reticulum
6. Cisternae
7. Golgi apparatus
8. Plasma membrane
9. Secretory vesicle
10. Vesicle containing plasma membrane components

Page 391   Cross Section of a Mitochondrion
1. Outer membrane
2. Inner membrane
3. Matrix
4. Cristae

Page 391   Cross Section of the Nucleus
1. Nucleolus
2. Nuclear pores
3. Chromatin
4. Nucleoplasm
5. Nuclear envelope

Bone Tissue
Page 392   Longitudinal Section of a Long Bone
1. Epiphysis
2. Diaphysis
3. Epiphysis
4. Articular cartilage
5. Spongy bone
6. Epiphyseal plate
7. Red marrow cavities
8. Endosteum
9. Medullary cavity
10. Compact bone
11. Yellow marrow
12. Periosteum

Page 392   A. Section of a Flat Bone
1. Compact bone
2. Cancellous bone

Page 392 B. Magnification of Spongy Bone Tissue
1. Trabeculae

Page 393 Longitudinal Section of a Long Bone and Magnification of Compact Bone Tissue
1. Osteons (Haversian systems)
2. Periosteum
2a. Inner layer
2b. Outer layer
3. Compact bone
4. Cancellous (spongy) bone
5. Medullary marrow cavity
6. Endosteum
7. Trabeculae
8. Haversian canals
9. Volkmann's canals
10. Osteon (Haversian system)
11. Blood vessels within Haversian or central canal
12. Lacunae containing osteocytes
13. Interstitial lamellae
14. Blood vessel within Volkmann's or perforating canal
15. Circumferential lamellae
16. Periosteum
17. Concentric lamellae

Muscle Tissue
Page 394 Structure of a Muscle
1. Muscle
2. Aponeurosis
3. Muscle
4. Fascia
5. Tendon
6. Bone
7. Myofibril
8. Myosin
9. Actin
10. Epimysium
11. Perimysium
12. Endomysium
13. Fascicle
14. Axon of motor neuron
15. Blood vessel
16. Fascicle
17. Muscle fiber (muscle cell)
18. Nucleus
19. Sarcolemma
20. Sarcoplasmic reticulum
21. Muscle fiber (muscle cell)
22. Endomysium
23. Perimysium

Page 394 Structure of a Muscle Illustrating a Sarcomere Unit
1. Muscle
2. Fascia
3. Tendon
4. Bone
5. Sarcoplasmic reticulum
6. Tubule
7. Z line
8. Sarcomere
9. Epimysium
10. Perimysium
11. Endomysium
12. Fascicle
13. Muscle fiber (muscle cell)
14. Myofibril
15. Z line

Page 394 Sarcoplasmic Reticulum and T Tubules of a Muscle Fiber
1. Sarcolemma
2. Mitcochondria
3. T tubule
4. Sarcomere
5. Myofibril
6. Sarcoplasmic reticulum

Page 395 Myosin and Actin Filaments
1. Actin
2. Myosin
3. Myosin arm
4. Thin myofilament
5. Thick myofilament
6. Myosin head

Page 395 Sliding Filament Action
No Labels

Page 395 Neuromuscular Junction
1. Motor neuron fiber
2. Schwann cell
3. Sarcoplasm
4. Acetylcholine receptor sites
5. Synaptic cleft
6. Myelin sheath
7. Synaptic vesicles
8. Sarcolemma
9. Motor endplate

Nerve Tissue
**Page 396   Types of Neurons
(nerve cells)**
First Illustration
1. Dendrites
2. Cell body
3. Axon
Second Illustration
1. Dendrites
2. Cell body
3. Axon
Third Illustration
1. Cell body
2. Dendrites
3. Axon
3a. Peripheral process
3b. Central process

Page 396   Types of Neuroglial Cells
1. Foot processes
2. Capillary
3. Astrocytes
4. Microglia
5. Cilia
6. Ependymal cells
7. Oligodendrocyte
8. Nerve fiber
9. Myelin sheath
10. Unmyelinated nerve fibers
11. Schwann cell

**Page 397   Myelinated Axon of the
Peripheral Nervous System**
1. Node of Ranvier
2. Neurilemma (sheath of Schwann cell)
3. Nucleus of Schwann cell
4. Myelin sheath
5. Plasma membrane of axon
6. Neurofibrils

Page 397   A. Convergence of Neurons
1. Cell body
2. Postsynaptic axon
3. Presynaptic axon

Page 397   B. Divergence of Neurons
1. Postsynaptic axon
2. Presynaptic axon
3. Cell body

**Page 397   A. Electrical Synapse
Between Neurons**
1. Electrical charges
2. Presynaptic cell
3. Tight junction
4. Conduction of action potential
5. Gap junctions
6. Tight junction
7. Postsynaptic cell

**Page 397   B. Chemical Synapse
Between Neurons**
1. Presynaptic cell
2. Synaptic vesicles
3. Mitchondrion
4. Postsynaptic cell
5. Receptor molecule
6. Neurotransmitter molecules
7. Postsynaptic membrane
8. Synaptic cleft

Joints
Page 398   Three Types of Fibrous Joints
1. Tibia
2. Fibula
3. Interosseous ligament
4. Ulna
5. Radius
6. Parietal bone
7. Frontal bone
8. Suture
9. Coronal suture
10. Periodontal membrane
11. Root of tooth in socket

**Page 398   Three Types of
Cartilaginous Joints**
1. Ribs
2. Costal cartilage
3. Sternum
4. Costosternal synchondrosis
5. Epiphyseal plate (synchondrosis joint)
6. Long bone
7. Symphysis pubis
8. Vertebral disk (symphysis joint)

**Page 399   Structure of a Typical
Synovial Joint**
1. Bone
2. Periosteum
3. Blood vessel
4. Nerve

5. Articular cartilage
6. Joint cavity
7. Fibrous joint capsule
8. Articular cartilage
9. Synovial membrane

Page 399   Various Types of Synovial Joints
1. Saddle joint (biaxial)
2. Pivot joint (uniaxial)
3. Hinge joint (uniaxial)
4. Condyloid joint (biaxial)
5. Ball and socket joint (triaxial)
6. Gliding joint (nonaxial)

Integumentary System
Page 400   Diagram of the Skin
1. Hair shaft
2. Stratum corneum
3. Stratum granulosum
4. Stratum germinativum
4a. Stratum spinosum
4b. Stratum basale
5. Dermal papilla
6. Tactile (meissner) corpuscle
7. Sebaceous (oil) gland
8. Hair follicle
9. Papilla of hair
10. Cutaneous nerve
11. Openings of sweat ducts
12. Epidermis
13. Dermis
14. Subcutaneous layer (hypodermis)
15. Sweat gland
16. Artery vein
17. Vein
18. Arrector pili muscle
19. Pacinian corpuscle

Page 400   Glands of the Skin
1. Epidermis
2. Dermis
3. Subcutaneous layer
4. Hair follicle
5. Sebaceous gland
6. Eccrine sweat gland (in subcutaneous tissue)
7. Apocrine sweat gland (in dermis)

Page 401   Hair Follicle
Left Illustration
1. Dermal root sheath
2. External epithelial root sheath
3. Internal epithelial root sheath

4. Germinal matrix
5. Papilla
6. Artery
7. Vein
8. Hair shaft
9. Medulla
10. Cortex
11. Cuticle
12. Hair root
13. Arrector pili muscle
14. Sebaceous gland
15. Hair bulb
16. Fat

Right Illustration
1. Germinal matrix (growth zone)
2. Papilla
3. Hair
3a. Medulla
3b. Cortex
3c. Cuticle
4. Hair follicle wall
4a. Dermal root sheath
4b. External epithelial root sheath
4c. Internal epithelial root sheath
5. Melanocyte
6. Stratum basale
7. Basement membrane

Page 401   Structure of a Nail
1. Free edge
2. Nail body
3. Lunula
4. Cuticle
5. Nail root
6. Stratum germinativum
7. Stratum granulosum
8. Stratum corneum
9. Nail body
10. Cuticle
11. Nail root
12. Nail matrix
13. Nail bed

Cardiac System
Page 402   Anterior View of the Heart
1. Superior vena cava
2. Pulmonary trunk
3. Right pulmonary veins
4. Auricle of right atrium
5. Right coronary artery and cardiac vein
6. Right cardiac vein
7. Right ventricle
8. Aorta

9. Auricle of left atrium
10. Left pulmonary veins
11. Great cardiac vein
12. Anterior interventricular branch of left coronary artery and cardiac vein
13. Left ventricle
14. Apex

Page 402 Posterior View of the Heart

1. Left pulmonary artery
2. Left pulmonary veins
3. Auricle of left atrium
4. Left atrium
5. Great cardiac vein
6. Posterior artery and vein of left ventricle
7. Left ventricle
8. Apex
9. Aorta
10. Superior vena cava
11. Right pulmonary artery
12. Right pulmonary veins
13. Right atrium
14. Inferior vena cava
15. Coronary sinus
16. Posterior interventricular branch of right coronary artery
17. Middle cardiac vein
18. Right ventricle

Page 403 Interior View of the Heart

1. Superior vena cava
2. Right atrium
3. Pulmonary valve
4. Tricuspid valve
5. Inferior vena cava
6. Aorta
7. Pulmonary artery
8. Left atrium
9. Bicuspid or mitral valve
10. Aortic valve
11. Endocardium
12. Myocardium
13. Pericardium
14. Space for pericardial fluid
15. Left ventricle
16. Septum
17. Right ventricle

Page 403 Systemic and Pulmonic Circulations of the Heart

1. Systemic capillaries
2. Lung
3. Lung
4. Systemic capillaries

Venous System
Page 404 Major Veins of the Body

1. Inferior sagittal sinus
2. Angular
3. Facial
4. Right brachiocephalic
5. Right subclavian
6. Superior vena cava
7. Right pulmonary
8. Small cardiac
9. Inferior vena cava
10. Hepatic
11. Hepatic portal
12. Median cubital
13. Superior mesenteric
14. Gastroepiploic
15. Common iliac
16. External iliac
17. Femoral
18. Great saphenous
19. Small saphenous
20. Dorsal venous arch
21. Superior sagittal sinus
22. Straight sinus
23. Transverse sinus
24. Cervical plexus
25. External jugular
26. Internal jugular
27. Left brachiocephalic
28. Left subclavian
29. Cephalic
30. Axillary
31. Great cardiac
32. Basilic
33. Median basilic
34. Splenic
35. Inferior mesenteric
36. Common iliac
37. Internal iliac
38. Digital
39. Femoral
40. Popliteal
41. Fibular (peroneal)
42. Anterior tibial
43. Posterior tibial
44. Digital

Page 405 Venous Drainage of the Brain

1. Straight sinus
2. Transverse sinus
3. Occipital sinus
4. Sigmoid sinus
5. Superior petrosal sinus
6. Inferior petrosal sinus

7. Internal jugular vein
8. Inferior sagittal sinus
9. Superior sagittal sinus
10. Cavernous sinus
11. Ophthalmic veins
12. Facial vein

Page 405 Creation of Venous Blood Flow from Capillaries
1. Artery
2. Arterioles
3. Capillaries
4. Venules
5. Vein

Page 405 Unidirectional Venous Valves
1. Normal vein/normal (unidirectional) valve
2. Varicose vein/incompetent (leaky) valve

Lymphatic System
Page 406 Major Organs of the Lymphatic System
1. Tonsils
2. Cervical lymph node
3. Right lymphatic duct
4. Peyer's patches in intestinal wall
5. Red bone marrow
6. Entrance of thoracic duct into subclavian vein
7. Thymus gland
8. Axillary lymph node
9. Thoracic duct
10. Spleen
11. Inguinal lymph node

Page 406 Principal Lymphatic Drainage of the Body
1. Right lymphatic duct
2. Thoracic duct

Page 406 Role of Lymphatic Capillary in Draining Intercellular Fluid
1. Arteriole (from the heart)
2. Intercellular fluid
3. Blood capillary
4. Lymphatic capillary
5. Venule (to the heart)
6. Tissue cells
7. Lymph fluid (to veins)

Page 406 Lymphatic Capillary Structure
1. Overlapping endothelial cells
2. Fluid entering lymphatic capillary
3. Direction of flow

4. Valve closed
5. Valve open
6. Anchoring fibers

Page 407 Lymph Node Structure
1. Capsule
2. Medullary cords
3. Medullary sinus
4. Hilus
5. Afferent lymph vessels
6. Lymph
7. Sinuses
8. Germinal center
9. Cortical nodules
10. Trabeculae
11. Efferent lymph vessel
12. Venules
13. Arteriole

Page 407 Role of a Lymph Node in a Skin Infection
1. Site of infection
2. Afferent lymph vessel
3. Lymph node
4. Efferent lymph vessel
5. Venule
6. Arteriole

Respiratory System
Page 408 Structures of the Respiratory System
1. Upper respiratory tract
2. Left and right primary bronchi
3. Lower respiratory tract
4. Bronchioles
5. Nasal cavity
6. Pharynx
6a. Nasopharynx
6b. Oropharynx
6c. Laryngopharynx
7. Larynx
8. Trachea
9. Alveolar duct
10. Alveoli
11. Capillary
12. Alveolar sac

Page 409 Lobes of the Lungs
1. Right upper lobe
2. Major (oblique) fissure
3. Horizontal (minor) fissure
4. Right middle lobe

5. Right lower lobe
6. Left upper lobe
7. Lingula
8. Oblique fissure
9. Left lower lobe

Page 409   Bronchi of the Lungs

1. Trachea
2. Right primary bronchus
3. Left primary bronchus
4. Segmental bronchi
5. Lobar bronchi

Page 409   Bronchiole and Alveoli

1. Bronchiole
2. Pleura
3. Alveolus

Urinary System
Page 410   Anterior View of the Structures of the Urinary System

1. Inferior vena cava
2. Kidney
3. Aorta
4. Ureter
5. Bladder
6. Urethra

Page 411   Lateral View of the Bladder and Urethra of a Male

1. Pubis
2. Penile urethra
3. Penis
4. Bladder
5. Prostate
6. Prostatic urethra
7. Membranous urethra
8. Scrotum
9. Navicular fossa

Page 411   Section Through a Kidney

1. Interlobular arteries and veins
2. Interlobar arteries and veins
3. Segmental arteries and veins
4. Renal artery
5. Renal vein
6. Ureter
7. Lobar arteries and veins
8. Renal pyramid
9. Arcuate arteries and veins

Page 411   Structures of a Nephron

1. Efferent arteriole
2. Distal convoluted tubule
3. Collecting tubule
4. Papilla of pyramid
5. Afferent arteriole
6. Proximal tubule
7. Glomerulus
8. Descending limb of Henle's loop
9. Ascending limb of Henle's loop
10. Henle's loop

Gastrointestinal System
Page 412   Anterior View of the Structures of the Gastrointestinal System

1. Parotid gland
2. Submandibular gland
3. Pharynx
4. Esophagus
5. Diaphragm
6. Transverse colon
7. Hepatic flexure
8. Ascending colon
9. Small intestine
10. Cecum
11. Vermiform appendix
12. Rectum
13. Tongue
14. Sublingual gland
15. Larynx
16. Trachea
17. Liver
18. Stomach
19. Spleen
20. Splenic flexure
21. Descending colon
22. Sigmoid colon
23. Anal canal

Page 412   Structures of the Gastrointestinal System

1. Oral cavity
2. Salivary glands
3. Liver
4. Gallbladder
5. Duodenum
6. Large intestine
7. Ileum
8. Appendix
9. Palate
10. Uvula

11. Pharynx
12. Tongue
13. Esophagus
14. Common bile duct
15. Stomach
16. Pancreas
17. Jejunum

Page 413 Accessory Organs of the Gastrointestinal System
1. Corpus (body) of gall bladder
2. Neck of gall bladder
3. Cystic duct
4. Liver
5. Lesser duodenal papilla
6. Greater duodenal papilla
7. Duodenum
8. Sphincter muscles
9. Right and left hepatic ducts
10. Common hepatic duct
11. Common bile duct
12. Pancreas
13. Pancreatic duct
14. Superior mesenteric vein
15. Superior mesenteric artery

Page 413 Divisions of the Large Intestine
1. Hepatic flexure
2. Ascending colon
3. Cecum
4. Appendix
5. Anal canal
6. Transverse colon
7. Splenic flexure
8. Descending colon
9. Terminal ileum
10. Sigmoid colon
11. Rectum

Page 413 Section Through the Abdominopelvic Cavity
1. Diaphragm
2. Liver
3. Stomach
4. Transverse mesocolon
5. Greater omental sac
6. Mesentery of small intestine
7. Small intestine
8. Uterus
9. Urinary bladder
10. Symphysis pubis
11. Lesser omentum
12. Pancreas

13. Duodenum
14. Retroperitoneal space
15. Sigmoid colon
16. Rectum

Immune System
Page 414 Organization of the Immune System
1. Bronchial-associated lymphoid tissues
2. Thymus
3. Spleen
4. Liver
5. Gut-associated lymphoid tissues
6. Appendix
7. Tonsils
8. Lymph nodes
9. Lymph nodes

Page 414 Creation of B Cells and T Cells by the Bone Marrow
1. Step cell
2. T cell
3. Red bone marrow
4. Thymus
5. Lymph node
6. B cell
7. T cell

Page 414 Activation and Effects of T Cells
1. Antigen
2. T cell activated
3. Cytotoxic T cells
4. T memory cells
5. Target cell
6. Cytotoxic T cell
7. Lysis

Page 415 Actions of Antibodies
1. Inactivates antigen
2. Binds antigens together
3. Facilitates phagocytosis
4. Antigen
5. Antibody
6. Phagocytic body cell
7. Mast cell
8. Activates complement cascade
9. Initiates release of inflammatory chemicals

Page 415 Types of Antibodies
1. IgM
2. IgG
3. IgA

4. IgE
5. IgD

Page 415 Action of Antibody-Activated Complement
1. Complement
2. Bacterial cell

Endocrine System
Page 416 The Major Endocrine Glands of the Body
1. Pineal
2. Parathyroids
3. Testes (male)
4. Hypothalamus
5. Pituitary
6. Thyroid
7. Thymus
8. Adrenals
9. Pancreas
10. Ovaries (female)

Page 416 The Thyroid Gland
1. Thyroid cartilage
2. Right lobe
3. Isthmus
4. Left lobe
5. Trachea

Page 416 The Adrenal Gland
1. Adrenal gland
2. Kidney
3. Adrenal cortex
4. Adrenal medulla

Page 417 The Hypothalamus and Pituitary Hormones
1. Hypothalamic nerve cell
2. Bone
3. Growth hormone (GH)
4. Anterior pituitary
5. Adrenal cortex
6. Adrenocorticotropic hormone (ACTH)
7. Thyroid gland
8. Thyroid-stimulating hormone (TSH)
9. Gonadotropic hormones (FSH and LH)
10. Testis
11. Ovary
12. Prolactin (PRL)
13. Posterior pituitary
14. Antidiuretic hormone (ADH)
15. Kidney tubules
16. Oxytocin (OT)

17. Uterus smooth muscle
18. Mammary glands
19. Mammary glands

Page 417 The Pancreas
1. Duodenum
2. Common bile duct
3. Head of pancreas
4. Pancreatic duct
5. Tail of pancreas

Sensory System
Page 418 Somatic and Stretch Receptors
1. Free nerve endings
2. Krause's end bulb
3. Pacini's corpuscle
4. Merkel endings (Merkel's disc)
5. Meissner's corpuscle
6. Ruffini's corpuscle (Ruffini ending)
7. Tendon
8. Muscle fibers (extrafusal fibers)
9. Intrafusal fibers
9a. Nuclear bag fibers
9b. Nuclear chain fibers
10. Neuromuscular spindle
11. Type Ib sensory fiber
12. Golgi tendon organ
13. Capsule
14. Perimysium of muscle fiber bundle
15. α Efferent motor fiber
16. Connective tissue capsule
17. Type II sensory ending
18. Type IA sensory endings
19. Type II sensory ending
20. α Efferent motor fiber

Page 418 Superior View of a Horizontal Section of the Eye
1. Lacrimal caruncle
2. Optic disc
3. Optic nerve
4. Central artery and vein
5. Fovea
6. Macula lutea
7. Pupil
8. Lens
9. Visual axis
10. Cornea
11. Anterior chamber (contains aqueous humor)
12. Iris
13. Lower lid
14. Ciliary body

15. Retina
16. Choroid
17. Sclera
18. Posterior chamber (contains vitreous humor)

Page 419 External, Middle, and Internal Ear
1. External ear
2. Middle ear
3. Inner ear
4. Auricle (pinna)
5. Temporal bone
6. External auditory meatus
7. Tympanic membrane
8. Semicircular canals
9. Auditory ossicles
10. Malleus
11. Incus
12. Stapes
13. Oval window
14. Facial nerve
15. Acoustic nerve (VIII)
16. Vestibular nerve
17. Cochlear nerve
18. Cochlea
19. Vestibule
20. Round window
21. Auditory tube

Page 419 Lateral View of the Internal Nose
1. Fibers of olfactory nerve
2. Cribriform plate of ethmoid bone
3. Olfactory tract
4. Nasopharynx
5. Olfactory bulb
6. Frontal bone
7. Nasal cavity
8. Nose
9. Palate

Page 419 Dorsal Surface of the Tongue, Cross Section Through a Papilla, and a Taste Bud
1. Palatine tonsil
2. Circumvallate papillae
3. Lingual tonsil
4. Taste buds
5. Gustatory cell
6. Oral epithelium
7. Nerve fibers
8. Supporting cell

Reproductive System
Page 420 Male Reproductive Organs
1. Rectum
2. Seminal vesicle
3. Levator ani muscle
4. Ejaculatory duct
5. Anus
6. Bulbocavernosus muscle
7. Urinary bladder
8. Symphysis pubis
9. Prostate gland
10. Corpus cavernosum
11. Corpus spongiosum
12. Urethra
13. Testis
14. Glans

Page 420 Male Perineum
1. Location of symphysis pubis
2. Urogenital triangle
3. Anal triangle
4. Location of ischial tuberosity
5. Anus
6. Location of coccyx

Page 420 Tubules of the Testis and Epididymis
1. Nerves and blood vessels (vas afferens) in the spermatic cord
2. Ductus (vas) deferens
3. Epididymis
4. Efferent ductules
5. Seminferous tubules
6. Testis
7. Rete testis
8. Tunica albuginea
9. Lobule
10. Septum

Page 421 Female Reproductive Organs
1. Sacral promontory
2. Uterine tube
3. Ureter
4. Sacrouterine ligament
5. Posterior cul-de-sac (of Douglas)
6. Cervix
7. Fornix of vagina
8. Anus
9. Vagina
10. Ovarian ligament
11. Body of uterus
12. Fundus of uterus

13. Round ligament
14. Anterior cul-de-sac
15. Parietal peritoneum
16. Urinary bladder
17. Symphysis pubis
18. Uretha
19. Clitoris
20. Labium minus
21. Labium majus

Page 421   Female Perineum
1. Mons pubis (without pubic hair)
2. Prepuce
3. Labia minora
4. Hymen
5. Vestibule
6. Labia majora (without pubic hair)
7. Perineal body
8. Anus
9. Clitoris
10. Orifice of urethra
11. Orifice of vagina

12. Opening of greater vestibular gland
13. Urogenital triangle
14. Anal triangle

**Page 421   Anterior View of Female
Reproductive Organs**
1. Fundus
2. Corpus
3. Fimbriae
4. Ovary
5. Uterus
6. Bartholin's gland
7. Fallopian tube (uterine tube)
8. Ovum
9. Graafian follicle
10. Perimetrium
11. Endometrium
12. Myometrium
13. Cervix
14. Vagina
15. Hymen

Credits

The Cell

Page 390
A typical cell. (From Thibodeau GA, Patton KT: *Anatomy and physiology*, ed 5, St Louis, 2003, Mosby.)

Page 390
Major components of a cell. (From LaFleur Brooks M: *Exploring medical language: a student-directed approach*, St Louis, 2002, Mosby.)

Page 390
The cytoskeleton. (From Thibodeau GA, Patton KT: *Anatomy and physiology*, ed 5, St Louis, 2003, Mosby.)

Page 391
The cell membrane. (From Thibodeau GA, Patton KT: *Anatomy and physiology*, ed 5, St Louis, 2003, Mosby.)

Page 391
The endoplasmic reticulum and golgi apparatus. (From Thibodeau GA, Patton KT: *Anatomy and physiology*, ed 5, St Louis, 2003, Mosby.)

Page 391
Cross section of a mitochondrion. (From Thibodeau GA, Patton KT: *Anatomy and physiology*, ed 5, St Louis, 2003, Mosby.)

Page 391
Cross section of the nucleus. (From Thibodeau GA, Patton KT: *Anatomy and physiology*, ed 5, St Louis, 2003, Mosby.)

Bone Tissue

Page 392
Longitudinal section of a long bone; both spongy and compact bone are illustrated. (From Thibodeau GA, Patton KT: *Anatomy and physiology*, ed 5, St Louis, 2003, Mosby.)

Page 392
A, Section of a flat bone showing both spongy and compact bone tissue. **B,** Magnification of spongy bone tissue. (From Thibodeau GA, Patton KT: *Anatomy and physiology*, ed 5, St Louis, 2003, Mosby.)

Page 393
A, Longitudinal section of a long bone showing both spongy and compact bone tissue. **B,** Magnification of compact bone tissue. (From Thibodeau GA, Patton KT: *Anatomy and physiology*, ed 5, St Louis, 2003, Mosby.)

Muscle Tissue

Page 394
Structure of a muscle. (From Thibodeau GA, Patton KT: *Anatomy and physiology*, ed 5, St Louis, 2003, Mosby.)

Page 394
Structure of a muscle illustrating a sarcomere unit. (From Thibodeau GA, Patton KT: *Anatomy and physiology*, ed 5, St Louis, 2003, Mosby.)

Page 394
Sarcoplasmic reticulum and T tubules of a muscle fiber. (From Thibodeau GA, Patton KT: *Anatomy and physiology*, ed 5, St Louis, 2003, Mosby.)

Page 395
Myosin and actin filaments. (From Thibodeau GA, Patton KT: *Anatomy and physiology*, ed 5, St Louis, 2003, Mosby.)

Page 395
Sliding filament action. (From Thibodeau GA, Patton KT: *Anatomy and physiology*, ed 5, St Louis, 2003, Mosby.)

Page 395
Neuromuscular junction. (From Thibodeau GA, Patton KT: *Anatomy and physiology*, ed 5, St Louis, 2003, Mosby.)

Nerve Tissue

Page 396
Types of neurons (nerve cells). (From Thibodeau GA, Patton KT: *Anatomy and physiology*, ed 5, St Louis, 2003, Mosby.)

Page 396
Types of neuroglial cells. (From Thibodeau GA, Patton KT: *Anatomy and physiology*, ed 5, St Louis, 2003, Mosby.)

Page 397
Myelinated axon of the peripheral nervous system. (From Thibodeau GA, Patton KT: *Anatomy and physiology*, ed 5, St Louis, 2003, Mosby.)

Page 397
A, Convergence of neurons. **B,** Divergence of neurons. (From Thibodeau GA, Patton KT: *Anatomy and physiology*, ed 5, St Louis, 2003, Mosby.)

Page 397
A, Electrical synapse between neurons. **B,** Chemical synapse between neurons. (From Thibodeau GA, Patton KT: *Anatomy and physiology*, ed 5, St Louis, 2003, Mosby.)

Joints

Page 398

Three types of fibrous joints. (From Thibodeau GA, Patton KT: *Anatomy and physiology,* ed 5, St Louis, 2003, Mosby.)

Page 398

Three types of cartilaginous joints. (From Thibodeau GA, Patton KT: *Anatomy and physiology,* ed 5, St Louis, 2003, Mosby.)

Page 399

Structure of a typical synovial joint. (From Thibodeau GA, Patton KT: *Anatomy and physiology,* ed 5, St Louis, 2003, Mosby.)

Page 399

Various types of synovial joints. (From Thibodeau GA, Patton KT: *Anatomy and physiology,* ed 5, St Louis, 2003, Mosby.)

Integumentary System

Page 400

Diagram of the skin. (From Thibodeau GA, Patton KT: *Anatomy and physiology,* ed 5, St Louis, 2003, Mosby.)

Page 400

Glands of the skin. (From Thibodeau GA, Patton KT: *Anatomy and physiology,* ed 5, St Louis, 2003, Mosby.)

Page 401

Hair follicle. (From Thibodeau GA, Patton KT: *Anatomy and physiology,* ed 5, St Louis, 2003, Mosby.)

Page 401

Structure of a nail. (From Thibodeau GA, Patton KT: *Anatomy and physiology,* ed 5, St Louis, 2003, Mosby.)

Cardiac System

Page 402

Anterior and posterior views of the heart. (From Thibodeau GA, Patton KT: *Anatomy and physiology,* ed 5, St Louis, 2003, Mosby.)

Page 403

Interior view of the heart. (From LaFleur Brooks M: *Exploring medical language: a student-directed approach,* St Louis, 2002, Mosby.)

Page 403

Systemic and pulmonic circulations of the heart. (From Thibodeau GA, Patton KT: *Anatomy and physiology,* ed 5, St Louis, 2003, Mosby.)

Venous System

Page 404

Major veins of the body. (From Thibodeau GA, Patton KT: *Anatomy and physiology,* ed 5, St Louis, 2003, Mosby.)

Page 405

Venous drainage of the brain. (From Thibodeau GA, Patton KT: *Anatomy and physiology,* ed 5, St Louis, 2003, Mosby.)

Page 405

Creation of venous blood flow from capillaries. (From LaFleur Brooks M: *Exploring medical language: a student-directed approach,* St Louis 2002, Mosby.)

Page 405

Unidirectional venous valves. (From Thibodeau GA, Patton KT: *The human body in health and disease,* ed 2, St Louis 1997, Mosby.)

Lymphatic System

Page 406

Major organs of the lymphatic system. (From Thibodeau GA, Patton KT: *Anatomy and physiology,* ed 5, St Louis, 2003, Mosby.)

Page 406

Principal lymphatic drainage of the body. (From Thibodeau GA, Patton KT: *Anatomy and physiology,* ed 5, St Louis, 2003, Mosby.)

Page 406

Role of lymphatic capillary in draining intercellular fluid. (From Thibodeau GA, Patton KT: *Anatomy and physiology,* ed 5, St Louis, 2003, Mosby.)

Page 406

Lymphatic capillary structure. (From Thibodeau GA, Patton KT: *Anatomy and physiology,* ed 5, St Louis, 2003, Mosby.)

Page 407

Lymph node structure. (From Thibodeau GA, Patton KT: *Anatomy and physiology,* ed 5, St Louis, 2003, Mosby.)

Page 407

Role of a lymph node in a skin infection. (From Thibodeau GA, Patton KT: *Anatomy and physiology,* ed 5, St Louis, 2003, Mosby.)

Respiratory System

Page 408

Structures of the respiratory system. (From Thibodeau GA, Patton KT: *Anatomy and physiology,* ed 5, St Louis, 2003, Mosby.)

Page 409

Lobes of the lungs. (From Mathers LH, Chase RA: *Clinical anatomy principles,* St Louis, 1995, Mosby.)

Page 409

Bronchi of the lungs. (From Mathers LH, Chase RA: *Clinical anatomy principles,* St Louis 1995, Mosby.)

Page 409

Bronchiole and alveoli. (From LaFleur Brooks M: *Exploring medical language: a student-directed approach,* St Louis, 2002, Mosby.)

Urinary System

Page 410

Anterior view of the structures of the urinary system. (From LaFleur Brooks M: *Exploring medical language: a student-directed approach,* St Louis, 2002, Mosby.)

Page 411

Lateral view of the bladder and urethra of a male. (From Mathers LH, Chase RA: *Clinical anatomy principles,* St Louis, 1995, Mosby.)

Page 411

Section through a kidney demonstrating blood flow and urinary output. (From Thibodeau GA, Patton KT: *Anatomy and physiology,* ed 5, St Louis, 2003, Mosby.)

Page 411

Structures of a nephron. (From Thibodeau GA, Patton KT: *Anatomy and physiology,* ed 5, St Louis, 2003, Mosby.)

Gastrointestinal System

Page 412
Anterior view of the structures of the gastrointestinal system. (From Thibodeau GA, Patton KT: *Anatomy and physiology,* ed 5, St Louis, 2003, Mosby.)

Page 412
Structures of the gastrointestinal system. (From LaFleur Brooks M: *Exploring medical language: a student-directed approach,* St Louis, 2002, Mosby.)

Page 413
Accessory organs of the gastrointestinal system. (From Thibodeau GA, Patton KT: *Anatomy and physiology,* ed 5, St Louis, 2003, Mosby.)

Page 413
Divisions of the large intestine. (From LaFleur Brooks M: *Exploring medical language: a student-directed approach,* St Louis, 2002, Mosby.)

Page 413
Section through the abdominopelvic cavity. (From Thibodeau GA, Patton KT: *Anatomy and physiology,* ed 5, St Louis, 2003, Mosby.)

Immune System

Page 414
Organization of the immune system. (From Thompson JM, et al: *Mosby's clinical nursing,* ed 4, St Louis, 1997, Mosby.)

Page 414
Creation of B cells and T cells by the bone marrow. (From Thibodeau GA, Patton KT: *Anatomy and physiology,* ed 5, St Louis, 2003, Mosby.)

Page 414
Activation and effects of T cells. (From Thibodeau GA, Patton KT: *Anatomy and physiology,* ed 5, St Louis, 2003, Mosby.)

Page 415
Actions of antibodies. (From Thibodeau GA, Patton KT: *Anatomy and physiology,* ed 5, St Louis, 2003, Mosby.)

Page 415
Types of antibodies (immunoglobulins). (From Thibodeau GA, Patton KT: *Anatomy and physiology,* ed 5, St Louis, 2003, Mosby.)

Page 415
Action of antibody-activated complement and death of bacterium. (From Thibodeau GA, Patton KT: *Anatomy and physiology,* ed 5, St Louis, 2003, Mosby.)

Endocrine System

Page 416
The major endocrine glands of the body. (From Thibodeau GA, Patton KT: *Anatomy and physiology,* ed 5, St Louis, 2003, Mosby.)

Page 416
The thyroid gland. (From LaFleur Brooks M: *Exploring medical language: a student-directed approach,* St Louis, 2002, Mosby.)

Page 416
The adrenal gland. (From LaFleur Brooks M: *Exploring medical language: a student-directed approach,* St Louis, 2002, Mosby.)

Page 417
The hypothalamus and pituitary hormones. (From Thibodeau GA, Patton KT: *Anatomy and physiology,* ed 5, St Louis, 2003, Mosby.)

Page 417
The pancreas. (From LaFleur Brooks M: *Exploring medical language: a student-directed approach,* St Louis, 2002, Mosby.)

Sensory System

Page 418
Somatic and stretch receptors. (From Thibodeau GA, Patton KT: *Anatomy and physiology,* ed 5, St Louis, 2003, Mosby.)

Page 418
Superior view of a horizontal section of the eye. (From Thibodeau GA, Patton KT: *Anatomy and physiology,* ed 5, St Louis, 2003, Mosby.)

Page 419
External, middle, and internal ear. (From Thibodeau GA, Patton KT: *Anatomy and physiology,* ed 5, St Louis, 2003, Mosby.)

Page 419
Lateral view of the internal nose. (From Thibodeau GA, Patton KT: *Anatomy and physiology,* ed 5, St Louis, 2003, Mosby.)

Page 419
Dorsal surface of the tongue, cross section through a papilla, and a taste bud. (From Thibodeau GA, Patton KT: *Anatomy and physiology,* ed 5, St Louis, 2003, Mosby.)

Reproductive System

Page 420
Male reproductive organs. (From Thibodeau GA, Patton KT: *Anatomy and physiology,* ed 5, St Louis, 2003, Mosby.)

Page 420
Male perineum. (From Thibodeau GA, Patton KT: *Anatomy and physiology,* ed 5, St Louis, 2003, Mosby.)

Page 420
Tubules of the testis and epididymis. (From Thibodeau GA, Patton KT: *Anatomy and physiology,* ed 5, St Louis, 2003, Mosby.)

Page 421
Female reproductive organs. (From Thibodeau GA, Patton KT: *Anatomy and physiology,* ed 5, St Louis, 2003, Mosby.)

Page 421
Female perineum. (From Thibodeau GA, Patton KT: *Anatomy and physiology,* ed 5, St Louis, 2003, Mosby.)

Page 421
Anterior view of female reproductive organs. (From LaFleur Brooks M: *Exploring medical language: a student-directed approach,* St Louis, 2002, Mosby.)